3295

LP

50¢

HEALTHY AGING FOR DUMMIES®

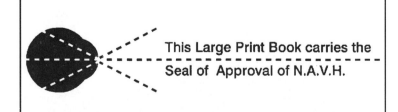

HEALTHY AGING FOR DUMMIES®

BRENT AGIN, MD,
AND SHARON PERKINS, RN

THORNDIKE PRESS

A part of Gale, Cengage Learning

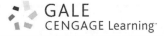

Detroit • New York • San Francisco • New Haven, Conn • Waterville, Maine • London

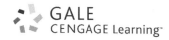

Thorndike Press, a part of Gale, Cengage Learning.

Thorndike Press® Large Print Healthy, Home & Learning.

The text of this Large Print edition is unabridged.

Other aspects of the book may vary from the original edition.

Set in 16 pt. Plantin.

Printed on permanent paper.

LIBRARY OF CONGRESS CATALOGING-IN-PUBLICATION DATA

Agin, Brent.
    Healthy aging for dummies / by Brent Agin and Sharon Perkins. — Large print ed.
      p. cm.
    ISBN-13: 978-1-4104-1454-0 (hardcover : alk. paper)
    ISBN-10: 1-4104-1454-X (hardcover : alk. paper)
    1. Aging. 2. Middle-aged persons — Health and hygiene. 3. Older people — Health and hygiene. 4. Physical fitness for middle-aged persons. 5. Physical fitness for older people. 6. Large type books. I. Perkins, Sharon. II. Title.
    RA777.5.A35 2009
    613'.0434—dc22
                                                                        2008056051

Published in 2009 by arrangement with John Wiley & Sons, Inc.

Printed in the United States of America
1 2 3 4 5 6 7 13 12 11 10 09

Dedication

We dedicate this book to all the readers who are going to make positive changes in their lives. In the book, we offer a lot of information and tips to improve your lifestyle and health; all you have to do is go for it! Feeling healthy is the goal, and this book is your motivation. To date, whether it's mental or physical health, neither of us has ever met a person who hasn't been able to get healthier if he or she tried. Conversely, the people who've really put their hearts and souls into the effort have beat odds time and again and have achieved amazing personal goals. So here's to you and to the rest of your healthy lives!

Authors' Acknowledgments

From Dr. Agin: I would like to thank the coauthor Sharon Perkins, my literary agent Barb Doyen, and the team at Wiley Publishing. With these folks' help I was able to accomplish a major goal in my life. For this, I acknowledge their guidance and patience and thank them dearly for the opportunity. I would also like to thank my family, friends, and co-workers for their support.

From Sharon Perkins: I think my list of people to thank grows longer with every book I write. I thank everyone who's had to help me through some tough times in the last year (you all know who you are), and I thank God and my agent, Jessica Faust, for the opportunity to write this book and take my mind off a difficult situation. Thanks also to Kristin DeMint, our Project Editor, to our Copy Editors — Pam Ruble, Carrie Burchfield, and Sarah Faulkner — and to the rest of the Wiley team; I always enjoy working with all of you. And to Brent, who made this job easy.

About the Authors

Brent J. Agin, MD, has been in private practice for the last five years and is recognized by the community as the go-to medical advisor in the field of healthy aging. He sees patients of all ages and maintains a diverse array of clientele, including professional athletes and celebrities. He's board certified in family medicine, receiving both his undergraduate degree and his MD at Michigan State University. He completed his internship and residency at the University of South Florida.

Dr. Agin offers family medicine, but his practice also provides aesthetics and weight loss assistance. He's the medical director of Novus Medical Detox, which provides private detoxification for multiple addictions. With a strong interest in nutrition, he's developed a supplement line and all-natural, rapid weight loss program, The TRIM Diet (www.trimlifestyle.com), while doing dietary and weight-loss consulting nationally.

In his free time, Dr. Agin enjoys golf, soccer, and fishing. He lives in Palm Harbor, Florida, with his wife Cindy and their two daughters.

Sharon Perkins is an RN with over 20 years of experience and an author of six *For Dummies* series books. She enjoys both jobs equally but enjoys her three grandchildren, five children, two daughters-in-law, one son-in-law, family, and friends more! She lives in New Jersey but spends a lot of time gallivanting around the country.

Publisher's Acknowledgments

We're proud of this book; please send us your comments through our Dummies online registration form located at www.dummies .com/register/.

Some of the people who helped bring this book to market include the following:

Acquisitions, Editorial, and Media Development
Project Editor: Kristin DeMint
Acquisitions Editor: Tracy Boggier
Copy Editors: Sarah Faulkner, Carrie A. Burchfield, Pam Ruble
Editorial Program Coordinator: Erin Calligan Mooney
Technical Editor: Philip G. Hays, MD
Senior Editorial Manager: Jennifer Ehrlich
Editorial Manager: Michelle Hacker
Editorial Assistants: Joe Niesen, Leeann Harney
Cover Photos: © Image Source/Corbis
Cartoons: Rich Tennant, (www.the5thwave.com)

Composition Services for Original Edition
Project Coordinators: Heather Kolter, Erin Smith
Layout and Graphics: Stacie Brooks, Reuben W. Davis, Alissa

11

D. Ellet, Melissa K. Jester, Christine Williams
Special Art: Kathryn Born, MA
Anniversary Logo Design: Richard Pacifico
Proofreaders: Broccoli Information Management, Jessica Kramer
Indexer: Potomac Indexing, LLC
Special Help
Vicki M. Adang

Publishing and Editorial for Consumer Dummies
Diane Graves Steele, Vice President and Publisher, Consumer Dummies
Joyce Pepple, Acquisitions Director, Consumer Dummies
Kristin A. Cocks, Product Development Director, Consumer Dummies
Michael Spring, Vice President and Publisher, Travel
Kelly Regan, Editorial Director, Travel
Publishing for Technology Dummies
Andy Cummings, Vice President and Publisher, Dummies Technology/General User
Composition Services
Gerry Fahey, Vice President of Production Services
Debbie Stailey, Director of Composition Services

Healthy Aging For Dummies®

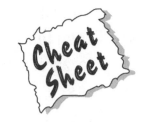

Ten Things You Can Do to Stay Healthy

Short on time? If you're a person who wants just the facts and not the small details, well, here they are. Tattoo this list on your forehead, follow it to the letter, and you'll be taking a big step toward healthy aging and disease prevention.

- ✔ If you smoke, stop. Seriously.
- ✔ Maintain a healthy body weight, as determined by your BMI (see Chapter 7).
- ✔ Exercise daily for 30 minutes.
- ✔ Eat five or more servings of fruits or vegetables daily.
- ✔ Avoid refined sugars and starches.
- ✔ If you drink alcohol, do so in moderation (no more than two drinks per day for men, one per day for women).
- ✔ Keep your blood pressure under control.
- ✔ Have your cholesterol checked yearly.
- ✔ Keep your blood sugar in normal range.
- ✔ Have a mammogram/prostate check yearly.

A Health-Promoting Grocery List

To read more about the health benefits of many foods, refer to Chapter 17. But for now, here's a list of good-for-you foods to guide you through the grocery store:

- ✔ Blueberries
- ✔ Broccoli
- ✔ Dark chocolate
- ✔ Egg whites (any way you like 'em)
- ✔ Extra virgin olive oil

13

- Fish with omega-3 fatty acids
- Green tea
- Mozzarella string cheese
- Nuts
- Oats
- Soy foods
- Strawberries
- Tomatoes
- Vinaigrette salad dressing
- Whole wheat pasta
- Yogurt

The Best Supplements for Specific Ailments

Your medicine cabinet doesn't need to have just medicine. Expand your healthful attitude to include a wellness cabinet full of dietary supplements for prevention. Try stocking up on these healthy supplements (see Chapter 8 for more details):

Supplement	Benefit
Fish oil	Lowers cholesterol
Probiotics	Support colon, intestinal, vaginal health
Saw palmetto	Promotes prostate health
Calcium	Strengthens bones
Glucosamine and chondroitin	Aid in joint health; lessen arthritis pain
Melatonin	Promotes sleep
Chromium	Helps manage insulin health and blood sugar levels
Calcium and magnesium	Control heartburn
Coenzyme Q10	Supports cardiac health
Zinc	Reduces the severity and duration of the common cold

Helpful Formulas to Remember

Refer to the following formulas as helpful reminders.

Cheat Sheet

To calculate the fat percentage of food

You want 30 percent or less of your total daily calorie intake to come from fat (less than 10 percent from saturated fats). To calculate the percentage of fat, you need to know the calories per serving and total grams of fat per serving. One gram of fat has 9 calories, and the total fat grams will be on the food label.

1. **Multiply the number of fat grams by 9.**

2. **Divide this number by the total calories per serving.**

3. **Multiply by 100.**

The result is the percentage of fat calories in the food.

Note: A food has to have less than 30 percent of its calories from fat to be considered "low fat."

To calculate your body mass index

Your body mass index (BMI) is an approximate measure of body fat based on your height and weight. The BMI is an approximation and is used as a tool to assess body weight and identify overweight and obese individuals.

1. **Calculate your weight in kilograms:** # of lbs $\times$ 0.454 (kg/lb) = # of kg

2. **Calculate your height in meters:** # of inches $\times$ 0.0254 (meters/inch) = # of meters

3. **Divide your weight (in kilograms) by your height (in meters) squared.**

To determine your basal metabolic rate

Your basal metabolic rate (BMR) is the amount of calories you'd burn if you stayed in bed all day. Calculations are different for men and women:

- **Adult male:** 66 + (6.3 $\times$ body weight in lbs.) + (12.9 $\times$ height in inches) − (6.8 $\times$ age in years)

- **Adult female:** 655 + (4.3 $\times$ weight in lbs.) + (4.7 $\times$ height in inches) − (4.7 $\times$ age in years)

Contents at a Glance

Table of Contents

Introduction

●●

If you're like many folks today, you realize that not only are people living longer than they used to, but also some of those people are living amazingly well while looking great. What's their secret to living such an independent, active, and radiant lifestyle? The answer lies in their healthy lifestyles — an approach to life we revisit multiple times in this book. The goal of this book is to educate you on the healthy choices you can make that reward you with a healthier, longer, happier life.

Some of the greatest threats to healthy aging come from disease and illnesses that cut your life short and the unhealthy choices that may have caused them. The good news is you can prevent many of these illnesses. Consider these facts:

✔ Nearly 80 million U.S. adults have some form of cardiovascular disease (CVD), and someone in the U.S. dies every 36 seconds from CVD.

✔ More than 20 million people have diabetes, and adults with diabetes die from heart disease at a rate two to four times higher than adults without diabetes.

✔ Heart disease and stroke account for about 65 percent of deaths in people with diabetes.

✔ Nearly 70 percent of Americans are overweight and more than 30 percent are obese.

These statistics focus on only a few health conditions, but we could give you similar numbers for many other ailments that people encounter as they get older. Wonder where all these statistics come from? In this book, many of the statistics we quote are from the World Health Organization (WHO), so if we don't cite a source, you can assume that WHO is it. So with this information in mind, take a look at some of the secrets to healthy aging. Here are a few keys to success:

✔ **Prevention:** By arming yourself with solid knowledge and making changes to your current lifestyle, you won't necessarily live longer (although you may), but you will live a better *quality* of life.

✔ **Moderation:** Easy does it and in small doses. Making small but significant changes in your life can make a difference over time.

✔ **Timing:** Start now! Whether you are 20-something or 70-something, you are the CEO of your body, and it's up to you to manage it.

✔ **Practice:** Much of the way you live is based on habits — some good, some bad — formed over a lifetime. Incorporating new routines in place of old habits takes some getting used to. In time and with consistent practice, these lifestyle changes can replace old habits and become second nature.

It's never too early or too late to start taking care of your body. The sooner you treat your body as if it's the only one you're going to get, the sooner you're on your way to healthy aging. Your body needs continuous respect and appreciation and if treated well can provide a wonderful, healthy life.

About This Book

This book is an excellent choice if you want to maximize your body's potential now and for as long as you own it. Whether you want to make a small adjustment, need some fine-tuning, or have to make a major overhaul, you find helpful advice in the pages of this book.

Our goal is to lay out the reasons why your body ages, explain the normal course of aging, and show you how aging is accelerated by your lifestyle choices. We've also given you information on how to prevent or reverse the effects of aging, disease, and illness.

You may be a 20-something looking for some tips on strength training and nutrition, while also wanting to know how to prevent illness while you're still young. On the other hand, you could be in early retirement or even beyond that point, looking to recreate the energy and great health you had when you were younger, while getting up to date on the important preventative health exams. Either way, we present you with useful material in an easy-to-follow fashion to help you achieve your goals. If you happen to be passionate about a particular topic (like muscles or nutrition), don't worry — we cover every subject in detail and even refer you to other *For Dummies* books in case you just can't get enough!

Conventions Used in This Book

To help you navigate easily through this book, we set up a few conventions used consistently throughout the book:

- ✔ Anytime we want to highlight new words or terms defined in the text, we *italicize* them.

- ✔ **Boldfaced** text is used to indicate the action part of numbered steps and the keywords of a bulleted list.

When this book was printed, some Web addresses may have needed to break across two lines of text. If you come across these instances, rest assured that we haven't put in any extra characters (such as a hyphen) to indicate the break. So, when typing one of these Web addresses in a Web browser, just type in exactly what you see, pretending as if the line break doesn't exist.

What You're Not to Read

That's right — you don't have to read this book cover-to-cover to find helpful information. Any text you find in a gray box is a sidebar. Sidebars contain interesting but unessential information. If you're in a hurry to get to the meat of the chapter, feel free to skip them and return to them later. Another area you can skip over, if you wish, are the places marked with a Technical Stuff icon. If you're the type who wants to know all the technical details, you'll enjoy these two areas; otherwise you can move on without missing essential information.

Foolish Assumptions

This book is for anyone who wants to live a healthier life, and we figure that means just about everyone! If you've picked up this book, we assume you fall into one or more of these categories:

- You're alive and want to stay that way for awhile, and you want to do so disease- and illness-free, as independent as possible, and with your mind as sharp as a tack.

- You're having some health issues and are willing to make some modifications to your lifestyle to be healthier but aren't sure what to do.

- You have no interest in reading a dry medical textbook; you want an easy-to-follow reference book with some helpful "how-to's" and "show-me-the-ways."

- You want a book that gives you the straight facts about what you need to know about how your body and mind work in order to make wise choices for healthy living, as well as how to adapt your lifestyle choices according to your age.

- You want to get a few laughs while you digest the information, because aging isn't always so easy to cope with.

How This Book Is Organized

Healthy Aging For Dummies is organized into six parts. Each part addresses a major area of the hows, whats, and whys of healthy aging. Because of this organization, it's simple to find the topic that you're looking for. Here's a quick overview of what you can find in each part.

Part I: So You Want to Look and Feel Young Forever . . .

If you want something badly enough, you must be willing to work for it. There's no Fountain of Youth, and there's no free lunch, either. In these chapters, you find out how to assess your current health, evaluate your challenges and strengths, and set your mark on what you desire most. More importantly, we show you how to achieve your goals.

Part II: Workin' on Your Framework

The chapters in this part discuss the fundamentals of caring for your permanent fixtures and structures, such your teeth, skin, and joints. As for your teeth, tooth loss is *not* solely a sign of aging — it's often a sign of poor dental hygiene, so we tell you what to do to keep those choppers for life. Your skin is your body's first line of defense against disease and illness, so protect it and care for it. We tell you how. We also fill you in on why bones become weak and brittle as the years pass, what lifestyle factors accelerate this process, and what you can do to prevent it.

Part III: Using Nutrition to Extend Your Expiration Date

Your body uses food as fuel to operate at maximum efficiency. The better the fuel, the better your body runs. While your body can survive on a diet of French fries, soda, processed meats, and cream-filled pastries, you pay a price. This part provides you with guidelines for using nutrition and supplements to help your body perform at its best for the long haul.

Part IV: Getting Physical

The human body is meant to move, and most people don't use their bodies to their full capabilities. Your muscles ache to be worked to the point of fatigue in order to rebuild and do it all over again. This part aims to get you excited about revving up your body to do what it craves. In turn, your body serves you well in the long run.

Part V: Sharpening the All-Important Mind and Spirit

For many folks, losing their memory (or their mind) is one of the biggest concerns of getting older. In this section, we explain the differences between normal memory loss and memory loss due to disease, how to improve your memory, and how maintaining an upbeat outlook on life positively influences your overall health and well-being.

Part VI: The Part of Tens

This part presents helpful information in lists of ten items each. You can read about ten myths and get the facts behind them. Find the ten proven most healthy foods, play ten mind games to stretch your brain power, and discover ways to make your home safer as you age.

In addition, we threw in a handy Appendix with a questionnaire to help you and your doctor determine your current state of health. From there, you can create a roadmap for healthy living.

Icons Used in This Book

This book uses icons — small graphics or images in the margins — to mark certain paragraphs of information that you may find useful. Here's the rundown of the helpful icons we use in this book.

 When you see this icon, you'll find a helpful hint about doing something to help you age gracefully.

 This icon denotes critical information that you need to take away with you. Be sure to read it.

 Once in a while, we go a bit deeper into the info on aging. This icon tips you off to that type of information. You can skip over these icons and still be able to age with perfection, but the info they contain enhances your understanding of healthy aging ever further.

 The Warning icon cautions you against something that's potentially harmful. Be sure to read and heed the information with these icons.

Where to Go from Here

You don't have to start at Chapter 1 and read straight through this book. Just like all *For Dummies* books, this one is set up so you can read any chapter, in any order, and still come out ahead. Sound good? Then keep on reading. (Starting wherever you want, of course.)

We're partial to this book and would love for you to read the whole thing, but if you don't have the time to do so (or just don't feel like it), we recommend that you make sure to read Chapter 3, because we believe it's one of the most critical chapters in the whole book. It covers what you should know about your family's health history, what checkups you need when, and how to create a plan for healthy aging. We encourage you to check out why setting goals and creating a plan is so vital. After you have your goals and an action plan in place, you can better use the information in this book. We'll be with you every step of the way.

Part I

So You Want to Look and Feel Young Forever . . .

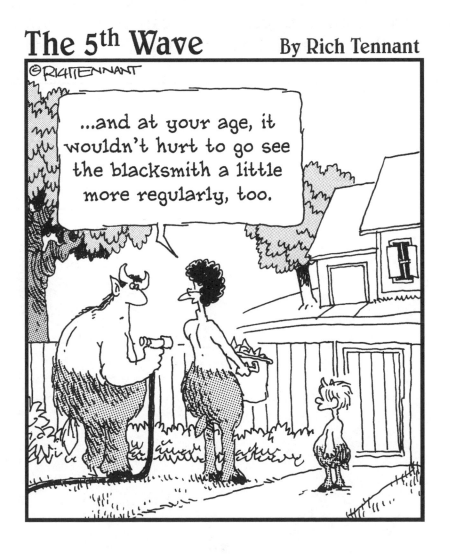

The 5th Wave — By Rich Tennant

...and at your age, it wouldn't hurt to go see the blacksmith a little more regularly, too.

In this part . . .

Why is 40 the new 30 or 60 the new 50? If people are actually looking and feeling younger today than they did 50 years ago, how are they doing it? What are the biggest road-blocks to living a longer, healthier life, and how can you maneuver around them?

In this part, we reveal the secrets to looking and feeling younger so you can evaluate your health, habits, and wellness goals.

Chapter 1

The Fountain of Youth, at Your Fingertips

In This Chapter

▶ Understanding the current life expectancy
▶ Uncovering proven methods to combat aging
▶ Looking at the staggering numbers of preventable deaths

Over the years, thousands of people have searched for the elusive Fountain of Youth, and although some have claimed to have found it, for most, it remains a hidden treasure. Great strides have been made in uncovering the secrets to aging healthfully and lengthening the lifespan, but there's still progress to be made. As much as you may wish otherwise, most people know there's no magic pill for good health and longevity. It takes commitment, work, and sometimes even denial of self — giving up poor eating habits, couch potato lifestyle, and the stressful schedules so many are addicted to — to stay healthy as you get older. You may be taking care of the externals but skipping over the basics of good health, which are also the basics of aging well.

You can't skip over the basics so easily, though. Balance is a big key in life, and healthy aging is no different. Skipping over essential healthcare is like ignoring routine maintenance on your car — the end result can be costly and dangerous.

Healthy aging is a current hot topic, and you can thank the baby boomer generation — the oldest of these people are now heading into their 60s — for today's emphasis on youthful, healthy aging. In this chapter, we discuss why people are living longer and better today than in previous generations, what impacted life expectancy a century ago, and what impacts our health and longevity today.

Life Expectancy in the 21st Century

The last 100 years have seen a tremendous change in the way people live and the ailments they fall prey to. The epidemics of yesterday have been wiped out in industrialized countries, and life expectancy has increased. But even though folks are living longer today, this life expectancy brings a whole new set of problems and solutions.

Today, many folks take for granted that they'll live into adulthood, while in the past, people were well aware of the unpredictable threats on their lives. Some of the most damaging health threats in the world today can be modified by lifestyle choices. Making healthy choices is the basis of healthy aging and the recurrent theme of this book.

To examine why people live longer lives today, you must first look at why people *didn't* live as long more than a century ago. This section focuses on the differences.

That was then . . .

Malnutrition, acute illnesses, infant mortality, and war were major contributors to shorter life expectancy 100 years ago.

In the period of 1918 to 1919, the influenza virus (the flu) infected more than 400 million people worldwide and killed nearly 40 million. Today people still die from the flu, but not nearly at the mortality rates common in the past.

Poor living conditions and poor sanitation were also major causes of death. Each incident people experienced had a negative cumulative effect on their health. Even diseases that didn't result in death left people more likely to develop chronic illnesses when they grew older and lead to poor life expectancy.

The statistical probability of a person 100 years ago going through life unscathed was extremely low. Here are a few of the problems that caused widespread disease and mortality then:

- ✔ **Crowded and unsanitary living conditions:** These scenarios resulted in multiple outbreaks of malaria, cholera, dysentery, typhoid fever, yellow fever, and flu. Survivors often faced lifelong health consequences.

- ✔ **War:** War caused death directly and also exposed soldiers to foreign disease. During the American Civil War between 1861 and 1865 there were twice as many deaths from disease associated with the poor health than from battle wounds. More than 200 million people died in the beginning of the 20th century from a combination of combat and disease.

- ✔ **Viral and bacterial infections with no medical treatments or vaccines:** Viruses and bacteria infections caused death in high numbers of both adults and children. Worldwide there have been many pandemics (affecting a large group, even the world) from the Spanish Flu in 1918 to the Asian Flu in 1957 that killed more than 50 million people.

Polio, smallpox, diphtheria, and measles killed many adults and children before the advent of vaccines and still do in third world countries.

- ✔ **Hazardous work environments and hard physical labor:** Starting as young as age 13, exposed to dangerous fumes and bacteria, and with minimal protective equipment, people worked 10- to 12-hour shifts. The number of work-related deaths peaked around 1900 and then started to improve with the formation of unions and other safety requirements.

- ✔ **Lack of certain nutrients:** People from soldiers to sailors as well as malnutrition in the poverty stricken suffered from lack of nutrients. These deficiencies included

  - **Pellagra:** A deficiency of niacin (b3) that may include symptoms of dermatitis, diarrhea, dementia, and death.
  - **Goiter:** Goiter is caused by a lack of iodine in a child's diet that can lead to hyperthyroidism (elevated thyroid hormone). Complications include heart problems, impaired mental function, and birth defects.
  - **Scurvy:** Lack of vitamin C led to scurvy, a condition where the body can't properly absorb iron, causing anemia.
  - **Rickets:** This affliction was due to a lack of vitamin D, which is necessary for bone mineralization. Children with rickets had bones that didn't fully develop and were deformed, often with the classic bowing of the legs. Kids were also more susceptible to whooping cough and measles.

... This is now

There has been a change in the major health concerns today versus 100 years ago, but globally, some similarities still exist. Worldwide, infectious disease is still a major cause of death, and the threat of newer strains of viruses and bacteria are always present. In addition, the mutation of "superbugs" that are immune to many antibiotics has been created by overuse of antibiotics.

Major medical discoveries and inventions have improved the outcomes of many conditions by earlier diagnosis and better medications and treatments, but lifestyle changes have resulted in the current prevalence of chronic and often preventable diseases, such as heart disease, cancer, respiratory illness, diabetes, and stroke, which have the highest mortality rates today (see Chapter 2 for more info).

Over the years, medical advances have fueled the changes that have overcome some major health threats to society. Here is the list of major contributors:

- ✔ **Infant vaccinations:** Today, over 80 percent of children age three or younger receive vaccinations. As a result, some of the deadly diseases, like smallpox and polio, are completely controlled in developed countries, while worldwide programs try to spread this success into the underdeveloped countries. Furthermore, new vaccines are available (like for chicken pox) that weren't available 30 years ago. People born in 1955 were the first to receive vaccinations in infancy, starting with polio. That factor alone significantly increased that generation's lifespan. In the years to follow, more childhood vaccines were added, such as measles in 1963, mumps in 1967, and rubella in 1969.

✔ **Antibiotics:** People have been receiving antibiotics since the 1940s for bacterial infections, such as syphilis, tuberculosis, malaria, and pneumonia. Penicillin was discovered in 1928 and first used medically in 1940. After the discovery of penicillin, the rate of development of newer antibiotics was paralleled by fear of emerging resistant bacteria. In the 1950s, new resistant bacteria emphasized the need to limit use of antibiotics to keep new resistant bacteria from emerging. Today, the improper use of antibiotics is widespread, leaving researchers nervous about the inevitable development of newer resistant bugs. Follow your doctor's recommendation about taking antibiotics seriously to help avoid further resistant strains from improper antibiotic use.

✔ **Medical technology:** Medical technology drives the improvements in modern medicine. To make better medications, vaccines, and diagnostic tests, there needs to be advances in equipment to identify and create them. Diagnosing disease in its early stages, which improves outcome, comes from better diagnostic imaging. Patients with disease that has advanced to a point where organs are failing are given hope from technology advancements in prosthetics, organ transplantation, and tissue repair. Here are a few of the major breakthroughs:

- The *artificial heart* can be used to keep heart failure patients alive until they can receive a donor heart.
- *Computer-aided tomography (CAT) scan* produces three-dimensional images of the body that can show doctors whether a tumor is present and how deep it is in the body, to guide diagnosis and treatments.

- *Magnetic resonance imaging (MRI)* is when magnetic fields and radio waves cause atoms to give off tiny radio signals, making it possible to detect cancer and other ailments early.

Despite these amazing advances, some diseases are still constant — cardiovascular disease (CVD) is still the leading cause of death in the world, and although cancer, respiratory illness, and diabetes all trail behind, they're still major health threats (see Chapter 2 for more info on cancer and CVD).

The Basics of Pro-Aging: The Best Actions You Can Take

You can't prevent the passage of time, but when you're *proactive* about your life choices, you can control some of the risk factors in your life associated with illness and disease. Being proactive doesn't automatically guarantee you won't develop a chronic disease or illness, but not doing anything or actively taking part in known risk factors that are linked to chronic disease or illness may lead to health problems.

You may not realize just how much control you have over how long you live — and we don't necessarily mean that in a good way. Seemingly casual choices you make every day may have the most profound impact on your health. In fact, it's estimated that if everyone in the United States led a healthy lifestyle (outlined in the list below), more than 50 percent of the cases of cardiovascular disease and diabetes could be avoided, and more than 50 percent of all cases of cancer prevented.

The earlier in life you choose to follow a lifestyle of disease prevention, the more you can lower your risks of developing chronic disease. Chronic disease and illness come from many different factors, some of which you can control — such as lifestyle choices — and others you can't — like your age and genetics.

The following tips show you how to avoid the most damaging and preventable threats to your health and aging:

- **Don't smoke — and if you already do, stop.** Really. Smoking increases the risks for the top three killers: heart disease, cancer, and cardiovascular ailments, including strokes. It also damages your lungs and other parts of your respiratory system. At least 60 chemicals in cigarette smoke cause cancer, and as a cigarette burns, it produces the poisons carbon monoxide, ammonia, formaldehyde, arsenic, and cyanide.

  Smoking raises your blood pressure and decreases the flow of oxygen to your brain and body. It's also a significant risk factor for other health concerns, including emphysema, chronic bronchitis, stroke, and osteoporosis. (See Chapter 2 for more info on smoking; Chapter 6 for osteoporosis.) In the year 2006, smoking resulted in 435,000 deaths or 18.1 percent of the total deaths (includes 35,000 deaths from secondhand smoke and 1,000 infant deaths due to maternal smoking).

- **Limit alcohol consumption.** If you drink alcohol, no more than two drinks a day are safe for men, and one or fewer drinks a day for women. (A standard drink is one 12-ounce bottle of beer or wine cooler, one 5-ounce glass of wine, or 1.5 ounces of 80-proof distilled spirits.) Women are more likely to have liver damage from drinking two or more drinks a day than men are, so it's especially important for women to keep alcohol consumption to one or fewer drinks a day.

Alcohol is a depressant and can exacerbate the symptoms of depression and other mental disturbances. Alcohol intoxication causes problems with coordination, speech, and decision making, leading to risky behaviors. At toxic levels of alcohol intake, vomiting, difficult breathing, seizures, and even death can occur. Alcohol has an addiction potential, with around 8 percent of adults having an alcohol use disorder. With addiction and chronic alcohol consumption, disease in the liver, pancreas, nervous system, and gastrointestinal system can occur. If you've had any history of addiction to alcohol or any other substance, you shouldn't drink at all.

Many studies have found that consumption of alcohol at these quantities can have protective measures in cardiovascular disease. Consumption of red wine may be particularly favorable, since red wine contains certain polyphenol antioxidants associated with cardiovascular health.

If you're pregnant, you should avoid alcohol altogether because researchers don't know how much alcohol will harm a fetus, but they do know that a certain amount can be extremely harmful.

✍ **Maintain a healthy, balanced diet.** We can't overstate the importance of a balanced and healthy diet as you age. A poor diet can lead to an increased risk of many health problems, including osteoporosis, heart disease, and impaired memory. Eating well, on the other hand, makes you feel and look better, keeps your body functioning optimally, wards off colds and sickness, and contributes to lowering

The high cost of free radicals

Free radicals can come from internal reactions or can be caused by external sources such as exposure to X-rays, cigarette smoking, air pollutants, pesticides, and other industrial chemicals. To understand free radicals, it helps to understand cell structure.

The human body is made up of cells. Cells are made up of molecules. Molecules consist of elements (water, calcium, iron), and elements are composed of atoms (made of a nucleus, neutrons, protons, and electrons). Atoms are bound by a chemical bond created by pairs of electrons that surround the atom. The number of protons (positive charge) in the atom's nucleus (center) determines the number of electrons (negative charge) that surround the atom. Electrons by nature are unstable and have a tendency to break away from the atom, leaving it with an unpaired electron. This unpaired electron turns the atom into a free radical, which becomes a scavenger looking for an available electron to stabilize itself. Free

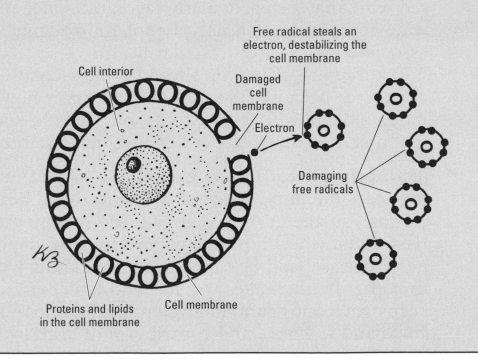

52

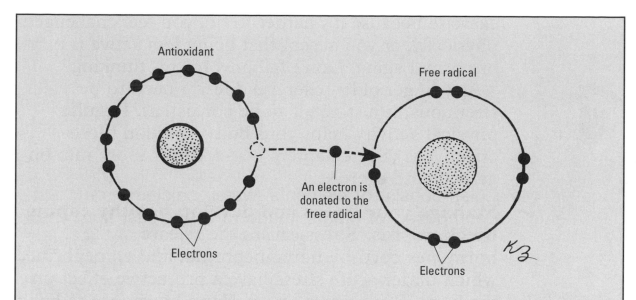

Antioxidant

Free radical

An electron is donated to the free radical

Electrons

Electrons

radicals steal electrons from other atoms, making these atoms, with missing electrons, become free radicals, and this sets off an ugly chain reaction (see figure on previous page). With time, free radicals cause damage to the cell structure and the cells die. Tissue that's continuously assaulted by free radicals leads to cell death, which leads to more rapid aging. Free radicals are known to be linked to cancer, heart disease, arthritis, and other disease.

Antioxidants work by targeting free radicals and donating one of their electrons to each free radical (a process called oxidation), neutralizing it, and preventing damage to the body's tissues (see figure above).

blood pressure and cholesterol levels, which in turn helps protect you against heart disease and stroke. (Chapter 7 tells more about good nutrition.)

✔ **Exercise regularly.** Over time, a sedentary lifestyle can lead to obesity, a preventable yet dangerous epidemic that poses a threat to people's longevity. And it's on the rise. As you age, regular exercise should be a cornerstone of healthy living. As your body slows down, you may be tempted to skip the exercise because it's harder to do, you feel challenged physically, or you accept that being less active is part of normal aging. Don't fall prey to this thinking!

As you get older, exercise doesn't need to be strenuous, it just needs to be consistent. Regular physical activity helps your body function more effectively. (See Chapters 9 and 10 for more info on activity and exercise.)

- ✔ **Manage your stress and develop healthy coping mechanisms.** Stress causes the release of the hormones cortisol, norepinephrine, and epinephrine, which under acute stress have a protective effect on the body. But *chronic* stress allows hormones to hang around longer than usual and cause the formation of free radicals. (See Chapter 13 for more information on the effects of stress.) Although these little buggers don't cause death directly, they do contribute to aging. Check out the nearby sidebar, "The high cost of free radicals."

- ✔ **Get enough sleep regularly.** You need sleep, both psychologically and physiologically. The body uses this time for healing and growth, and your body produces many hormones essential for proper functioning during the deepest sleep stages. Sleep irregularity can have a direct impact on some disorders, such as epilepsy and migraines, and has been associated with diseases, such as cardiovascular disease, clinical depression, diabetes, and other serious conditions. (See Chapter 14 for more on sleep.)

- ✔ **Visit your doctor for the recommended screening tests for your age.** Several important tests can help protect against cancer, heart disease, stroke, diabetes, and osteoporosis. Some of these tests find diseases early, when they're most treatable, while others can actually help keep a disease from developing in the first place. (See Chapter 2 to find out which tests you should have and when.)

If Staying Young and Healthy Is So Easy, Why Isn't Everyone Doing It?

There's nothing terribly complicated about living a healthy, life-prolonging lifestyle. So why are more people falling prey to partially preventable diseases every year? In this section, we explore what we think are the biggest reasons behind the staggering numbers of preventable death. Take these pointers to heart, so you can recognize any that may be present in your own life and make the modifications to effectively enhance the quality of your life, both now and in the future, no matter what your age.

Short-sighted thinking

We're going to let you in on a little secret, everyone is mortal. Despite this being common knowledge, few people think about the inevitability of their own death and the things they can do to prevent it from happening prematurely. If they did, there would be far fewer accidents of every type, no one would ever break their hip falling off a ladder they shouldn't have been on in the first place, and cigarette sales would plummet.

The idea that death can be postponed leads to thinking that "tomorrow" is a good time to start a dietary overhaul, an ambitious new exercise regimen, and, of course, tomorrow is the best time to quit smoking and drinking. For many people, tomorrow is also a good time to finally call and set up the routine physical or breast exam they've been avoiding for the past five years.

We're not advocating that you get out the sackcloth and ashes and carry a sign that states "The End is Near," but a little realism can go a long way toward a new way of living that can literally save lives — at least for a few more years.

How can you inject enough realism to make you want to change but not so much that you feel it's all too futile anyway? The following ideas may help:

- **Take a quiz.** There are online sites that allow you to input your health information and get a prediction of how long you'll live. Seeing your projected timeline in black and white may be enough to get you motivated to make changes. One such site is www.livingto100.com.

- **Pay attention to how you feel.** Often the little nagging symptoms that can signal something big brewing are ignored. One way to keep track of what's going on with your health is to keep a journal. Don't do this if you're already obsessed with your health — most likely you already keep track of your symptoms. Do this only if you're the type of person that ignores warning signs like shortness of breath, chest pain, or headaches. You may see a pattern that needs to be addressed.

- **See your doctor.** Make it clear when you make the appointment that this isn't a "sick" visit but rather a consultation, so more time is allotted. Ask him what you can do to improve your health, and then *do it.*

Many people have joined a "managed care" system where there are limitations on treatments and a focus on cutting costs, often leaving individuals managing their own care. The plethora of health information on the Internet (not all accurate, but abundant) leads people to self-diagnosing or making their own clinical decisions based on information they find on the Internet. It's not bad to be informed, but it can be dangerous if this information is replacing doctor visits.

Confusing what feels good with what is good

Making healthy food choices can have a major impact on health and aging. Most people know some of the fundamental eating habits that should be avoided such as eating fried foods and high sugar content snacks. Those same people also know that fruits and vegetables are good for you. Then why are so many people unable to make the decision to eat the way they know they should?

Could it be that some people's inability to stop eating poorly is an addiction, similar to addictions to tobacco and alcohol? More likely, it's the cavalier attitude many people have about their health that keeps them eating poorly, until they're slapped in the face with the reality of poor health. You may have heard the saying "cancer is the cure for smoking." Well, you would think diabetes and heart disease would be the cure for obesity . . . but sadly, they often aren't. This battle is never ending in the medical profession. Moving to healthy eating habits is difficult. Eating what's good for you just doesn't feel as good as eating what's bad for you, in many cases. It's not that you can't ever eat a fast food meal again — you can. You can't, however, eat fast food or packaged food all or even most of the time and stay healthy.

The desire for a quick (and easy) fix

Given a choice, most people will take the quick fix over hard work every time. Lose 25 pounds in a week, guaranteed? Sign me up! Quit smoking overnight? Here's my money! Build a beautiful body in only two minutes a day — and you don't even have to stand up? That's for me!

It's human nature to want something for nothing, but when it comes to living longer, you have to put in the time and effort — hours in the gym, self-control in the grocery store, and discipline in your lifestyle choices. And make no mistake, it takes time and effort to eat healthier foods, exercise, and maintain a focused, balanced low-stress lifestyle. You have to give up things — horribly unhealthy foods that taste so wonderful as well as time you feel short on anyway — to get yourself in a positive aging routine.

Some of the more recent "quick fix" ideas have involved getting hormone supplements to stay young. Here's the real story on some of the most often touted anti-aging hormones:

- **Human growth hormones (HGH):** These are produced by your pituitary gland and are required for growth and cell repair. They start dropping at around age 40, and by age 70, HGH production may have dropped as much as 75 percent. So, HGH supplementation sounds like the perfect way to reverse the effects of aging. But does it work?

  Some studies have shown an increase in muscle mass and decrease in body fat in patients with a documented deficiency who received injections several times a week. The studies didn't, however, demonstrate an increase in strength along with the increase in muscle mass in those that didn't have a deficiency in the hormone. Evidence supports that HGH use in those who have a deficiency does offer benefits, but doesn't appear to be the simple answer for those without deficiency but are looking for a short cut.

✔ **Dehydroepiandrosterone (DHEA):** DHEA is a hormone produced by the adrenal glands and is converted into the hormones estrogen and testosterone. Levels of DHEA drop as you get older, and it's been theorized that raising DHEA levels may increase muscle mass and bone density, boost the immune system, and delay aging symptoms, such as joint pain, decreased muscle, libido, and lower energy.

  However, a study of 144 people over age 60 conducted by the Mayo Clinic over a two year period showed no increase in muscle strength, bone mass, endurance, or quality of life. An earlier, smaller, and shorter study did show some reduction in body fat and insulin resistance in those taking DHEA. Based on the evidence, use of DHEA without diagnosed deficiency doesn't seem to offer much benefit. As with other hormones, DHEA can help those who have a deficiency.

✔ **Testosterone therapy:** Like many hormones, testosterone production starts to decrease around age 30. Low testosterone levels can cause impotence in men and decreased sex drive, bone loss, muscle loss, and low energy levels in both men and women.

  • **Men:** In men with low testosterone, supplementation can increase all the above, so the interest in testosterone as a way to keep older men "young" developed. However, using testosterone supplements if you have normal testosterone levels already can be risky; very high levels of testosterone have been linked to breast cancer in men and can cause prostate enlargement, which can accelerate already present prostate cancer.

- **Women:** Women with low testosterone can have improvements in weight management and libido, but they may also develop male characteristic side effects such as increased facial hair and deepened voice. These won't occur if you're truly deficient and monitored correctly.

While hormone supplementation can be valuable, it's only valuable if you have a hormone deficiency. If you're having symptoms of fatigue, erectile dysfunction, inability to lose weight, muscle wasting despite exercise, or decreased libido, supplementation with hormones may help, but you need to discuss testing with your doctor instead of grabbing a bottle off the health store shelf. People who don't have a deficiency and are using it as a short cut to improve strength, endurance, and energy may have adverse reactions. Also, athletes have been using this for enhancement without a true deficiency or understanding of what the long-term consequences are.

Modifying Your Lifestyle: The One True Source of Hope

Wading through the mire of information, articles, products, and research on aging is enough to leave you feeling conflicted and confused. Medicine is starting to center on the behavioral modification that effectively helps people practice healthy lifestyles. So familiarize yourself with the truth — which we provide for you in the pages of this book — and resolve to let it guide your decisions.

In the end, living a healthier lifestyle is nine-tenths attitude change and one-tenth real effort. If you change your attitude about food, eating healthy will no longer seem like a punishment. Changing your exercise attitude makes exercise a pleasure rather than a pain. Getting rest is the energy for tomorrow. This type of attitude pushes you forward through the rest of this book and educates you further about the dangers and rewards of better lifestyles and healthier aging. And we're happy to take the first leg of your journey to healthful living and aging with you.

Chapter 2

The Four Major Health Concerns about Aging (And How to Prevent Them)

. . . .

In This Chapter

▶ Looking closely at cancer's most common forms
▶ Gauging the effects of diabetes, heart disease, and osteoporosis

. . . .

If you were a fine wine, you could honestly say, "I'm not getting older, I'm getting better" and mean it. You may not be aging like fine wine, but you can help yourself age well, especially when it comes to avoiding the four biggest health risks of aging: cancer, diabetes, cardiovascular disease, and osteoporosis. You have the benefit of technology and research providing the tools to carry you further in life, with fewer health problems than any generation before you. Your job is to pick up the tools — the information, screening techniques, and recommendations for healthier living — and use them.

Life is full of choices and every one of them influences health in some form. Because you can't look into the future, the best thing to do is to live as if every lifestyle choice you make has health ramifications down the road. The key phrase we repeat often throughout this book is *modify your lifestyle.* We hope this chapter convinces you that everyday changes can add up to healthier years — for years to come.

Cancer: The Four Most Common Forms

Few health diagnoses strike as much fear as the words, "You have cancer." But today, like at no other time, cancer can be conquered or kept under control in many cases. Cancer is one of the top causes of death worldwide, responsible for 13 percent of all deaths in 2005. If projections are accurate, this number could reach 9 million by 2015. Cancer cells exist and thrive in two ways:

- **Metastasize:** This term means that abnormal cells in a part of the body grow and can spread rapidly to other areas of the body. Metastasis is the major cause of cancer death, but in most cases, metastasis occurs later in the course of the disease . . . hence the importance of early detection.

- **In situ:** The term *in situ* means that the cancer cells haven't spread beyond the sites where the cancer began; it's still contained in the ducts or lobules.

The chance of developing cancer increases with age; 76 percent of all cancer is diagnosed in people over the age of 50. Although some of the risk factors for cancer, such as age, ethnicity, and family history, are beyond your control, you can still prevent 40 percent of cancers by modifying lifestyle choices, eating a healthy diet, staying physically active, and steering clear of tobacco products.

In this section, we cover the four most commonly diagnosed cancers — breast, colon, lung, and prostate — as well as their specific risk factors and preventive measures. We chose these particular cancers to discuss in detail not only because they're common cancers, but also because they're among the most easily diagnosed through routine examinations, which can increase cure rates. And in the case of lung and colon cancer, they're the most preventable by lifestyle modification and/or early treatment. (Many other cancers, such as liver and stomach, can't be diagnosed through routine testing and often aren't diagnosed until symptoms develop.)

Lung cancer

About 1.3 billion people worldwide smoke, even though it's no secret that smoking can kill you. If you aren't convinced to quit, what will it take? Check out the following statistics of lung cancer:

- ✔ Is the most common cancer worldwide, with 1.2 million new cases diagnosed in 2007 alone

- ✔ Is the deadliest cancer and has the highest worldwide mortality rate

- ✔ Three million people diagnosed with lung cancer worldwide

- ✔ Causes more deaths than the other three most common cancers combined (colon, breast, and prostate)

The good news? Most lung cancer is preventable, because 90 percent of cases are caused by smoking. Imagine how quickly new cases of lung cancer would drop if everyone quit lighting up.

Differentiating among the different types

Lung cancer falls into two general categories, small-cell lung cancer (SCLC), also called *oat cell cancer,* and non

64

small-cell lung cancer (NSCLC). NSCLC is much more common — around 80 percent of lung cancers are NSCLC. SCLC grows more quickly than NSCLC and is almost entirely caused by smoking.

NSCLC can be divided into three different types:

- **Adenocarcinoma:** These cancers account for about 40 percent of lung cancers and have a better prognosis than other types of lung cancer. Adenocarcinomas are often found in the outer regions of the lungs and initially develop in the mucus producing cells.

- **Large cell carcinoma:** Around 10 to 15 percent of lung cancers fall into this category; large cell carcinoma has characteristically large, rounded cells, grows rapidly, and has a poor prognosis.

- **Squamous cell carcinoma:** This cancer accounts for about 25 to 30 percent of all lung cancers and most commonly occurs near the center of the lung in one of the bronchus (one of the two main branches of the windpipe). Smoking is the main cause.

Understanding your risk

Unlike some cancers, doctors know what causes lung cancer. Take a look at the risk factors:

- **Smoking:** Cigarette smoking is the number one cause of lung cancer. Ninety percent of lung cancer cases occur in people who smoke. The more cigarettes you smoke, the higher your risk of developing lung cancer. Cigarette smoke contains over 4,000 chemicals, many of which are proven to be cancer-causing substances called *carcinogens.*

Carcinogens cause irreversible damage to your body's DNA cells and increase the chance of cancerous change.

✔ **Radon inhalation:** Radon is a gas not detected by sight, taste, or smell. Radon is the second most common cause of lung cancer. Radon gas causes between 15,000 and 22,000 lung cancer deaths each year in the United States. Radon gas comes up through the soil and in through cracks in your home or a building's foundation. It tends to build up in unventilated basements, pipes, drains, or walls. Home sales in many places now require radon testing — call the Environmental Protection Agency (EPA) or the National Environmental Health Association for more info.

✔ **Workplace chemicals:** People (mine workers, pipe fitters, and shipbuilders) who are exposed to certain workplace materials, such as asbestos, (see the sidebar "When the culprit is fibers, not nicotine") have a higher risk of lung cancer because inhaled fibers and dust can become embedded in the lung cells, causing a chronic inflammatory reaction that can eventually result in cancerous cell changes. Workers' risks are much higher if they smoke in addition to having these types of chemical exposures.

✔ **Secondhand smoke:** The EPA has classified secondhand smoke as a known cause of cancer in humans. Secondhand smoke is also known as environmental tobacco smoke and is classified as any mixture of smoke given off by the burning end of a cigarette, cigar, pipe, or smoke exhaled from a smoker's lungs. Secondhand smoke causes approximately 3,400 lung cancer deaths in the U.S.

every year. Some of the carcinogens in secondhand smoke include formaldehyde, benzene, vinyl chloride, arsenic, ammonia, and hydrogen cyanide. These agents have an immediate effect on your cardiovascular system.

✔ **Age:** As with many cancers, your risk for developing lung cancer increases with age. The longer you smoke and the more cigarettes you smoke, the greater your chances of developing lung cancer. Less than 1 percent of lung cancer cases occur in people under age 40. The development of lung cancer increases thereafter, with the average patient age at diagnosis around 60.

✔ **Family history:** People who have a *first-degree* relative (mother, father, brother, or sister) with lung cancer have a higher incidence of lung cancer because some lung cancer is linked to mutations in the genetic cells that can be passed on to blood relatives.

Playing your part in prevention

If you want to reduce your risk for lung cancer, stop smoking, never start smoking, stay away from those who do, and avoid exposure to asbestos or chemicals (like radon and chromium) that can cause lung cancer. Eliminating these risks of lung cancer and lung disease and getting thorough medical evaluations for any exposures can almost completely eliminate the risk of lung cancer.

People with certain exposures may need to have yearly x-rays or other imaging due to the duration that some cancers take to develop. Some of the cancers can be missed with x-rays alone while computed tomography (CT) scans can be more sensitive, so see your doctor to establish the proper testing.

What if you used to smoke, but don't now? Your risk for developing lung cancer starts to decline approximately five years after you kick the habit. After ten years, your risk of lung cancer is about 50 percent lower than a smoker's, and the risk continues to decrease with time. It takes nearly 20 years for your lungs to return to "almost" normal, but some damage always remains. For people who've quit smoking and do develop lung cancer, studies show they usually respond better to treatment and may live longer than those who continue to smoke.

Recognizing the symptoms

In the early stages of lung cancer, you may not experience symptoms. Many of the cases of lung cancer are found when doing screening tests or diagnostic tests for something else and then identifying lung cancer. By the time any symptoms develop, lung cancer is most likely in advanced stages and has metastasized. For these reasons, the mortality rate for lung cancer is so high. The following are the most common lung cancer symptoms:

When the culprit is fibers, not nicotine

Two other types of cancer are mesothelioma, usually found in asbestos exposed workers, and carcinoid tumors. Asbestos is a naturally occurring fibrous mineral, which is used in many industrial building materials because it's durable and resistant to heat. Mesothelioma cancer takes 35 to 40 years to develop and grows in the lining of the lungs. It produces copious amounts of fluid, which needs frequent draining from the lungs. Carcinoid tumors are rare, benign tumors accounting for only 1 to 2 percent of lung cancers. They can be removed, or chemotherapy or radiation can be used to shrink them.

- ✔ Cough that persists or worsens without any particular reason

- ✔ Hoarseness

- ✔ Fever or night sweats

- ✔ Coughing up blood

- ✔ Weight loss and loss of appetite

- ✔ Shortness of breath, wheezing, or chest tightness

- ✔ Chronic infections such as bronchitis or pneumonia

Talk to your doctor if you experience any of these cancer symptoms.

Treating lung cancer and considering the prospects

Lung cancer treatments are based on the type of lung cancer, how advanced the disease, and your underlying general health. If the cancer is found to be treatable and your health supports treatment, doctors usually use some combination of chemotherapy, radiation, and surgery:

- ✔ **Chemotherapy:** Chemotherapy is used to shrink tumors, keep tumors from spreading, or simply to help relieve pain from some of the tumors when someone is receiving comfort measures only. Chemotherapy drugs damage healthy cells as well as cancerous cells and can have severe side effects that may seem worse than the cancer symptoms themselves. These types of reactions depend on the type of agents used; some chemotherapy agents cause fewer symptoms than others. A cancer doctor can determine the best option for your specific cancer situation.

✔ **Radiation:** Radiation uses x-rays to kill cancer cells. This procedure can be accomplished by shooting the radiation through the outside of the body or directly inserting radiation into the cancer or area of the cancer by needles or catheters. The delivery method depends on the type of cancer, stage, and location of the cancer, with the goal of destroying cancer cells with minimal harm to the surrounding healthy tissue. Radiation can damage normal tissues, so make sure to discuss radiation treatment with a doctor specializing in radiation therapy.

✔ **Surgery:** Lung cancer treatment may involve removing a portion, a lobe, or a whole lung. Lymph nodes surrounding the cancerous area may be removed during surgery to determine whether treatment options are needed.

Regardless of the treatment, lung cancer can have a poor prognosis if not found early. The following statistics apply to lung cancer:

✔ Only one in eight lung cancer patients survives five years after their diagnosis.

✔ The five-year survival rate is almost 50 percent for patients with localized tumors; unfortunately, less than 25 percent of cases are diagnosed that early.

✔ After the cancer metastasizes, the five-year survival rate is less than 2 percent.

✔ Approximately six out of ten lung cancer patients die within one year of their diagnosis; between seven and eight out of ten people die from their disease in two years.

Breast cancer

Many young women state that their biggest health fear when growing older is breast cancer. Even though lung cancer has a higher mortality rate and heart disease is a greater health risk (see respective sections in this chapter), breast cancer is still what many women worry most about. On the flip side, many women don't worry about breast cancer because it doesn't run in their families. This false sense of security can be a costly mistake if it keeps you from having preventative testing.

Consider the following breast cancer facts:

- Globally, breast cancer is the most commonly diagnosed cancer among women and is the second leading cause of cancer death for women.

- About 1.2 million people worldwide are diagnosed with the disease each year with approximately 502,000 global deaths.

- Breast cancer also affects about 1,600 men worldwide each year.

- Breast cancer is more common among women over the age of 40 and is rare in women under age 25.

- Fifty percent of diagnosed breast cancer is in women over age 65.

You can't completely prevent breast cancer — everyone is at risk. Great strides have been made in breast cancer awareness in recent years, with more women aware of the symptoms and utilizing self-exam and diagnostic techniques regularly.

Differentiating types of breast cancer

Breast cancer is classified in different ways according to its location and whether it's metastasized. The following list describes other terms you may hear used to describe breast cancer:

- **Adenocarcinoma:** Most breast cancers start in the glandular tissue (lobes and ducts) of the breast; cancers of glandular tissue are called adenocarcinoma. There are two types of adenocarcinoma:

  - **Ductal carcinoma in situ (DCIS):** DCIS means the cancer is contained within the walls of the ducts and hasn't spread to other breast tissue or metastasized. This is the most common type of noninvasive breast cancer, accounting for around 20 percent of newly diagnosed cases. Almost all women diagnosed at this stage can be cured.

  - **Lobular carcinoma in situ (LCIS):** LCIS begins in the lobules of the breast but hasn't invaded through to surrounding breast tissue. LCIS isn't a true cancer; it may be the early stage of cancer or may simply increase a woman's risk of getting cancer later. Everyone agrees that at a minimum having LCIS increases your risk and that it's important to follow the screening guidelines for breast cancer closely if you have LCIS.

- **Invasive ductal carcinoma (IDC):** IDC, which starts in a duct and then breaks through to the fatty part of the breast, accounts for 80 percent of all invasive breast cancers. After the cancer breaks through, it can metastasize through your blood stream or lymphatics.

- ✔ **Invasive lobular carcinoma (ILC):** Ten percent of invasive breast cancers are ILC, which begins in the lobules (milk producing glands). ILC is harder to feel on examinations and harder to detect on mammograms than IDC, but can metastasize in the same way, through lymphatics and blood vessels.

- ✔ **Inflammatory breast cancer (IBC):** This cancer is an uncommon type of breast cancer accounting for only 1 to 3 percent of cases. Instead of containing a single lump or tumor, the entire breast becomes warm and red, with the skin taking on the appearance of an orange peel. This condition occurs because the cancer cells are blocking the lymph vessels in the skin. IBC is more likely to spread (metastasize) than ductal or lobular cancers (see previous bullets).

- ✔ **Paget disease of the nipple:** This cancer is rare and accounts for only 1 percent of all breast cancers. The upside of this cancer is that it has an excellent prognosis (meaning that there are good cure rates) in most cases. The disease starts in the breast ducts and then spreads to the skin of the nipple and then to the areola, the dark circle around the nipple. You may feel itching or burning and notice crusted, scaly, and red areas, which may ooze or bleed.

Understanding your risk

You can control some risks for developing breast cancer. Unfortunately, with breast cancer, the risks you can't control outweigh the ones you can. For these reasons, early detection is important. The following are major risk factors for breast cancer:

✔ **Gender:** Both men and women can develop breast cancer:

- Women are far more likely to develop breast cancer than men. The ratio of women to men with breast cancer is 100 to one. The National Cancer Institute predicts that one in eight women born today will develop breast cancer in her lifetime.
- Risk factors for men include age (the average age for breast cancer in men is about age 67), obesity (obese men have higher levels of estrogens in their body), testicular and liver disease, and a disease called Kleinfelter's syndrome, which occurs in men who are born with two or more "x" chromosomes. Exposure to high levels of radiation also increases men's risk.

✔ **Age:** As your age increases, so does your chance for developing breast cancer. This is due to exposure to estrogen over your lifetime and the fact that there has been a longer time for cells to have cancerous changes. According to the National Cancer Institute, for women age is a factor as follows:

- Age 30 to 39 — 1 in 233 probability of breast cancer
- Age 40 to 49 — 1 in 69 probability of breast cancer
- Age 50 to 59 — 1 in 38 probability of breast cancer
- Age 60 to 69 — 1 in 27 probability of breast cancer

✔ **Family history of cancer:** A woman's risk of developing breast cancer increases if she has a *first-degree* relative (mother, sister, or daughter) diagnosed with breast or ovarian cancer before the age of 40. Other combinations of family history risk factors are moderate risks, such as having two close relatives from the same side of the family diagnosed with breast cancer (one must be mom, sister, or daughter, while the other can be an aunt, grandma, or even Uncle Bob).

Scientists have found that women with genetic mutations (random structural changes) to genes *BRCA1* and *BRCA2* (short for Breast Cancer 1 and Breast Cancer 2) have up to an 85 percent chance of developing breast cancer in their lifetime. Less than 10 percent of breast cancer cases are related to inheritable genes, however. If you do have a strong family history, your doctor may want you to have earlier or more frequent testing done.

✔ **Long-term estrogen exposure:** A strong correlation exists between breast cancer development and the hormone estrogen. Estrogen stimulates cancer cells to grow and divide rapidly. A woman's estrogen levels rise during puberty, then decrease during menopause. The longer a woman's breasts are exposed to estrogen, the greater her risk for developing breast cancer. Therefore, breast cancer risk may be higher in women who started menstruating before age 12 or in women who went through menopause after age 55. Research has also implicated hormonal birth control — whether oral, injected, or implanted — as a risk, especially if used for more than five years. Hormone replacement therapy after menopause may be a risk factor as well, but studies are inconclusive.

✔ **Drinking alcohol:** Around one in fifty cases of breast cancer may be attributed to alcohol consumption in the U.S.; in countries where alcohol consumption is higher the risk may be as much as one in six cases. You can control this risk by watching your alcohol intake.

✔ **Poor nutrition and being overweight:** Evidence suggests that animal fat can increase the risk of breast cancer, but being overweight holds a much stronger correlation to the development of breast cancer and has an adverse effect on survival in post menopausal women. (See Chapter 7 for tips on nutrition.) You can curb this risk by taking better care of yourself.

Playing your part in prevention

"Know thy breasts" should be the defining statement for early detection of breast cancer. Breast cancer prevention starts with regular breast self-exams, beginning when you're in your 20s. Using a step-by-step approach on a specific schedule (see the next section, "Recognizing abnormalities"), women can be aware of how their breasts normally look and feel.

Monthly self-exams provide you with a baseline; if anything changes from month to month, you're the first to know. Report any breast changes to a health professional as soon as they're discovered. Remember that a breast change doesn't mean you have cancer!

The best time for a woman to examine her breasts is one week after her period is over, when her breasts aren't tender or swollen, so she can feel any abnormalities or lumps that may be present. This examination is no small task at times; some women have very lumpy breasts and the lumps may change from month to month. (See the nearby sidebar, "All lumps aren't created equal," for more info.)

All lumps aren't created equal

There are a lot of fibrous tissue, glands, and ducts in the breast that can feel like lumps. Lumpy breasts, more scientifically known as fibrocystic breast disease (FBD), are experienced by as many as 60 percent of all women. The cause isn't completely known, but most feel that hormones are the front runner. Fortunately, women with FBD notice a reduction in lumpiness after menopause due to the decrease in female hormones. The lumps are benign, sometimes painful, and may change at different points of your menstrual cycle. Caffeine is thought to make FBD worse, but whether there's a true link is controversial. It's still advisable to stop caffeine if you have FBD, but consult your doctor for the specifics.

Women who are pregnant or breastfeeding should still keep examining their breasts regularly, even though the breasts may be tender. Women with breast implants should ask their surgeon to help them differentiate between breast tissue and the implant. To ensure proper technique, women should review their self breast exam (SBE) process with their healthcare professional during their clinical breast exam.

Clinical breast exams should be done at every yearly gynecologic exam. At age 40, women need to have the first of their recommended annual mammograms as well as yearly breast exams, unless they had an abnormal breast exam or there's a strong family history of breast cancer. Mammograms are currently the best and most reliable screening method, although it may take as many as six to ten years for breast cancer tumors to be detected by mammography. Your doctor may recommend an earlier screening if you have a personal or family history with breast cancer.

77

Sometimes ultrasound is used and is good for distinguishing whether a detected lump is a cyst (likely to be benign) or a solid mass (which could indicate a tumor). This technique is good to use in women with breast implants and dense breasts because a mammogram sometimes has difficulties "seeing" through dense tissue or implants. Ultrasound is also a great method for guiding physicians to do needle biopsies of suspicious lumps.

In 2007, the American Cancer Society recommended that women at high risk (such as a previous history of breast cancer or a strong family history) for breast cancer should have a magnetic resonance imaging (MRI) scan in addition to their mammograms (not in lieu of). MRIs are more sensitive, picking up more spots than a mammogram, and may result in more false positive results. The two tests together give better data to evaluate a woman for breast cancer. If your doctor detects any abnormalities, he may schedule a follow-up biopsy or some other doctor-recommended procedure.

Recognizing the symptoms

When feeling for a lump in your breast, keep in mind the following things:

- Cancer cells are an abnormal overgrowth — meaning *irregular* in shape. The lump will be hard and have a bumpy texture.

- The lump may not move during your self breast exam, but because it may be small and covered with healthy tissue, you may have a hard time telling if it moves or not.

- Although cancerous masses have some particular characteristics, any lump no matter what it feels like should be checked out by a healthcare professional.

✔ Look for dimpling of the skin, retraction of the skin or nipple, thickening of the skin, or nipple discharge.

The technique recommended for self breast exams has changed. There's evidence that the woman's position (lying down), area felt, pattern of coverage of the breast, and use of different amounts of pressure increase the sensitivity of the self-exam.

To perform a SBE, use these steps (see Figure 2-1):

1. **Standing in front of a mirror, look at your breasts for any changes of size, shape, contour, dimpling, pulling, redness, or flaking skin around the nipple or surrounding skin.**

2. **Lie on your back and place your right arm comfortably behind your head.**

   When you lie on your back, your breast tissue spreads more evenly and thinly over your chest. This position makes feeling for lumps or abnormalities easier.

3. **Place the three middle fingers of your left hand on your right breast.**

4. **Using the pads of your fingers, make small circular motions over your breast tissue to feel for lumps.**

   You should circle the tissue three times and use varying levels of pressure before moving on to the next area.

   • Start lightly to feel the skin's surface.
   • Use medium pressure to feel the tissue just under the skin, and then
   • Press more firmly to feel the tissue closest to your chest and ribs.

Use enough pressure to feel all the breast tissue, but don't cause yourself pain.

5. **Manipulate your fingers over the entire breast area in an up and down pattern starting from under your arm and across your breast to the middle of the chest bone (sternum) making a large square.**

    Use this pattern to help:

    • Draw an imaginary square (from just under your arm along your neck to your collar bone, then down your breast bone and over your rib cage and back up).

    • Using the pads of your fingers, walk them up and down imaginary rows of the square like a BINGO card, feeling the breast tissue for any abnormalities or lumps.

        This up-and-down pattern is the most effective method for not missing any tissue.

6. **Now repeat the process of Steps 2 to 5 on your left breast, using the fingers on your right hand.**

7. **When you're done examining your breasts from a reclining position, stand up.**

8. **Standing in front of the mirror, place your hands on your hips and look at your breasts for any changes of size, shape, contour, dimpling, pulling, redness, or flaking skin around the nipple or surrounding skin.**

    The act of pressing down on your hips contracts the muscles in your chest. This makes any changes in your breast more apparent.

9. **Place your arms by your side and look; raise**

your hands above your head and press your palms to one another and look again.

This completes your monthly exam. Report any lumps or abnormalities to your doctor.

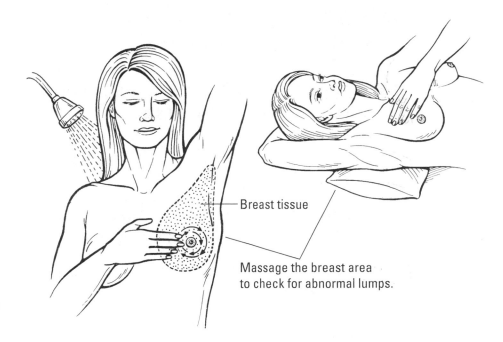

Breast tissue

Massage the breast area to check for abnormal lumps.

Figure 2-1:
How to perform a self breast exam.

Following up on a lump

Most of the lumps that you can feel are benign (not cancer); most often the first sign of breast cancer is abnormalities found on a mammogram when it can't be felt on SBEs or by a medical professional. In fact, the American Academy of Family Physicians indicates as many as 90 percent of breast lumps are benign. Have any lumps or changes evaluated by your doctor.

After you find a lump in your breast, here's what happens during a typical physician evaluation:

✔ You give a full health history, including the mention of an immediate family member with breast cancer (mother, sister, daughter).

- ✔ You have a full breast exam, with the doctor palpating your breasts for any lumps or abnormalities.

- ✔ You schedule a mammogram, ultrasound, or breast MRI (one or more of these may be done).

If the physician workup reveals any suspicious lumps you may be scheduled for one of the following procedures:

- ✔ A needle to remove cells from the lump to test for cancer

- ✔ A core biopsy to remove part of the lump for evaluation

- ✔ A lumpectomy to have the lump surgically removed and tested

If your lump is breast cancer, the earlier you can begin treatment, the better your survival rate.

Treating breast cancer and considering the prospects

Treatment options for breast cancer include surgery, chemotherapy, hormone therapy, and radiation. The five-year survival rate for localized breast cancer is 98 percent. Unfortunately, advanced *metastatic* cancer has a higher mortality rate. If the cancer has spread regionally this survival rate drops to 81 percent and those with distant metastases have a 26 percent five-year survival rate. After the five-year mark, the overall survival rate drops to 80 percent.

We don't go into treatment details here, but for more info, check out *Breast Cancer For Dummies* (Wiley) by Ronit Elk, PhD, and Monica Morrow, MD.

Prostate cancer

The prostate plays a vital role in the male reproductive system. A healthy prostate is about the size of a peach pit and the shape of a walnut. It's located underneath the bladder, in front of the rectum, and surrounds the urethra, which carries urine and seminal fluid (not simultaneously). Blood vessels and nerves also travel through the prostate tissue.

Prostate cancer is cancer inside this small gland and is quite common. This cancer is treatable when caught early and is usually found during routine screening. Despite the excellent cure rate, men are particularly frightened of prostate cancer because they see it as a huge threat to their manhood. Many already feel uncomfortable with the screening procedure and are really reluctant to have biopsies and possible surgery.

Male hormones (androgens) can cause the prostate to grow, and many men develop benign enlargement of the prostate as they age. An enlarged prostate squeezes the urethra, vessels, and nerves and can cause symptoms similar to the symptoms of prostate cancer. Enlargement is a very common condition, but don't assume prostate symptoms are just age-related prostate enlargement. The symptoms are so similar to prostate cancer that you should see your doctor to rule out cancer.

Understanding your risk

Prostate cancer is the most commonly diagnosed cancer, other than skin cancers, and the second leading cause of cancer death in American men. The good news, though, is that 90 percent of prostate cancers are diagnosed early, while still in the prostate (or close by) and carries a five-year survival rate for these men of nearly 100 percent.

While the exact cause of prostate cancer isn't known, there are certain identifiable risks:

✔ **Age:** Some clinicians feel that every male would develop prostate cancer if they lived long enough, but most men die of a different cause before this happens. It's an interesting thought. Although many men are now being diagnosed as early as their 40s, the majority, about 65 percent, of diagnoses are made in men over age 65. Here's the age breakdown:

  - Under age 40: You have a 1 in 10,000 chance
  - Ages 40 to 59: You have a 1 in 39 chance
  - Ages 60 to 69: You have a 1 in 14 chance

✔ **Ethnicity:** African-American men are nearly 60 percent more likely to develop prostate cancer than Caucasian men. They are also two and a half times more likely to die from the disease and are ranked with the highest percentage of prostate cancer cases in the world. Researchers haven't been able to explain these racial differences.

✔ **Family history:** Men with a single first-degree relative (think father, brother, or son) diagnosed with prostate cancer have a greater risk of developing prostate cancer. A man with a family history of two or more relatives with prostate cancer is four times more likely to develop the disease himself. The risk is highest in men whose family members were diagnosed before age 65.

✔ **Western-Hemisphere lifestyle:** A diet high in calories from unhealthy fat, refined carbohydrates, and animal protein, coupled with low physical activity contributes to a variety of diseases, including cancer. The WHO specifically attributes the development of prostate cancer to this "Western lifestyle."

Playing your part in prevention

In order to diagnose prostate cancer early, you need to take an active part in your healthcare. Just as women should perform monthly self breast exams and receive mammograms starting at age 40, men need to start having these annual screening exams at age 40:

- **Digital rectal exam (DRE):** This rectal exam is administered by a doctor. The doctor inserts a lubricated, gloved finger into the rectum to check the prostate for lumps, nodules, or masses. The prostate should be smooth, uniform in shape, and symmetrical.

- **Prostate-specific antigen (PSA):** This test measures the level of PSA in the blood. PSA is an enzyme produced mostly by the prostate to liquefy semen and normally enters the bloodstream in small amounts.

When the two tests are done in conjunction with each other cancer detection is improved. Doing these tests singularly may increase the chances of a missed diagnosis in a cancer that already doesn't produce many symptoms.

Recognizing the symptoms

The symptoms of prostate cancer are easily misinterpreted as other problems, so here are some of the most common signs and symptoms of prostate cancer:

- Rectal pressure or pain in the space between the anus and the scrotum

- Frequent or painful urination

- Frequent urination at night (nocturia)

- Difficulty getting the urine stream started
- Blood in the urine or ejaculate
- Painful ejaculation
- Loss of appetite and weight
- Bone pain caused from local cancer spread into the bones

Treating prostate cancer and considering the prospects

Your prostate cancer treatment options may involve surgery, radiation therapy, or hormone therapy. Discuss your best course of action with your doctor. Your doctor monitors your health closely for any changes in your symptoms, if you develop new symptoms, or if any worsen.

The survival stats for men with the cancer without having metastasized to other organs or tissues are as follows:

- 99 percent survive at least 5 years
- 92 percent survive at least 10 years
- 61 percent survive at least 15 years

Colorectal cancer

Colorectal cancer is located in the colon *or* in the rectum but is more commonly referred to as simply colon cancer. The colon is the first 4 to 5 feet of the large intestine while the rectum, the connector between the colon and the anus, is the last 5 to 6 inches. The areas are both extensions of each other and cancers in these areas are handled similarly. Colorectal cancer is the third most-common type of cancer in the world with 940,000 new cases diagnosed annually. In the U.S., colon cancer has the second highest mortality rate of all cancers, but many deaths can be prevented with proper screening and risk reduction.

Understanding your risk

There's no single known risk factor for developing colon cancer, but rather a group of risk factors:

✔ **Polyps:** Polyps are small, fleshy bumps or nodules attached to the wall of the colon or rectum, and they're the biggest risk factor of colorectal cancer. Almost all cases of colorectal cancer develop from polyps. These bumps that aren't removed may grow abnormally and eventually becoming malignant.

The process of going from a benign polyp to a malignant tumor can take several years. Many colon polyps are benign, but all polyps have the potential to become cancerous, some more aggressively than others. When cancer grows within a polyp, in time it can infiltrate the wall of the colon, spreading into blood vessels or lymph nodes. After metastasis has occurred the cure rate drops significantly, which is why detection and removal of polyps before they become cancerous are important.

✔ **Age:** Over 90 percent of cases are diagnosed in people over the age of 50 with the average age at diagnosis around 70. Your chance of being diagnosed with colorectal cancer is 50 times higher if you're age 60 to 79 than if you're younger than age 40.

✔ **Family history:** Colorectal cancer is more likely to occur among people with a first-degree relative (mother, father, sister, son) diagnosed with colorectal cancer, especially if the cancer was diagnosed at a young age. Between 2 and 5 percent of people with colorectal cancer inherit abnormal genes: One is called familial adenomatous polyposis

(FAP) and the other hereditary nonpolyposis colorectal cancer (HNPCC). If you have one or more relatives diagnosed with colorectal cancer before the age of 50, consider having a blood test to determine if you have the gene mutation and then take the appropriate preventative measures.

✔ **Chronic inflammatory bowel disease:** People who suffer from *Crohn's disease* (inflammatory condition of the gastrointestinal tract) or *ulcerative colitis* (inflammatory bowel disease) for at least eight to ten years have a higher risk of colorectal cancer. Constant inflammation of the colon can cause cell turnover and can also speed up the growth of polyps. Your doctor may suggest doing more frequent colonoscopies.

Playing your part in prevention

The incidence of colon cancer has gone down in the last 15 years due to the fact that, in many cases, colorectal cancer can be prevented by removing precancerous polyps. Early detection with regular exams after age 50 is the biggest factor in early detection and treatment of colorectal disease, but less than 50 percent of eligible people have been screened for colorectal cancer.

There are a few types of screenings you can have done to test for colorectal cancer:

✔ **Digital rectal examination (DRE):** This exam begins at age 40 (some doctors start at age 50) and continues annually. During a rectal exam, your doctor may be able to detect polyps in the rectum. If older than 50, at no time does this test replace the need for a colonoscopy.

✔ **Fecal occult blood test (FOBT):** This screening

starts at age 50 and continues annually. FOBT tests for hidden blood in three consecutive stool samples. As a doctor, Brent likes to have people start at age 40 because the test is simple, non-invasive, and helpful. This test is also helpful for people that are suspicious of blood in the stool but aren't sure.

✔ **Double-contrast barium enema:** This test consists of a series of X-rays of the colon and rectum after being given an enema containing barium dye and an injection of air into the bowel. This test isn't done as frequently as colonoscopy because the barium enema isn't as effective as the colonoscopy at detecting polyps smaller than a half an inch. But the barium enema is still an acceptable, low-cost alternative when a colonoscopy can't be performed.

✔ **Colonoscopy:** A colonoscopy is an internal examination of the colon using a flexible lighted instrument called a colonoscope. The whole purpose of the colonoscopy is to find polyps, remove them, and then follow proper monitoring after removal. Colonoscopies can be used as screening tests or as follow-up diagnostic tools when the results of another screening test are positive. Colonoscopy screenings start at age 50 and if anything is found then the frequency is increased. If nothing's found, doctors may wait up to ten years for your next scope (depending on the doctor).

Recognizing the symptoms

Early colorectal cancer may not cause many symptoms. The most common symptoms are associated with changes in bowel habits, which includes one or more of the following:

✔ **Rectal bleeding:** This bleeding occurs with visible

Having a colonoscopy . . . it's not so bad!

Most people feel that the prep to clean out the colon (which is necessary) is worse than the colonoscopy itself. To clean the colon properly, you need to use laxatives and/or enemas, as well as not eat solid foods for 24 to 48 hours prior to the test.

Note: Because there's a risk of bleeding with this procedure, people taking blood thinner medication or supplements should consult with their doctor prior to examination.

A colonoscopy procedure can be performed with or without a sedative and pain reliever for comfort, although most people elect to have medication. To begin, you lie on your left side with your knees drawn up toward your chest. The colonoscope is then inserted through the rectum and gently advanced to the lowest part of the small bowel. Air and water pass through the scope to remove anything obstructing the doctor's view, and suction is used to remove debris as needed. If the doctor finds any abnormalities, tissue samples are taken with instruments that can be inserted through the scope.

blood in the stools, on toilet paper, or in the water.

✔ **Microscopic blood:** This blood isn't visible to the naked eye. This is why fecal occult blood testing is important (see preceding section).

✔ **A change in usual bowel patterns:** Having constipation or diarrhea for more than 7 to 10 days can indicate a problem.

✔ **Nausea or vomiting:** These symptoms are common complaints from people with certain cancers of the gastrointestinal tract due to the location of the cancer. Some other cancers can also effect appetite and indirectly induce some nausea.

- ✔ **Lower abdominal pain:** Pain from either gas, cramping, or bloating that lasts longer than a week or feeling that your stomach is distended or full should be discussed with your doctor.

- ✔ **Shape of the stool:** Thinning of your stool into "thin pencil shapes" could indicate an obstruction in the intestine that is pressing on the stool creating the thinner form.

- ✔ **Unexplained weight loss:** Cancer can use up much of the body's energy and sometimes can release substances that can alter metabolism. Furthermore, people with cancer often develop loss of appetite that develops so slowly that it's not recognized as a problem.

Never ignore rectal bleeding, because early detection of colon cancer can save your life. Get a second opinion if a doctor doesn't appear to be taking your case seriously. When treating patients with blood in the stool, Dr. Agin always remembers the tragic situation of a nurse's 30-year-old husband. Over a five-year period, the husband was evaluated by several doctors who told him the bleeding was most likely from hemorrhoids, although no one sent him for a colonoscopy. By the time he found a doctor who sent him for a colonoscopy, he had advanced colon cancer and died from it within four years. If your doctor isn't taking continuing rectal bleeding seriously, get another opinion!

Treating colorectal cancer and considering the prospects

Surgery is the most common form of treatment for colorectal cancer. Surgical removal of a portion of the bowel can increase a person's survival rate by 75 percent. Some small, malignant polyps can be removed with the colonoscope, but many patients with colorectal cancer need to undergo bowel resection — the removal of the portion of bowel that contains the cancerous cells. In most cases each side of the colon can be reattached after the cancerous section is removed, but sometimes the patients have to have a colostomy (the bowel is attached to an opening in the abdominal wall, a stoma, for excretion or waste). Most of the time this solution is temporary to allow the bowel to heal and then the bowel is corrected. A secondary bowel resection may be necessary in approximately 25 percent of those patients who have a recurrence. Twenty percent of those people remain colorectal cancer free.

Colon cancer has decent cure rates, depending on the stage:

- ✔ The 5 year survival is greater than 90 percent for localized stage.

- ✔ The 5 year survival rate is 65 percent for regional stage.

- ✔ The 5 year survival rate is less than 10 percent for distant stage.

Diabetes

Diabetes is a chronic illness that if not diagnosed or treated properly can have a number of complications. People with diabetes have problems managing the amounts of glucose (sugar) in the blood. When glucose levels build up in your blood instead of being delivered to your cells as fuel, your cells become starved for energy. Over a long period of time, high blood sugar levels lead to kidney failure, cardiovascular disease, nerve damage, and arteriosclerosis. Other complications that come from diabetes and poor blood sugar control include blindness and severe infections. Diabetics also have a higher risk for certain cancers, like pancreatic and uterine cancer. Unfortunately, diabetes isn't curable — it is, however, manageable.

 Diabetes is one of the top ten causes of death worldwide, with approximately 171 million people having diabetes. This number is expected to increase by 150 percent in the next 20 years due to the increase in obesity, poor nutrition, and sedentary lifestyle.

For the complete rundown on diabetes, read *Diabetes For Dummies,* 2nd Edition (Wiley) by Alan L. Rubin, MD.

Differentiating among the types of diabetes

Diabetes can show up in different forms:

- ✔ **Type 1 diabetes:** Type 1 diabetes, the unpreventable form, is typically diagnosed in childhood or young adulthood and is formerly known as juvenile diabetes. In people with type 1 diabetes, the insulin producing cells in the pancreas (beta cells) stop functioning. Type 1 diabetes requires insulin administration for survival and can't be controlled with diet and exercise. Possible causes of type 1 include autoimmune disease, genetic disease, and environmental agents.

- ✔ **Type 2 diabetes:** Type 2 diabetes is the most common form accounting for 90 to 95 percent of people with diabetes. People with type 2 diabetes make some insulin, but either it's not enough or their cells become resistant to insulin. Many people with type 2 diabetes can control their blood sugar with diet, exercise, and oral medication, but some people still require insulin injections.

On average, people with type 2 diabetes die 5 to 10 years before people without diabetes, mostly due to cardiovascular disease. However, and this is a big *however,* many of these cases are preventable.

🗸 **Gestational diabetes:** This form is a type of glucose intolerance that occurs in approximately 3 to 5 percent of pregnant women, and should be tested for during the 24th to 28th week of pregnancy. There's an increase risk for pregnant women if they have a strong family history of diabetes or are obese. Women who have gestational diabetes are then at an increased risk for developing type 2 diabetes later in life (up to 20 years).

Understanding your risk

You can't prevent type 1 diabetes, and gestational diabetes has limited preventable causes, but you can control the risk factors for type 2 diabetes:

🗸 **Obesity:** This is the single greatest risk factor for developing type 2 diabetes, because being overweight can inhibit the body from making or using insulin efficiently. People with a body mass index (BMI) of 30 or higher have an 80 to 90 percent greater incidence of developing type 2 diabetes than people who maintain a healthy weight.

🗸 **Age:** Most people who develop diabetes are over age 40 with the risk increasing as a person ages; however, the obesity epidemic in children is resulting in more type 2 diabetes being diagnosed in children.

🗸 **Family history of diabetes:** If you have a first-degree relative with type 2 diabetes, you're at a higher risk.

✔ **Gestational diabetes:** If you had gestational diabetes, your risk for developing type 2 diabetes increases. According to the National Diabetes Education Program (NDEP) between 5 to 10 percent of women with gestational diabetes develop type 2 diabetes.

✔ **Physical inactivity:** You can prevent up to 80 percent of type 2 diabetes cases by adopting a healthy diet and increasing physical activity.

Check with your doctor about a healthy diet and exercise plan to decrease your sugar levels and get back on track to a healthy weight.

Playing your part in prevention

By taking an active role in modifying your lifestyle choices, you can significantly reduce your risk for developing diabetes. Check out the following changes:

✔ **Maintain a healthy weight:** People who lose an average of 10 pounds of weight through diet and exercise can reduce their risk of developing diabetes by nearly 60 percent. The healthy combination of weight management and exercise not only reduces the risk of diabetes, but for those already diagnosed with diabetes, this combo also can reduce symptoms and improve management of your blood glucose levels. (See Chapter 9 for specific guidelines.)

✔ **Get regular exercise:** It's no secret that regular physical activity is good for you. By exercising for 30 minutes five or more days a week, you significantly reduce the risk of developing type 2 diabetes. (Chapters 10 and 11 can get you going.)

✔ **Eat a healthy diet:** Because diabetes is an illness affecting blood glucose levels, you can help control and moderate those levels with the foods you eat and how often you eat them. (Check out Chapters 7 and 8.)

✔ **Have your fasting blood sugar tested:** The American Diabetes Association recommends that if you're age 40 or older, have your healthcare provider check your fasting blood sugar once every three years. Testing for diabetes is done by a simple blood test or urinalysis.

If you experience any of the symptoms listed in the preceding section and you're under age 40, notify your doctor immediately to schedule a blood sugar test — these symptoms can be serious no matter your age.

Recognizing the symptoms

Over 6 million Americans have diabetes and don't know it. Diabetes can be effectively managed, but it has to be diagnosed first. Many people with diabetes don't have recognizable symptoms, while others have symptoms but don't know they're indicative of diabetes. Some of the most major symptoms associated with diabetes are:

✔ **Excessive thirst:** When glucose builds up in your bloodstream, fluid gets pulled from your tissues and may make you feel thirsty. As you drink fluids to quench your thirst, you also urinate more frequently.

✔ **Extreme hunger:** If insulin is unable to move the glucose from your blood into your cells, you feel hungry, even if you just ate.

✔ **Unexplained weight loss:** Even if you eat more

because you're hungry, you may keep losing weight because the energy from glucose isn't getting to your muscle tissues and fat stores, so they diminish.

- **Tiredness and fatigue:** Without energy from food in your cells, you get tired, weak, and irritable.

- **Blurred vision:** When blood sugar levels are too high, your body takes fluid from body tissue, including your eyes. This makes it hard to focus.

If you experience one or more of these symptoms and think you may have diabetes, check with your doctor for an accurate diagnosis.

Managing diabetes and considering the prospects

If you have diabetes, it's imperative that you keep your blood sugar under control. Whether you take insulin, oral medications, or control your diet, the key to minimizing complications from diabetes is to keep your blood sugars within the parameters your doctor sets for you. Taking insulin or oral medication doesn't mean you can eat whatever you want.

Here are a few pointers to keep in mind:

- Watch what you eat, eliminating refined sugars and empty calories as much as possible.

- Choose the right types of carbohydrates to stabilize blood sugar.

- Use the glycemic index (rates carbohydrates by the affect on blood glucose levels) to better understand what foods or food combinations you can eat to keep your blood sugar levels steady. (See Chapter 7 for more about the glycemic index.)

✔ Another key factor in management of the insulin and blood sugars is to incorporate a weight management and exercise program.

If you're diabetic, you need to check your blood sugar several times a day. Your doctor can give you a prescription for a glucometer, lancets, and a log book to keep track of your blood sugars. A nurse can show you how to use your glucometer and record the readings and have you give a demonstration to make sure you're doing it correctly. Your doctor has you check your blood sugar a certain number of times per day based on your blood sugar readings and other health concerns.

Cardiovascular Disease

Cardiovascular disease (CVD) is the leading cause of death in the world and is responsible for one third of all deaths. The deadly combination of heart disease and stroke kills 17 million people every year, particularly those in poor countries. This death rate is projected to climb to a staggering 24 million by 2030. The increase is based on increasing trends in obesity, poor diets, smoking, and physical inactivity, particularly in the younger population.

Cardiovascular disease is *not* a normal part of healthy aging. The lifestyle choices you make directly impact the health of your heart and vascular system and whether you develop CVD.

Understanding the components of the cardiovascular system is a good start to understanding the problems that occur when abnormalities arise in different areas. The cardiovascular system consists of the pump (heart), hoses (vessels), fluid (blood), and the nozzle (valves); if any one of them isn't working properly you can have problems. (See Figure 2-2 for a working diagram.)

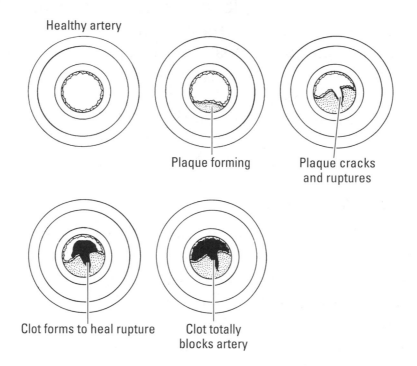

Healthy artery

Plaque forming

Plaque cracks and ruptures

Clot forms to heal rupture

Clot totally blocks artery

Figure 2-2:
How heart disease forms.

Differentiating among the various heart diseases and illnesses

Cardiovascular disease is a broad term to describe a mix of many diseases and illnesses that affect heart health. It's not only possible but common to have more than one of these illnesses simultaneously, which further increases your chance of dying from heart disease. We explain the major forms of heart disease in the following sections.

There's really no cure for heart disease, but prevention and screening are the best tools for delaying the onset or minimizing the damaging effects.

Coronary artery disease (CAD)

Coronary artery disease (CAD) is also known as *coronary heart disease* or *ischemic heart disease,* and it kills more than 7 million people in the world each year. CAD results from *atherosclerosis* (narrowing of the arteries). In atherosclerosis, *plaque* deposits build up in the arteries. Plaque is made up of fat, cholesterol, calcium, and other substances from the blood.

According to the American Heart Association, CAD's damage is caused by elevated levels of blood cholesterol and triglycerides, high blood pressure, and tobacco smoke.

High blood pressure

High blood pressure is the result of your heart working harder than normal to pump blood out into the arteries. The blood pressure is at the highest when it pumps blood out (systolic pressure) and the lowest in between pumps (diastolic pressure). The higher a person's blood pressure measures, the greater that person's risk of heart attack, stroke, heart failure, kidney disease, and eye damage (retinopathy).

For more info on high blood pressure specifically, check out *High Blood Pressure For Dummies,* 2nd Edition (Wiley) by Alan L. Rubin, MD.

Stroke

A person suffers a stroke when blood flow to part of the brain is blocked or if a blood vessel breaks and you bleed into the brain, causing brain cells to die. Over 15 percent of people who have a stroke die within 30 days. Of the people who survive a stroke, 15 to 30 percent suffer from some type of permanent disability. The major risk factors for stroke are high blood pressure and tobacco use. There are three main types of strokes:

- **Ischemic stroke:** This stroke is the most common type accounting for over 80 percent of all strokes. During an ischemic stroke a clot forms, usually caused by atherosclerosis, which blocks a blood vessel that's supplying blood to various areas of the brain.

- **Hemorrhagic stroke:** This type of stroke results from a blood vessel that breaks and bleeds into the brain. It's usually much more damaging and has a higher mortality rate than ischemic stroke (see preceding bullet). The cause of this stroke is either high blood pressure or an *aneurysm* (a weak spot on the artery wall that balloons with blood and may eventually burst from pressure).

- ***Transient ischemic attack* (TIA):** This type of stroke is often referred to as a *mini stroke* because it only causes a short interruption of blood flow to the brain. The symptoms of a TIA last less than 24 hours and are considered warning signs, because about one-third of people who have a TIA will suffer from a stroke in the future.

For more info on strokes, pick up a copy of *Stroke For Dummies* (Wiley) by John R. Marler, MD.

Understanding your risk

Cardiovascular disease is a major problem and is related to many choices you make every day. Some factors are even out of your control (such as being male). Here are some of the most common risk factors:

- **Smoking:** Smoking has been linked to plaque buildup and high blood pressure. Smoking also causes your blood to be thicker, which increases the risk of a stroke. Even if you have smoked for years, stroke is one condition that can still be reduced if you quit.

- ✓ **Poor diet:** Reducing the intake of saturated fats, trans fats, and cholesterol decreases plaque buildup and risks of ischemic strokes (see the preceding section). A diet high in vegetables and fruit can reduce your risks, too (see Chapter 7 for more info on nutrition).

- ✓ **Inactive lifestyle:** Physical activity is decreasing in all age groups. This lack of movement increases risk for diabetes, high blood pressure, elevated cholesterol, and therefore strokes.

- ✓ **Obesity:** Being overweight is associated with elevated cholesterol levels, high blood pressure, and an increased risk of coronary artery disease. Excess fat increases the heart's work which over time can lead to heart disease.

- ✓ **Gender and age:** Men have a higher risk of heart attack than women. Even though the difference narrows after women reach menopause, men still have a higher risk. Most of heart disease related deaths occur after the age of 65, although the disease likely was present at an earlier age.

- ✓ **Heredity:** Heart disease does tend to run in families. Children of parents with heart disease are more likely to develop it also. Certain ethnic groups, such as African Americans and Hispanics, tend to have a higher prevalence of cardiovascular disease.

Risk factors starting at younger ages are setting the stage for a surge in cardiovascular disease. Childhood obesity and smoking rates are rising and so are the rates of diabetes and high cholesterol. These two diseases were once thought of as diseases of middle-age, but are now being diagnosed in younger populations. Even some autopsies have found plaque in the aorta and coronary arteries of children that have died in accidents.

Playing your part in prevention, and managing cardiovascular disease

Cardiovascular disease isn't an inevitable part of aging; there are things you can do to greatly reduce your risk of becoming a heart attack or stroke statistic. If you already have CVD, take immediate steps to reduce the chances of your disease worsening. The key to preventing as well as managing your CVD is modifying your lifestyle choices. Here's how:

- ✔ Avoid using tobacco products.

- ✔ Maintain healthy cholesterol levels, and have your physician check your cholesterol levels at each routine checkup visit.

- ✔ Reduce your blood pressure (BP). Stop in to your doctor for a quick BP check, or take advantage of the free machines at your local pharmacy or grocery store.

- ✔ Eat a healthy diet (see Chapter 7).

- ✔ Maintain a health weight (refer to Chapter 9).

- ✔ Control your diabetes. If you have diabetes, make sure that you keep your blood glucose under excellent control. Poorly controlled diabetes is a major risk factor for heart disease.

✔ Increase your physical activity. You should be getting a minimum of 150 minutes of aerobic exercise a week.

✔ Figure out how to manage stress (check out Chapter 13). There are many ways to reduce stress, and some of them involve activities that are also helping reduce risks, such as exercise!

Recognizing the symptoms of coronary artery disease

You may look right past the first warning signs of coronary artery disease (CAD), and for many people, there are no warning signs at all. Their first sign that something's wrong is a heart attack. That's scary! Although not all cases of CAD are preventable — heredity plays a part in who gets it — you *can* modify or eliminate many risk factors by visiting your doctor regularly and being aware of potential early warning signs. The main symptoms of CAD are as follows:

✔ **Angina (chest pain):** *Angina* refers to chest pain and/or discomfort, with or without pain in one or both arms or in the left shoulder, neck, jaw, or back.

✔ **Shortness of breath:** This may occur when the coronary arteries become narrower due to the buildup of plaque (atherosclerosis).

✔ **Irregular heart beats or palpitations:** If your heart starts to skip beats or you feel it beating irregularly.

If a full evaluation by your doctor shows that you have

CAD, your doctor may be able to control the disease with medications while monitoring for any changes in symptoms. In some instances you may need invasive tests and procedures to open up blocked arteries prior to medication therapy.

 The tricky situation with CAD is deciding when to call your doctor versus calling 911 when you experience symptoms of CAD. Each case is different, and your doctor, who knows your case best, can discuss how you should approach the onset of chest pain or other symptoms. If you've established CAD but haven't discussed a plan with your doctor, any new, changing, or worsening symptoms are reasons to call 911. If you have the onset of CAD symptoms and have never experienced any in the past, you also need to treat those symptoms as a possible heart attack and call 911.

 Not all heart attacks look like they do on TV or in the movies. You may have multiple symptoms at the same time that increase in intensity, or just one symptom that doesn't seem very intense. Here are some symptoms:

- A feeling of overwhelming exhaustion; unable to do anything

- A feeling of anxiety along with shortness of breath that doesn't let up

- Feeling winded when exerting very little effort, which subsides when you stop

- Experiencing terrible heartburn, possibly with nausea and vomiting or feeling like you have the flu

- Feeling of pressure, pain, or discomfort, through the chest or back

- A feeling of discomfort, numbness, tingling and/or pain in jaw, upper back, shoulders, neck, arms

(usually on the left side of your body)

✔ Getting the "cold sweats" and pale skin

Right after calling 911 if you think you're experiencing a heart attack, go to your medicine cabinet for a lifesaver everyone should have on hand — plain aspirin (if you're not allergic to it!). Chew a 325 milligram tablet of plain aspirin; aspirin helps reduce platelet formation around the ruptured plaque. Platelets can form a larger clot, which further decreases blood flow. Chewing aspirin speeds its absorption — you'll get over the taste later.

Osteoporosis

Osteoporosis is a progressive disease in which the bones become weak and lead to an increase risk of fractures. Any bone can be affected by osteoporosis, but the most common bones that break are in the hip, back, and wrist. Often people don't know that they have osteoporosis until a bone actually breaks and further evaluation reveals poor bone density. Osteoporosis affects more than 75 million men and women worldwide. To discover more about your bones and osteoporosis, refer to Chapter 6.

Understanding your risk

Osteoporosis is a risk factor for women, mainly. Women have an increased risk of osteoporosis because of their hormonal influences. There are several other risk factors:

✔ **Age:** In both men and women, the risk of osteoporosis increases with age, with bone loss usually starting around age 30. Women can experience up to a 20 percent loss of bone mass in the 5 to 7 years following menopause (average age is 51), due to estrogen loss. Women usually show signs of osteoporosis around age 65. Men's bone loss tends to occur gradually and they don't usually show signs until age 75.

✔ **Gender:** Women are four times more likely to have osteoporosis than men. Women's bones are thinner and less dense than men's, and in addition, men tend to have more muscle, which serves to protect the bone.

✔ **Smoking:** The role of smoking and osteoporosis isn't clearly understood, but smoking is thought to decrease the amount of calcium absorbed from food as well as reduce the production of bone cells (osteoblasts).

✔ **Nutrition:** People with a very low calcium intake have a higher risk of developing osteoporosis because calcium plays such a vital role in bone development.

✔ **Physical activity:** Bone remodeling (new bone formation) occurs in response to activity. Weight bearing exercises are the best form of activity to improve lean muscle mass and strengthen your bones (see Chapter 10 for strength-training tips).

Playing your part in prevention

Many cases of osteoporosis are preventable, and the earlier you start making healthy lifestyle choices the better. The best way to prevent breaking a bone due to osteoporosis is to stop osteoporosis before it starts! Take the following steps to reduce your risk:

✔ **Get regular weight-bearing exercise.** Getting started at an early age helps prevent osteoporosis or at minimum slow the progression. By strengthening your muscles, you're also strengthening your bones. When you lift weights, the stress on the bone causes the body to increase the calcium into your bones for added strength. (See Chapter 10 for ideas.)

✔ **Make sure you get enough calcium, vitamin D, and vitamin K.** All these vitamins and minerals make your bones strong. A diet rich in calcium is essential for bone strength. Because you need vitamin D to absorb calcium, it also plays a vital role in maintaining bone density (see Chapter 8 for info on vitamins and minerals).

✔ **Talk to your doctor about available treatments if you're at high risk of osteoporosis or already experiencing bone loss.** Medications are available to slow the rate of bone loss and even help rebuild bone. Talk to your doctor to see what type of treatment option is best for you.

Recognizing the symptoms

Osteoporosis has been called the silent thief because it can take decades to slowly increase the size of the holes in your bones, weakening them enough to break. Unfortunately, the first sign that a person has osteoporosis is often when a fracture occurs. Other symptoms may be severe back pain, loss of height, or spinal deformities such as *kyphosis* (hump back) that occur as a result of collapsed vertebrae.

Managing osteoporosis

Osteoporosis doesn't have a cure, but current treatments and newer treatments exist that can slow the rate of bone loss and increase bone density.

Hormone therapy used to be the main treatment, but after a large study showed that the benefits of hormones on the bones didn't outweigh the cardiovascular risks, doctors started using alternative therapies.

Medications such as bisphosphonates are helpful in certain cases. These therapies can help people keep living their daily lives without the constant fear and worry that every little bump, twist, or turn will result in a fracture.

The quality of life for people with osteoporosis is improving. Other strategies such as fall-prevention techniques should be incorporated into a fracture-prevention program. See Chapter 6 for more on medications and Chapter 19 for fall-prevention tips.

Chapter 3

Evaluating Your Health and History and Setting Goals for Wellness

People used to go to the doctor only when they were sick or had broken a bone. And plenty of people still cower or scoff at the idea of visiting the doctor when they're ill, let alone getting a checkup if they're feeling just dandy — you know, the *if it ain't broke, don't fix it!* rule.

Well, we don't happen to prescribe to that philosophy as a recipe for longevity or even good health. Today more than ever before, you have the power of healthy living and early detection to help prevent debilitating — and possibly fatal — illnesses and diseases.

In this chapter, we discuss the general measures you can implement to prevent the most threatening illnesses and diseases today (and throughout the rest of the book, we discuss the specifics of keeping yourself healthy as you get older). Because your body doesn't come with an owner's manual to tell you when it's time for a tuneup, we tell you what to look for, what age to start looking, and what tests or screenings to schedule with your healthcare provider. We also give you some gender-specific disease-related information. Then we help you put your goals down on paper and devise a plan that will keep you from giving up when the going gets tough. Last but not least, we look at ways to have fun while you're getting healthy.

Investigating and Writing Down Your Medical and Family History

Staying healthy as you age actually consists of two parts: knowing what your general health risks are now, and knowing what inherited tendencies can lead to disease in the future. Although your healthcare provider can give you the most accurate depiction of your overall health (more on that topic in the next section), this section helps you take the first steps in assessing your present health so that you can provide the information your doctor needs. That info plus an understanding of potential inherited health problems puts you in a much better position to create personal health goals and to devise a plan (with your doctor, if appropriate) for reaching them.

Taking stock of yourself

Standing back and taking an objective look at yourself from a healthy living perspective isn't always easy. Self-evaluation is, however, one of the first, easiest, and most effective steps you can take toward eliminating behaviors that may keep you from living your best as you age.

Although seeing your doctor is important, she can go by only what you tell her when it comes to diet, exercise, and other important health factors in your life. You may be a perfect size six, but if you stay that way by eating two candy bars a day (and nothing else), by skipping dinner in lieu of three glasses of wine a night, or by smoking instead of eating, your health is going to suffer. You may look okay on the outside (at least for a while), but the one person you really can't fool when it comes to your lifestyle is yourself.

In the appendix, we provide a comprehensive self-assessment to help you identify strengths and weaknesses in your lifestyle and to pinpoint any health risks. (We put it at the end of the book so that you can easily make a copy of it — or tear it out, if you like — fill it out, and take it to your next doctor's appointment, especially if you're planning to improve the quality of your health and well-being.)

Is it really necessary to let your doctor know that you've decided to give up ice cream bars and start walking two miles a day? Possibly not, if you're perfectly healthy with no family risk factors at all. But if there's anything at all concerning in your history or in your physical exam that would preclude major changes in lifestyle, you may save yourself a lot of health complications by discussing your plan with your doctor first. Besides, she may have suggestions to help make your transition into a healthier you an easier one.

The depth of information you need to gather varies from doctor to doctor; however, many of the basics (allergies to medications, current medical conditions, and so on) are fairly standard, and we include assessment questions for all that info in the appendix.

Looking down the family line

Do you have a family? Yes, you do, even if you don't always

like to claim them. With your family comes a family health history. Although having a sibling with cancer or a grandparent who died of heart disease doesn't mean that you're going to suffer the same fate, many disease tendencies can be inherited, and knowing your family history can give you a blueprint of potential health landmines in your genetic makeup.

Your doctor needs to know about any family history of illness, such as cardiovascular disease, cancer, and so on, because it can change prevention, testing, and treatments due to certain familial links. In addition to the self-assessment in the appendix, plan to research your family history and bring pertinent info to your doctor's appointment.

When compiling a family health history, start with your immediate family — brothers, sisters, mom, and dad. You can start by asking questions of your parents, such as:

- ✔ **How long did your parents live and what did they die of?** You may not get a straight answer on the cause of your grandparents' deaths, because often cause of death wasn't accurately recorded a generation or so ago. Even deaths recorded as accidents may not be accurate; a "car accident" may have been caused by a sudden heart attack.

- ✔ **Did they have any health problems?** Try to get specifics; "bad blood" could be anything from anemia to syphilis! Some of the more common conditions with genetic links are heart disease, cancer, addiction, and diabetes.

- ✔ **What do you remember about them?** They may remember that grandma was blind and had only one leg without making the connection that these conditions may have been caused by diabetes.

113

✔ **Do you have any pictures of relatives?** One look at a series of pictures of great grandma and grandma at different ages can make it evident that osteoporosis runs in the family — they kept getting shorter!

✔ **Did any diseases or defects "run in the family"?** Expect some waffling on the answer if mental conditions or birth defects were common in the family. Explain your need to know as a desire to understand your family medical history rather than pure nosiness.

✔ **What about your brothers and sisters and their families?** Make sure that you're recording health issues only from blood relatives, not their spouses or their in-laws.

After picking mom and dad's brain, talking to your aunts and uncles may yield new information or a different slant on things. Always start with your most talkative/nosy family members first, but remember that they may also be the most likely to embellish the family history! To dig a little deeper, particularly if your immediate ancestors have passed on or don't have the info you need, try to access death certificates, obituaries, and family medical records from extended family members or library newspaper files. If anyone in your family is a pack rat or a genealogy buff, he may have already done much of the legwork for you, and would probably be flattered if you asked for a copy of his research.

After you gather enough data to make up a cohesive family history, write it all down. You can get fancy, drawing an elaborate tree with actual branches, or you can write it down in simple linear fashion. The U.S. Surgeon General considers your family history recording important enough to have devised a personalized form that you can use to record pertinent info; you can find it at www.familyhistory.hhs.gov. Some other helpful Web sites to consider are www.birthrecords.ws and NGSgenealogy.com.

 If you're adopted, you may not be able to delve into your family history to any great degree. Adoption agencies often do have some family medical history on file. Your adoptive parents may or may not have this information available for you, but the agency they used may. It's worth a phone call or visit to get any bits of information they have.

Regardless of whether you're adopted, you may be unable to come up with any concrete past family medical information. If that's the case, don't worry about it. Doctors can use this info as a tool to help in some situations, but medical personnel will use their expertise regardless of having any pertinent family history.

Visiting the Doc

Some people would rather have a tax audit than go to the doctor. The main reason? Fear — and fear of the unknown only perpetuates the problem. The scenario of *what ifs* may run through your head like a freight train on rocket fuel until you scare yourself into staying away from the doctor and convincing yourself that nothing can be done about your less-than-healthy condition.

Note: This line of thinking may become a self-fulfilling prophecy. If you avoid the doctor for years and suffer with an ache or pain long enough, it just may turn into something serious. So when a person finally can't take it anymore and goes to the doctor, the news is bad. "Well, Mr. Jones, if you had come to me 12 years ago, we could have caught this thing in time. With the right medication, lifestyle changes, diet, and exercise, you'd live another 20 years." Then the patient says, "Gee, Doc, with all the medical advances and technology and your expertise, isn't there anything you can do?" In a case like this, nothing works better than prevention.

Taking your body to the doctor for regular checkups is an important part of living long and well. To make sure that you cover your bases, we devote this section to those appointments.

Having regular checkups: What should happen

Remembering to schedule regular maintenance visits for your car is usually easier than remembering to do it for your body. At least your car gets a sticker that reminds you when to get an oil change or a warning light that indicates a need for service. But as long as you're feeling okay, you probably don't think about getting a physical exam — not good for two reasons:

✔ Prevention is the key to reducing your risks of developing disease and illness, so if you don't take advantage of your doctor's insight regarding your risks, you're missing out on a key component of aging healthfully.

✔ When you do visit the doctor regularly, you can immediately address any health concerns the doctor may find; if you don't, you may not know about those health concerns soon enough to combat them before they take their toll on your body. For example, if your bad cholesterol levels are too high, your doctor may suggest modifications to your diet and lifestyle, or she may start you on a medication to lower cholesterol.

For folks ages 40 and older, we highly recommend health examinations every one to two years. (Younger adults don't need the exam this often — every three to five years is good.)

During the annual exam, your doctor performs the assessments in the following sections.

Discussing current medical complaints

The first part of the exam is an opportunity to discuss your current medical situation so that it can be further evaluated throughout the rest of the examination. You should discuss your medical complaints one at a time, mentioning all the symptoms that you're having. Your medical practitioner will ask some directed questions, but this is your time to speak. A lot of valuable information can be obtained in the history, often enough for clinicians to formulate a strong differential diagnosis.

The review of your body systems is a way for the doctor to assess your overall health quickly (and sufficiently). You'll be asked a number of questions to gather information to direct the diagnosis, treatment, and prevention, such as the following:

- **Overall well-being:** Have you had unintentional weight loss or weight gain? Do you generally feel well? Are you able to complete activities of daily living?

- **Skin:** Do you have any rashes, itching, dryness, redness, or changes in hair or nails?

- **Eyes, ears, nose, mouth, and throat:** Do you have any blurred, loss of, or double vision? Do you feel any pain in the eyes? Do you have dizziness, loss of hearing, ringing in the ears, bloody nose, bleeding gums, tooth pain, sore throat, hoarseness, lumps in the neck, or stiffness of the neck?

117

- ✔ **Cardiovascular system:** Do you have any chest pain, irregular heartbeat, shortness of breath on exertion or during the night, or pain in the lower legs with exertion?

- ✔ **Respiratory:** Do you have shortness of breath, cough, wheezing, bloody sputum, or recurrent bronchial infections?

- ✔ **Gastrointestinal:** Any changes in appetite, pain with swallowing, heartburn, nausea, vomiting, bloody vomit, diarrhea or constipation, blood in stool, increased gas, or pain with bowel movements?

- ✔ **Genitourinary:** Any increased frequency of urination, pain with urination, blood in urine, problems urinating, history of kidney stones, recurrent infections, erectile dysfunction (male), or sexually transmitted diseases? Females, what was the age of onset of menses? Are your periods regular? What was the date of your last period? Do you have any pain with menstruation, heavy or light bleeding, or pain with intercourse?

- ✔ **Musculoskeletal:** Do you have any pain in the joints, cramping, muscle weakness, or decreased range of motion?

- ✔ **Neurologic:** Any seizures, tremors, numbness, tingling, paralysis, memory loss, problems with coordination, anxiety, depression, or speech difficulty?

Although routine medical examinations are supposed to be just that — routine — they're often a time when patients divulge all the medical issues they've experienced or been concerned about since their last medical exam. Many patients come to routine examinations with multiple items to discuss, or they answer "yes" to many of the questions in the preceding list. We want to stress that if you have issues to be addressed, don't wait until your routine examination to address them. If the steering on your car is off, you don't wait until your 12-month inspection to have it evaluated; you shouldn't ignore symptoms affecting your most expensive possession — your body — without having them checked out.

Reviewing past medical information

At this stage of the examination your doctor will want to go over past medical information that may pertain to your current medical complaints. He'll also see whether any past medical issues need to be readdressed or further evaluated. Your doctor may revisit the same question each year to make sure that nothing has changed. Many past occurrences can be very important with current medical ailments and future preventative examinations. Here are a few of the main categories covered in this section of the examination:

- ✔ **Medications:** Tell your doctor about all the medications you're taking and about any recent changes in medications. Your medication includes over-the-counter meds, herbal supplements, and anything you take for allergies. Bring in the bottles or copy their info onto a piece of paper if you don't know all your medications off the top of your head.

- ✔ **Past medical conditions or current ongoing conditions:** These conditions may include high blood pressure or diabetes and should date back to childhood.

- ✔ **Hospitalizations:** Tell your doctor about any hospitalizations in the past five years, and have all the details handy if you've been hospitalized in the last 6 months.

- ✔ **Surgical history:** This category includes all surgeries in your life. Your doctor won't want to send you to the hospital to have your appendix evaluated if it was surgically removed a year ago.

- ✔ **Immunizations:** See the Immunization section later in this chapter.

- ✔ **For women, menstrual cycle and reproductive history:** This info includes all live births, the age of the children, and any miscarriages.

- ✔ **Occupational history:** This one helps the doctor evaluate any potential hazardous exposures, such as asbestos or other chemicals, or hearing loss if you work with loud machinery or guns. Jobs with intense labor may explain pains in the back and joints or past head injuries.

- ✔ **Relationship status:** Talking about your relationship can help your doctor understand the home environment if you're experiencing stress or any potential abuse situations. Knowing what kind of support network is at home is also helpful for some ailments and treatment modalities.

- ✔ **Alcohol and illicit drug use:** Let your doctor know about past or present use. This includes tobacco and even the abuse of prescription medications.

At this point, you can also whip out your comprehensive family history (see the section "Looking down the family line," earlier in this chapter) to help your doctor assess for possible inherited problems and tendencies.

Checking your vitals

Vital signs are a group of measured tests that help give a quick assessment of a patient's basic bodily function. These functions include blood pressure, pulse, respirations, and temperature. A few other measurements can be thrown into this mix, including height, weight, pulse oximetry (a noninvasive measure of the oxygenation in your blood), and pain. Your doctor may check your vitals herself. Or other medical personnel may do it before the doctor even sets foot in the room. That way, she already has that info when she looks at your chart. Sometimes this step happens at the beginning of your appointment, and sometimes it happens after you go over all the history (see the previous section). Scan this list for additional info:

✔ **Blood pressure measurement:** Blood pressure is a measurement of the force that's applied to the heart and vessels as blood is pumped into the heart chambers and out into the vessels of the body (not to be confused with *pulse,* which is the number of times the heart beats in a given period of time). In a blood pressure measurement, the first number (systolic) is the rate at which the blood flows through your arteries during a contraction of the large chambers of the heart (ventricles), and the second number (diastolic) is the pressure measured at rest when the ventricles are filling. For example, a typical blood pressure reading is 120/80 mmHg (millimeters of mercury).

By checking blood pressure regularly and following your care provider's advice regarding diet, exercise, medication, and risk-factor reduction, you can help control your blood pressure and stave off heart disease.

✔ **Temperature:** You may think that everyone's "normal" temperature when taken by mouth is 98.6 degrees Fahrenheit or 37 degrees Celsius. Some research suggests that "normal" oral temp actually falls in a range between 98 to 99 degrees Fahrenheit. Elevated body temperature of over 100 is called a *fever.* Fever can be caused by a number of things, such as infection, some medical diseases, or heat stroke. Low body temperatures occur with some infections and metabolic diseases, such as underactive thyroid and diabetes. Abnormally low temperature is called *hypothermia.* Most of the time, symptoms or pertinent medical history explains abnormal temperatures. If not, the doctor does testing that may include an examination, blood testing, urinalysis, and possibly X-rays.

✔ **Pulse rate:** The pulse is the pressure felt in the arteries as a result of the heart pumping. It's most commonly felt on the neck or wrist and is calculated as the number of pulses per minute. The normal pulse rate is between 60 and 100 for adults and is higher in young children. The pulse rate increases with exercise and can reach rates of greater than 200. In addition to pulse rate, you can check for the strength of the pulse and the rhythm — is it regular or irregular? A simple pulse check helps assess potential problems with the cardiovascular system.

✔ **Respiratory rate:** This is the number of breaths a person takes per minute. The rate is usually assessed when the person is at rest and can be measured easily by observing the chest's rise and fall while breathing. The normal adult rate is between 12 and 20 breaths per minute and is higher in children. Abnormal respiratory rates can be a result of medical conditions such as fever, respiratory infections, or other systemic diseases such as congestive heart failure and thyroid disease.

✔ **Height and weight:** These measurements are important. Changes in height as you age may signify changes in your spine or posture. Weight loss that's unintentional can be related to numerous diseases. Weight gain is becoming a norm and has numerous risks involved. Try to pick up on changes in height and weight so that you can take action early. (See Chapter 9 for more info on weight gain.)

At last, undergoing the physical exam

Sooner or later, you have to put on that skimpy gown and sit on the crinkly-paper-covered exam table to get checked out. Your doctor examines you from head to toe, checking most of your orifices, squeezing muscles, and pointing out any abnormalities to discuss and possibly test further:

✔ **General appearance:** You'd be surprised what you can assess just looking at someone. Mobility, mood, skin color, and hygiene can all be evaluated within a minute or two of general conversation.

✔ **Skin:** Doctors check the skin for any suspicious rashes or moles.

✔ **Head, ears, eyes, neck, throat (HEENT):** Examination of the head basically consists of checking the ears, mouth, and nose. Evaluating the visual fields and papillary reaction, and testing with an eye chart are included in an eye exam. To examine your throat, a doctor checks for neck stiffness, thyroid enlargement, and lymph node swelling.

- ✔ **Cardiovascular:** The doctor checks your vital signs by listening to the heart for any abnormal rhythm or sounds, checking for any swelling of the extremities or varicose veins, and listening to the carotid arteries of the neck for any signs of blockage.

- ✔ **Respiratory:** After checking the respiratory rate, your doctor listens to the lungs for any wheezing, lack of breath sounds, or other sounds suggestive of disease.

- ✔ **Gastrointestinal:** Your doctor listens for bowel sounds, and presses on the abdomen looking for pain, masses, hernias, or abdominal distention.

- ✔ **Genitourinary and rectal:** For men this includes evaluation of the penis and scrotum, including evaluating the testicles for any masses. The female exam is discussed in the next list (see the Pap smear bullet). Patients start getting rectal exams at age 40 unless otherwise needed; doctors use this exam to check for hemorrhoids and to evaluate the prostate for any enlargement or masses.

- ✔ **Musculoskeletal:** Your doctor evaluates range of motion and muscle strength, and checks the spine for straightness and any tenderness. Your doctor also listens for *crepitus,* a creaking sound, when your joints are moved.

- ✔ **Extremities:** Your doctor evaluates your extremities for swelling and any abnormalities in the muscles. He feels the pulses in the knee and foot, and looks for any enlarged lymph nodes in the groin.

- ✔ **Neurological:** The doc checks reflexes of the knees, feet, and elbow by tapping them with a small hammer. Your doctor may check your gait by watching you walk, and then check your feet and hands for sensory defects.

Other tests are often done at the time of routine examinations and are just as important, but not all these tests are done at every annual examination. A few of these important tests are done at different set times or when other circumstances arise. Here are a few tests to expect at some point, whether annually or not:

- ✔ **Pap smear:** From the time you become sexually active or turn 18 (whichever comes first), you should have a yearly Pap smear until age 30. After age 30, women have Pap smears every three years after three yearly negative tests in a row. Sexually active women ages 18 to 25 should also be screened for sexually transmitted diseases (STDs), including HIV (human immunodeficiency virus) and HPV (human papillomavirus), every year. The vaccine for HPV can reduce the risk of cervical cancer and genital warts (see the nearby sidebar on immunizations). Pap smears may be discontinued after age 65 if previous screenings (a minimum of three negative Pap tests in the last ten years) are normal and documented.

    Multiple sexual partners, early onset of sexual activity, current use of oral contraceptives, and smoking are increased risk factors for cervical cancer. However, even without these factors, you should be tested to help detect cervical cancer. Early diagnosis and treatment greatly increase the success rate against it.

- ✔ **Clinical breast exams and mammograms:** Because breast care is one of the most important aspects of women's healthcare, clinical breast exams should begin at age 20. Women age 40 and older should have a mammogram every year. Detecting changes in the breast through clinical exams and regular mammograms is the key to early diagnosis, effective treatment, and high success rates against breast cancer.

A clinical breast exam involves palpating for lumps or bumps in each breast. A mammogram is an X-ray of your breast that shows tissue changes; your breast is flattened and compressed for the exam because breast tissue is normally dense. This can be mildly uncomfortable.

✔ **Prostate cancer screening:** Prostate cancer is the second leading cause of cancer deaths among men. Each year, men age 40 and older should have:

- **A prostate specific antigen (PSA) screening test.** The PSA is a simple blood test that in some cases can detect cancer in the prostate before signs and symptoms are present. The only problem is that it isn't always accurate. A man can have prostate cancer and still have a normal PSA. The PSA can also be abnormal when cancer isn't present thanks to certain infections, inflammation, and benign enlargement of the prostate. Therefore, the PSA shouldn't be used as a diagnostic tool, but it can be helpful to monitor the treatment of prostate cancer.
- **A digital rectal exam.** This test is done to assess the size of the prostate and palpate for any other abnormalities, such as pain or masses.

You must have both of these tests — a blood test alone isn't a definitive diagnostic test. Trust the doctor — if the PSA blood test was accurate enough, doctors would be the first to tell you that you don't need to have a rectal exam. Unfortunately, that isn't the case. Have both tests. Early diagnosis and treatment greatly increase the success rate of a cancer cure.

When you visit the doctor, you complete some general forms, one of which should be a health assessment form or medical history — refer to the first section in this chapter for more info on that topic.

Less frequent exams

Some tests need to be done only when you reach a certain age, have certain risk factors, or are having problems in a particular area. The following list describes some of the tests that fall into this category:

- **Cholesterol screening:** Every five years, all adults should have a *lipid profile,* a cholesterol test done after you've had nothing to eat or drink for 12 hours (called a "fasting" test) that assesses all the components of cholesterol: total, HDL or good cholesterol, LDL or bad cholesterol, and triglycerides.

  The link between high cholesterol and the increased risk of heart disease is well established, so these tests can help determine your risk.

- **Eye exam:** Plan to have an eye examination at least once from age 18 to 29, at least twice from age 30 to 39, every two to four years from age 40 to 64, and every one to two years thereafter.

  Many significant eye problems — like glaucoma (increased pressure in the eye) and macular

Immunizations

You may think immunizations are just for kids, but some immunizations are as important for adults as they are for children, especially if you have certain risk factors. According to the Center for Disease Control (CDC), the following vaccinations should be on your to-do list if you fall into any of the categories described here:

✔ **Influenza:** If you're age 50 or older or if you have a weakened immune system, you should have these yearly flu shots. The influenza vaccine can also be given to anyone who requests it because it may benefit the healthy working adult. Influenza can lead to pneumonia, dehydration, and death in people who are debilitated, and can worsen heart disease, diabetes, and asthma. Around 36,000 Americans alone die from the flu and its complications each year.

✔ **Tetanus Diphtheria Pertussis (Tdap):** You need this series of combined vaccinations if you're an adult who didn't receive the primary series as a child. In addition, all adults under age 65 should receive a *booster* (an injection given to make sure the levels of protection in the blood stay high) of Tdap at least every ten years thereafter. Adults over the age of 65 should receive a booster of Td (tetanus and diphtheria only) every ten years. Tetanus is a preventable disease caused by a bacteria introduced into a wound, and it's fatal in around 30 percent of cases. Diphtheria, fatal in 5 to 20 percent of cases, is a highly infectious preventable disease seen only rarely today in developed countries due to high vaccine rates. Pertussis, also known as whooping cough, is a highly contagious, serious disease seen most recently in those aged 11 to 19 when their immunity wears off. New recommendations for booster shots in children and adults are needed and currently in the works.

✔ **Pneumonia:** If you're 65 or older, or if you have medical conditions that increase the risk of pneumonia — such as chronic lung diseases (asthma, bronchitis, emphysema), chronic heart conditions, diabetes, kidney disease, or liver disease — you should have a one-time pneumonia vaccination (*pneumococcal vaccine* or *pneumovax*). In some cases, a second vaccine after five years may be prudent; ask your doctor whether you fall into this category.

✔ **Human Papillomavirus (HPV):** This relatively new vaccine is recommended for young females (starting at age 9 and up until age 26) to decrease the risk of cervical cancer and genital warts due to HPV. Ideally, you should receive this vaccine before becoming sexually active, but women who are sexually active should still be vaccinated. A complete series of this vaccine consists of three doses. At this time the vaccine is known to be effective for at least five years; further research will determine whether or not booster injections will be required.

✔ **Meningitis:** Although meningitis is rare, outbreaks on college campuses or other areas where large numbers of people live in close contact, such as military bases and institutions, can occur. Therefore, the following people should receive the meningitis vaccine (called the meningococcal vaccine): college students, military recruits, people with immune problems, people with damaged or removed spleens, people traveling to countries where meningitis is common, and anyone who has been exposed to someone with meningitis.

✔ **Hepatitis B:** Hepatitis B is a virus that can cause serious damage to the liver. Vaccination consists of a series of three vaccines. The following people, among others, should receive the hepatitis vaccine: medical personnel; people with HIV, kidney disease, or liver disease; and people who receive blood products on a regular basis, such as hemophiliacs.

degeneration (deterioration of the macula, the central part of the retina) — go undetected in adults until serious damage is done. Certain health conditions like diabetes and high blood pressure increase your risk of eye problems.

✔ **Fasting blood sugar screening:** Fasting blood sugar should be measured every three years, starting at age 45, to screen for *diabetes mellitus,* one of the most commonly undiagnosed diseases.

Certain risk factors such as family history, excess weight, and inactivity raise your chances of developing diabetes. Untreated, the complications can be serious; diabetes can cause severe kidney, nerve, eye, heart, and blood vessel damage. But early diagnosis and treatment can greatly reduce risks of complications, improve your health, and control the diabetes.

✔ **Colorectal cancer screening:** A complete colonoscopy and examination of the intestines are done using a flexible lighted scope while you're under mild sedation. People age 50 and older should have this test done every ten years — and more frequently if you have a family history of colon cancer or a previous abnormal colonoscopy.

Colorectal cancer is the third-leading cause of cancer deaths among all adults, and a colonoscopy offers the best opportunity to detect cancer at an early stage, when successful treatment is likely. Some cancers may be prevented by detection and removal of polyps.

✔ **Bone-mineral density exam:** Women age 65 and older should have a bone mineral density measurement at least once to check for *osteoporosis,* a disease in which bones become fragile and more likely to break.

Because osteoporosis isn't visible, the information from a bone density test enables your healthcare provider to identify your risk of fractures.

✓ **Hearing test:** Adults over the age of 64 should have at least one hearing assessment. Your healthcare provider will ask about your hearing, and if you're having difficulty or noticing small changes, he will probably recommend a hearing test. Proper treatment, including cleaning or treating infections, can greatly improve your ability to hear.

Determining Your Goals and Putting Them on Paper

To achieve goals, you need plans. No architect creates a building and no engineer creates a computer without a written plan. You're the architect and engineer of your lifestyle, and you need a plan when building for healthy aging. Your *plan of action* acts as a set of blueprints for the changes you want to create for your health and well-being. The plan turns your major goals into a multitasked project with clear milestones and deadlines and specific tasks in a specific order.

The simpler the plan, and the less disruption it causes to your daily life, the more likely you are to stick to it. Think of your body as a machine that needs certain maintenance. Plan on the regular, routine maintenance and if any signs of breakdown appear, get to the doctor sooner rather than later to prevent any worsening of the situation. The body is complex and therefore is somewhat unpredictable, so accept that you have to adapt to changes and make adjustments to keep the body aging well. Have you ever seen a set of blueprints that didn't have changes before the final construction was complete? Your plan will also have modifications along the way.

Developing your goals

When determining and implementing your goals, follow a few guidelines to make them effective:

- ✔ **Develop your goals as clearly as possible.** Your goals should be deliberate and well thought out. Each goal should be defined as a specific task that's action oriented. If it's action oriented, you can actually do something to accomplish it. Having a goal of "losing weight" isn't as clear as "losing five pounds a month by cutting out afternoon and after dinner snacks and walking two miles a day." The second goal has specific, action oriented tasks for you to work on.

- ✔ **Make sure that your goals are measurable.** This factor is critical. If you can measure your goals, you can manage them. Just like in a game of sports, if you don't assign a point value to a score, how do you know who's winning? With goals, if you can't measure them, how do you know whether you've accomplished them? The difference between a goal and a wish is as simple as these two statements:

  - I want to lose weight.
  - I want to lose 25 pounds.

  The second statement is actually a goal.

- ✔ **Set firm but realistic deadlines.** There isn't much

132

point of having a goal if you never set a time frame to reach it.

☑ **Own your goals.** Many people don't stick to their goals because they don't really take ownership of them. Your goals must be a burning desire for *you* — not for someone else. If you're a smoker and the loved ones in your life want you to give it up and you know that you should (but you're trying to do it for their sake), you aren't really owning this goal. Feeling the conviction and desire for your goal is essential because you'll encounter obstacles, challenges, and temptations that try to sabotage your attempts. Whether your goal is going to the gym four days a week, eating healthy food to lose weight and maintain it, choosing a positive attitude over a negative one, or protecting your skin from sun damage — every goal has obstacles. Choose goals that you're passionate about. You're much more likely to achieve them.

Keep these guidelines in mind and start fine-tuning your goals by letting the following questions and considerations guide you:

1. **What's your current state of health?**
   - Weight
   - Medical conditions
   - Exercise and physical activity
   - Nutrition and diet
   - Mental, emotional, and spiritual

2. **Where would you like to be with regards to your health and well-being?**

3. **How did you get where you are today regarding your current state of health?**

    - What did you do right?
    - What would you do differently?

4. **What do you do next to get from where you are to where you want to be?**

5. **What should you be doing more or less of?**

6. **What should you start doing that you aren't?**

7. **What should you stop doing altogether?**

8. **Can you set realistic timeframes for each of your goals?**

9. **Where do you want to be in one year in relation to your goals?**

Change is good, although for many people it can be uncomfortable. Discomfort often comes from fear of the unknown or fear of failure. If you notice a gap between where you want to be and where you are now, see it as an opportunity for improvement, rather than an insurmountable obstacle or a failure; don't let fear keep you rooted in the same old spot.

Recording your goals

Plenty of research supports the effective correlation between writing down your goals and achieving them. Here's why we also believe in the power of this process:

- ✔ Writing down your goals forces you to organize your thinking.

- ✔ Thinking about what you must do to accomplish

your goals helps you to plan your tasks more thoughtfully.

✔ A well-written plan provides the ability to review it for flaws as well as to identify strengths and weaknesses.

✔ A written plan allows you to focus on just a few key objectives.

✔ Writing your plan ahead of time instead of flying by the seat of your pants saves time, energy, confusion, and mistakes.

You may want to keep your plan in a notebook or a three-ring binder that's easy to refer to on a daily basis. As you write your plan

✔ **List every task and activity.** For example, if you want to start exercising, list the activity you want to begin, the time you want to allot, the time of day you're going to exercise, and where you're going to exercise. You also need a schedule for starting slow and increasing your exercise time and intensity.

✔ **Prioritize your goals.** What's the most important thing you hope to accomplish? If you're losing weight because you're diabetic, changing your diet to decrease your blood sugar may be more important than how many pounds you lose.

✔ **List your goals sequentially.** You may want to increase your aerobic exercise to a certain point first, and then start using weights. Or you may want to start with one weight, and then increase to another level.

✔ **Identify your limitations.** Limitations aren't

failures, and should be built into any plan. For example, you may have a chronic foot injury. If you know that the injury flares up from time to time, have an alternate plan for those times, such as switching from walking to swimming for exercise.

✔ **Expect failure and remain flexible, keeping your focus on the solution.**

✔ **Have measures and standards for tracking your progress and deadlines.** For example, "I will be walking three miles daily at a speed of 4 miles an hour on the treadmill."

 All successful people work from *written* plans. Action without planning is the number one reason for failure.

Pushing for Persistence to Successfully Reach Your Goals

Making plans and setting goals is fun; carrying them out can be less enjoyable, especially over the long run. Yet few things are as rewarding as completing goals, so the effort is well worth it.

You may not always feel like keepin' on, but by starting small and gradually increasing your efforts and goals, you can achieve great changes that can impact the way you age for years to come. The road to the top seems much easier if you take your goals one step at a time, stay realistic about what you can do, and find support along the way.

In this section, we focus on the mental side of carrying out your goals — especially when the ruts and bumps start to rattle your confidence.

Staying focused — and optimistic

Few things in life are more motivating than a realistic positive attitude. Referring to your plan and rechecking it to make sure that your goals are realistic and attainable can keep you from giving up because your goals aren't being met. Being both realistic and positive is essential: Being positive may tell you that you're going to be 30 pounds thinner in a month; being realistic may tell you that's not likely and that 4 to 8 pounds (1 to 2 pounds a week) may be a better goal.

Sometimes, despite your most upbeat efforts, pessimism starts to worm its way into your daily routine. "What's the use? I'll never get there" becomes your new mantra, and it can become a self-fulfilling prophecy.

To be successful at goal-setting and attainment, the most successful people use a powerful tool called *visualization.* Imagine yourself as your ideal self and keep that focus. For example:

- ✔ See the action-oriented goals you need to accomplish in order to become that healthy person you want to be.

- ✔ See the obstacles in your way and visualize removing them from your path.

- ✔ See yourself where you want to be and who you want to be and lock in on those images.

The more often you visualize your ideal, the closer you come to attaining it. You can even write down a detailed description in your notebook of what you see to help reinforce the images. As you review your goals every day, visualize yourself acting them out and accomplishing them. Be sure you refer to this list when you're stuck or off track.

137

As we mentioned earlier, the process of goal-setting takes practice. The most successful people in the world fail more times than unsuccessful people do. And successful people have failed at meeting a goal on time. You're the boss of your own body, and it's counting on you not to quit. If you don't meet a goal or deadline, set a new one! If you have a big goal, break it down into smaller, more manageable tasks. Just don't give up!

How often should you review your goals? It depends on how quickly you want to achieve them. Some people review their goals daily, and we think this is a good plan. The more often you use your goals *and* act on them, the better you get at creating goals, solving problems, and achieving the results you want.

Measuring your progress

Almost nothing is more satisfying than a written record of success. Forgetting how far you've come is easy when you don't have a tangible record of it. By setting specific measures on your goals and accurately tracking your performance each day, you reinforce the changes to your health and well-being (like incorporating healthy choices and maintaining a positive mental attitude) and make it easy to refer to when you need to revise goals.

Jotting down notes related to your activity is also helpful. For example, did you feel especially hungry on a given day? Tired? Angry? Were certain exercises extremely difficult to do, or was a certain activity impossible to continue because of fatigue? Knowing what worked for you and what didn't can help you plan a more realistic and successful plan.

One easy way to keep track of your diet and exercise is online at a Web site like www.fitday.com or www.my fooddiary.com, which is only $9 per month. The Web site www.mapmyrun.com allows you to map your biking or jogging routes and change them and save them according to the distance. If you want something that you can hold in your hand that's already laid out for you, a company called BodyMinder sells journals for recording anything related to exercise and diet. Look in the fitness section in any bookstore for different choices to see what fits your needs best.

Removing obstacles and getting back on track

On your course to a healthier lifestyle, you're going to experience detours, potholes, bottlenecks, and of course, the occasional flat tire. All the more reason to set goals; they can't prevent obstacles, but when they're written clearly, action-oriented, and measurable, they can help you get up and going again. To minimize the obstacles that may block your path, we recommend a three-step approach:

1. **Identify your obstacles.**

   Don't take it personally — goals aren't about perfection but reality. Building failure into your plan just makes sense.

   For example, maybe your goal is to improve your lean muscle mass by 20 percent in six months with strength training. You plan to work out with weights four days a week, one hour each session. Three months into your goal, you're in a car accident and in the hospital for a week. Your recovery period puts you behind schedule and you can't make it back to the gym for three months. You failed to meet your goal. What do you do? Set a new goal.

   Your roadblocks can come from work, family, or financial obligations, or they can be less tangible factors like motivation. When you can identify them, you can prepare for and overcome them when they occur. You can have a Plan B.

2. **Prioritize the obstacles in the order you need to overcome them.**

   By prioritizing and writing them down on paper in your planning notebook, you can see what's standing between you and your goals. No matter how challenging the obstacle, write it down. For example, if your biggest obstacle to exercising is that your fitness center's hours no longer fit your schedule, list *Look for ways to change schedule to get to gym* as a priority, with *Look for a new gym* as a second priority if the first fix isn't possible.

   The more you practice problem-solving skills, the better you become at resolving these roadblocks and the more quickly you achieve your goals. You also realize just how often obstacles come across your path and you become more confident at setting larger or more challenging goals.

3. **Rewrite a new goal to address each obstacle.**

   In Step 2, a person who can't find time for exercise may need a new, more specific goal. He may have to write *find 30 minutes three times a week to exercise by cutting out XYZ* (replacing XYZ with a real event). This suggestion may sound simple, but change isn't always easy. He may have to eliminate 90 minutes of something he enjoys, like watching TV or spending time on the computer.

To overcome obstacles, your goals must be desirable *and* you must be committed to them.

Finding support

Unless you're a Lone Ranger type (and even he had a side-kick!), you're likely to find lifestyle changes like dieting, quitting smoking, and starting an exercise program much easier if you have company along the way. A good friend or a whole support group of people can encourage you, help you get back on track when you waver, and cheer you on when you succeed. Plus, a little healthy competition may spur you all on to success. The beauty is that you can find people who specialize in helping you achieve your goals if you find it hard to go it alone.

Finding support for specific goals can be simple. Want to quit smoking? Find a friend or relative to team up with, or join a group like Nicotine Anonymous, a spinoff organization of Alcoholics Anonymous. Diet plans? You can find dozens, both online and live, to choose from. Not interested in baring your problems in public? Look for the hundreds, if not thousands, of online support groups for every type of issue under the sun, including support for specific diet plans and forums that discuss exercise videos made by different groups or individuals.

Just making your goal known to someone else — even if it's just your mom or best friend — increases the likelihood that you'll stick with it. Want to make the stakes higher? Organize a group where each person contributes a monetary amount and the person closest to his or her goal after a set time wins the pot. Or make your own personal reward system; put money toward something you really want and then hand the money to someone else to "keep" for you until you reach your goal.

"Going it alone" can be successful, but it can be a lonely road. Team up with friends or make some new ones and the journey toward your goals will seem much shorter — and a lot more fun, too.

Part II

Workin' on Your Framework

The 5th Wave

By Rich Tennant

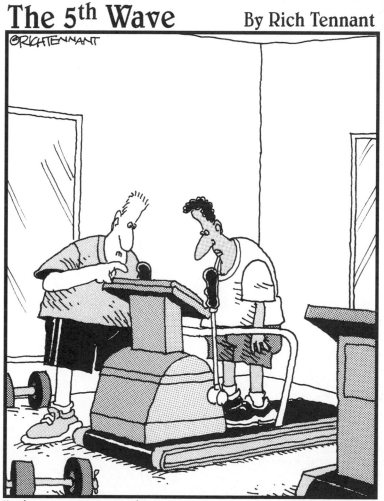

"This readout shows your heart rate, blood pressure, bone density, skin hydration, plaque buildup, liver function, and expected lifetime."

In this part . . .

Proper care of your body's mainframe, such as your teeth, skin, and bones, helps you withstand the test of time. Some people are very hard on their bodies and push them to the limit. When body parts wear out, they aren't so easily replaced. The chapters in this part help you understand your body parts and explain what you can do to keep them in tiptop shape.

Chapter 4

Putting Your Best Face Forward

In This Chapter

▶ Discovering the means of good oral health
▶ Figuring out ways to keep your ears healthy
▶ Keeping clear and healthy eyes

Your face is the first thing people relate to when they meet you. Are your eyes bright, your teeth gleaming, your ears open, and your breath fresh? While making a first impression is important, leaving a lasting impression on your health as you age is even more important. Letting your eyes, ears, mouth, and teeth fall into disrepair can have far reaching consequences for your general health, especially as you age. Periodontal disease is seen in a majority of the adult population, and age-related hearing and vision loss are both in the top eight most prevalent chronic conditions in older Americans. These areas of the body are very common sources of medical visits and many of the problems related to them could be avoided with preventative measures.

In this chapter, we look at your face, and we talk about

145

keeping your eyes, ears, mouth, and teeth healthy.

Your Mouth, from Cradle to Golden Years

Think a healthy mouth is all about straight teeth or whitening strips? Even worse, do you think having a healthy mouth consists of making sure your dentures stay in place while you eat corn on the cob? Sure, these things are important, but they don't have a long lasting effect on your health. Taking care of teeth, mouth, and gums takes more than cosmetic effort.

In elementary school, you were taught to brush and floss your teeth twice a day to avoid getting cavities. You were also told to avoid the kinds of foods that cause cavities (like sugary snacks and sticky foods that get stuck in your teeth). Armed with this important knowledge, you were off to face the world with a milky-white smile and the confidence that you could remain cavity- and infection-free for life.

Twenty (or more) years later, you're sitting in that very comfortable dental chair as the hygienist pokes around your gums and measures the depth of those pockets around your teeth. And you're cheerfully told that you have periodontal disease, a condition where the bacteria in plaque (the sticky, colorless film that covers your teeth) causes your gums to become inflamed.

Your cheerful hygienist (sure, she's cheerful — these aren't *her* teeth) tells you that some of your pockets are deep enough that they've become infected. They need to be treated with an injection or you're at risk of bone loss and eventually losing your tooth. She tells you that you also need to

- Brush and floss more
- Swish with antiplaque/antigingivitis rinse

146

✔ Add an anticavity, high-fluoride rinse

✔ Keep regularly scheduled checkups

You can't imagine how you're supposed to have time to earn a living, take care of a family, and keep up with all this tooth work at the same time. (Read more about periodontitis in the section "Open Wide! What You Need to Know about Oral Health.")

Moving into your 60s and 70s, you have other concerns about your mouth, like how you're going to pay for dental care and food at the same time. Or you may have other medical concerns that overshadow your oral healthcare. The ability to brush and floss is often difficult for seniors because of physical limitations. Getting to dental appointments can also be a challenge for seniors who lack access to transportation.

The point is that at any point in life, taking care of your teeth can be a pain. But teeth are around for a long time — or should be. What you do when you're young has long-term consequences on your future mouth health, but all isn't lost if you didn't own a toothbrush until you were 36. Understanding what can go wrong with your mouth can help keep problems from happening.

Open Wide! What You Need to Know about Oral Health

From periodontal disease to cancer, your mouth can be a source of pain and disease ranging from a mild nuisance to a disabling condition. Dentures are becoming routine practice, but the sad part is that it can often be prevented.

Grab your toothbrush and dental floss and throw away your cigarettes and sweets, not just for your teeth, but because brushing and flossing can also prevent diseases in other parts of your body. In fact, some studies link the same bacteria that cause mouth disease with other chronic conditions such as heart disease and diabetes.

Outlining the top two oral health concerns

Two common oral health concerns that are often not discussed are tooth decay and periodontal disease. *Tooth decay* is the most common chronic childhood disease, and it continues on as you age. *Periodontal disease* effects your gums. This disease is also very common and potentially dangerous. Both are preventable, but with poor lifestyle choices starting with the younger population, these problems are becoming an uphill battle.

In this section, we provide information for you to face this battle, so don't rush and grab your toothpaste and floss just yet.

Tooth decay

You may not know it, but your mouth is continually trying to wear down your teeth. The bacteria that occur naturally in your mouth mix with your saliva and bits of food in your mouth to form a coating (dental plaque) that sticks to your teeth. When this plaque hardens, it becomes tartar.

The acids in both the plaque and the tartar wear away the teeth's enamel. These acids can get inside the teeth and create holes or cavities. Tartar forms a rough area on the teeth and can be stained much more easily than healthy enamel. Everyone is at risk for getting cavities throughout life. By the time they're adults, 85 percent of people will have had a cavity! Here are a few activities that increase your risk of tooth decay; we're sure you'll recognize a few:

- **High sugar and carbohydrate diet:** These types of foods attract the bacteria that cause tooth decay. Combine poor diet with poor dental hygiene and presto, you have tooth decay.

- **Lack of dental care:** Regular cleaning is needed to remove plaque and bacteria from the teeth and gums. Dental care includes both your own daily regimen and routine follow-up with your dentist.

- **Smoking:** Smokers have more tooth decay than nonsmokers. One reason is that smokers produce less saliva, which cleans the teeth and inside of the mouth. Smokers also have a higher incidence of gum disease, because smoking decreases blood flow to the gums.

- **Fluoride deficiency:** Fluoride helps teeth ward off the acids that can erode the enamel. Some water supplies don't have fluoride added in so check with your local water company and then pick up some fluorinated toothpaste!

As people age, they produce less saliva allowing more bacteria to accumulate in their mouths making the teeth even more susceptible to tooth decay and fractures. These bacteria don't stop at the teeth and if allowed eventually wreak havoc on your gums and become a major instigator of bad breath.

Periodontal disease

Periodontal disease, a chronic bacterial infection of the gums and the area between the teeth and gums (the *sulcus*), is a common problem affecting about 80 percent of the adult population. It begins when the bacteria and other food particles that cause tooth decay move down into the

149

gums. If left untreated, this condition can turn into mild gum inflammation and then into serious gum disease that can affect not only the gums but also the teeth and supporting bone. When periodontal disease advances, the infection infiltrates the bone structures that hold the teeth in place and ultimately can lead to tooth loss. Early stages of the disease can be painful and, if not approached aggressively, the disease can be destructive and costly.

Periodontal disease is classified according to the severity of the disease as gingivitis or periodontitis. *Gingivitis* is reversible, but when left untreated, it can lead to the more serious periodontitis. *Periodontitis* is the most common cause of tooth loss among adults. Here are some additional facts about the two:

- ✔ **Gingivitis:** Your gums can become inflamed and reddened. They may even bleed, especially when you floss. Most of the time, you have no associated pain. This condition is reversible if you seek dental treatment and initiate good dental hygiene at home.

- ✔ **Periodontitis:** If you fail to treat your gingivitis, you may end up with this more serious inflammatory condition. The inflammation causes the gums and bone to start receding leaving small pockets around the teeth for more bacteria and plaque to congregate. This continues the disease process and eventually the bone may extend where the teeth are anchored and tooth loss may result.

Some risk factors for periodontal disease include

- ✔ **Smoking:** Cigarette smoke contains thousands of chemicals including formaldehyde, carbon monoxide, ammonia, arsenic tar, and nicotine. These

Grappling with the effects of tooth loss

Losing teeth isn't just a social embarrassment. You may not know that when you lose your teeth, you also lose bone in your jaw, and eventually your face starts to sag. The aging process accelerates at a rapid pace whether you lose your teeth at 45 or 75. Bone loss can also make dentures loose and difficult to wear. The more jawbone that's worn away, the less available bone you have to secure the dentures.

Dental implants can help prevent bone loss following a tooth extraction. As common replacements for missing or fractured teeth, dental implants are permanent fixtures of titanium posts that are anchored to the jawbone and topped with individual replacement teeth or a bridge that screws or cements into the posts. Implants may replace one tooth, be a combination of several implants (a bridge), or work in combination with dentures.

chemicals affect gum healing by decreasing blood flow and also causing inflammation of the gums.

✓ **Dry mouth:** Dry mouth (*xerostomia*) is decreased production of saliva. Saliva is needed in the mouth to wash away food particles and bacteria. Saliva can neutralize acids and therefore deter plaque formation. See the sidebar later in this chapter, entitled "Coping with a dry mouth: More than just a nuisance."

✓ **Hormonal changes in females:** Hormonal shifts that cause elevated levels of progesterone increase your risk of gum disease. Pregnancy, parts of the menstrual cycle, and possibly some birth control pills can all result in elevated progesterone levels. Progesterone dilates blood vessels and can block collagen, which can lead to swelling and inflammation. Gum disease is a common complaint during pregnancy and right before periods begin.

✔ **Diabetes:** Research supports that diabetics with poor control of their blood sugars are more likely to develop gum disease. Because diabetes affects immune function and increases risk of infection, it's more difficult for diabetics to fight off the bacteria that causes periodontal disease.

✔ **Medications:** A few medications are implicated in gum disease. Oral contraceptives, antidepressants, and some blood pressure medicines are found to cause dry mouth. Other medications, such as anti-seizure and some heart medications, can cause the gums to enlarge, which can increase inflammation and increase collection of plaque.

✔ **Genetic susceptibility:** It isn't clear what the genetic link is, but it's estimated that about 30 percent of the population have an increased susceptibility to periodontal disease. This requires these people to pay more attention to preventative measures and regular dental care.

Understanding how an unhealthy mouth may affect the whole body

Unfortunately, periodontal disease doesn't stop at your teeth and gums. Many researchers have a particular interest in these pesky oral bacteria and possible links to other diseases, such as heart disease and respiratory infections. Numerous studies link heart disease to common bacteria associated with periodontal disease. (See the sidebar "Conjecture or link?" in this chapter for more info.) The American Academy of Periodontology states that people with periodontal disease have nearly twice the risk of coronary artery disease. Research is ongoing, but for now, aggressively treating periodontal disease may help you reduce the risks of some common and serious diseases such as the following:

- ✔ **Heart disease:** Patients with valvular heart disease (rheumatic heart disease, congenital valve problems, previous endocarditis or infection involving a heart valve, and previous valve replacement) are at risk of valve infection. Bacteria can enter the tiny scrapes and cuts that are inevitable during dental or surgical procedures and end up on the heart valves. If you have any of these conditions, or if you're not sure, see your medical doctor before having dental work done, because you may need to take antibiotics prior to dental work.

  A study published in *Circulation: Journal of the American Heart Association* studied 657 people without known heart disease. It found that people who had higher blood levels of certain disease-causing bacteria in the mouth were more likely to have atherosclerosis in the carotid artery in the neck.

- ✔ **Diabetes:** The Center for Disease Control estimates that 95 percent of Americans with diabetes have periodontal disease due to the increased susceptibility of diabetics to infections. Diabetic infections can be more serious and harder to treat, so diabetics need to be especially diligent about seeing their dentists every six months.

- ✔ **Respiratory infection:** Researchers have found that bacteria that inhabit the oral cavity can be aspirated into the lung, causing respiratory diseases such as pneumonia. People with periodontal disease are especially susceptible, and this risk could be preventable for those already weakened by other diseases or those prone to respiratory infection.

Recognizing a quiet but increasing threat: The oral cancer epidemic

Oral cancer is the 6th most common cancer in men and 14th in women with more than 30,000 new cases occurring each year. Many types of cancer are frequently publicized in the news, increasing people's awareness of their risk factors and symptoms, but oral cancer doesn't get much press. What's most disconcerting is that the number of new cases *and* the death rate from oral cancer is up 11 percent from 2006. The Center for Disease Control estimates that 75 percent of the cases of oral cancer are associated with smoked and smokeless tobacco use.

If oral cancer isn't diagnosed and treated in its early stages, it can spread, leading to chronic pain, loss of function, irreparable facial and oral disfigurement following surgery, and even death. If found early, oral cancer has a promising survival rate, but a lack of dental care and the vagueness of the symptoms can lead to delay in diagnosis. Many people discover oral cancer only when it has metastasized to another location, most likely the lymph nodes of the neck and beyond, at which point the prognosis is poor.

Risk factors for oral cancer

Unlike some cancers, oral cancer doesn't have a large list of related risk factors. We can sum up the majority of the risk of oral cancer with two words and neither should be of any surprise — tobacco and alcohol. The good news is you have the choice to remove these major risks and the bad news is too many seldom do.

154

Conjecture or link? Heart disease and gum disease

The potential link between heart disease and gum disease is a topic of much debate in the medical and dental community. Whether gum disease is actually the direct cause of heart disease isn't crystal clear; however, the fact that medical science and researchers keep looking for links and finding them is enough to warrant mention. Read on for some of the proposed mechanisms of the gum disease (periodontitis) and heart disease association.

First, the researchers stress that this possible link between certain bacteria in the mouth and heart disease isn't yet fully studied. But here's what they found: Several strains of bacteria that cause periodontal disease can enter the bloodstream and travel to the heart, where they can cause thickening of the arteries. Thickened arteries reduce blood flow to the heart, increasing the risk of heart attack. Thickened carotid arteries (arteries that lead to the brain) can raise the risk of stroke. To connect the dots, researchers have to find out which came first, the thickened arteries or the nasty bacteria in the mouth.

Studies show that the oral bacteria Streptococcus sanguis does cause the clumping of blood platelets. This clumping can be the first stage in the development of a blood clot — the cause of a heart attack. The periodontal infection reduces the health of the lining of the gum tissues, which, in turn, allows bacteria from the mouth to enter into the underlying tissues.

Patients with periodontitis have significantly higher levels of inflammatory products (fibrinogen and white blood cells), which are well-known risk factors for acute heart attacks. Dental bacterial components affect the body's response to infection and can play a role in the development of atherosclerosis.

New development in medical research is raising further concerns that bacteria can cause heart attacks. One bacteria, Chlamydia pneumoniae, has been found in the walls of the blood vessels of patients who have had heart attacks.

Here are the risks in detail:

✔ **Tobacco use:** The main risk factor for oral cancer is tobacco use. Smoking and the cancer connection is a popular theme that you pick up on in this book.

✔ **Excessive alcohol consumption:** An estimated 75 to 80 percent of people with oral cancer consume alcohol. A large number of smokers also drink heavily, making a direct connection between alcohol and oral cancer harder to prove. Studies at this point indicate a higher risk for those who both smoke and drink heavily.

✔ **Sun exposure:** Lips are also an area where oral cancer can occur; sun exposure is definitely a risk factor for cancer of the lip. Block those rays with sunscreen and/or a large brimmed hat.

✔ **Age and gender:** Another risk factor for oral cancer is age, with greater than 90 percent of cases occurring in people over the age of 45. The average age is around 60. Forty years ago, oral cancer had a 5 to 1 male to female ratio, but now, the ratio is just 2:1. This is directly linked to the increased rate of smoking in women.

Common symptoms of oral cancer

The most frequent oral cancer sites are the tongue, the floor of the mouth, and soft palate tissues in back of the tongue, lips, and gums. Your dentist probably performs a thorough screening for oral cancer each time you see him — another good reason not to miss your dental appointments!

Now that we've brought oral cancer out into the light, here are a list of some of the most common oral cancer symptoms:

- ✓ **Non-healing sores:** If you have a sore, blister, erosion, or bleeding in the mouth or on your lip that doesn't heal in 2 to 3 weeks, have it evaluated by a medical doctor.

- ✓ **Discolored patches:** Any white or red patches on the tongue, lips, gums, or lining the mouth should raise suspicion of cancer. These patches require immediate attention.

- ✓ **Lumps:** Even if you don't see discoloration, a lump needs to be evaluated. If you have any lumps in the lip or mouth, have them looked at so that the doctor can decide whether they need further evaluation.

- ✓ **Difficulty swallowing:** Any pain that you may have — whether it's in the throat, mouth, or when you move your tongue — should be evaluated.

 Monitor your mouth for any of these symptoms and discuss them with your doctor or dentist as soon as possible, particularly if you use tobacco products or drink alcohol.

Tending to Your Oral Cavity — Your Mouth, That Is

We don't know of anything more motivating toward improving your oral hygiene than the sound of the infamous dental drill. We're not asking you to spend 45 minutes a day on each tooth; just a few minutes of attention goes a long way. Your mouth deserves it, so now is the time to get out your mouth cleaning tools and start cleaning.

Doing away with tooth decay

When you're ready to do away with tooth decay, grab your

tools — your toothbrush, some dental floss, a good dentist's phone number. This section touches on the basics, but you may discover a thing or two about tooth care that ultimately may keep you from hearing the dreaded dental drill. Most important of all: Don't think that dentist visits and cavities are just for kids; the older you get the more important good dental care is.

Here are the basics of dental hygiene:

✔ **Brush your teeth.** Use a toothbrush with soft enough bristles that it does not cause bleeding. Use short strokes and make sure that you get the back teeth and the gums. Plan on getting a new tooth brush about every four months or when the bristles are bent. It is hard to pick a brushing time limit, but you should brush for 3 to 4 minutes. This routine is not only to give you fresh breath, but also is the opportunity to get rid of the plaque and bacteria that adhere to your teeth and gums. Don't forget to brush your tongue, but remember you have this thing called a gag reflex at the back of the throat which doesn't like toothbrushes.

Use a fluoride toothpaste because fluoride has been found to strengthen the enamel on the teeth therefore making it more resistant to acids. If possible, drink water that is fluorinated. If your teeth are particularly vulnerable to cavities, use a fluoride mouth rinse at home — you just swish once daily after brushing your teeth.

✔ **Floss.** There are several areas of the teeth that your brush won't get and the only way to get to those areas is to floss daily. Flossing gets out plaque and food pieces from between your teeth that the bristles from your toothbrush just can't reach. If you aren't flossing then you aren't taking care of your teeth . . . period!

✔ **Schedule regular dental visits every six months.** Yes, it's a pain; you dread it all week, but it's important to get regular cleanings. The dental hygienist is able to scrape away some of the plaque buildup and scan for cavities. They can also check for gum disease or erosion and screen for suspicious lesions. Just do it.

✔ **Eat the daily recommended intake of foods high in calcium to help support strong teeth.** Calcium poor diets can lead to bone loss and

Fixing a broken tooth

Teeth are coated with the hardest substance in your body — enamel. Breaking a tooth is no small feat, yet it's possible and occurs more often then one may think. Fractured teeth may crack a long time before they actually break, they may or may not hurt, and they can't heal like bones do.

So what should you do if your tooth just breaks? Chances are good that the tooth that broke was already cracked and under stress — the weakest link, if you will. It may have been weakened by a filling, or it may have already had a small crack. Because it didn't have the ability to heal itself like bone, it was just a matter of time (and it usually happens just as you're headed on vacation).

If one of your teeth breaks, cover it with a sterile gauze pad (pressing it firmly to keep it in place and stop any bleeding), and call your dentist immediately. Don't have a sterile gauze pad handy? Try a paper towel or napkin. Also, avoid sweet, hot, crunchy foods and liquids until your dentist fixes the tooth. Instead, try foods that are soft and are mild in flavor and temperature.

Coping with a dry mouth: More than just a nuisance

Dry mouth, called *xerostomia,* is a common occurrence and complaint with aging. It's more than just an annoyance, though; it can have harmful side effects. Chronic dry mouth can lead to sores in the mouth and cracking of the lips and corners of the mouth, which can lead to infection. It can also increase the risk of tooth decay from lack of saliva to help wash away bacteria and food particles. Dry mouth can cause bad breath, burning of the tongue, dryness in the throat, and a chronic hoarse voice.

Saliva glands often produce less saliva as you age. Hundreds of medications, many prescribed for age-related conditions, can cause dry mouth, mostly due to the effects that the drugs have on the parasympathetic nervous system. Drugs that are known to cause dry mouth include the following:

- Allergy medications (antihistamines)
- Antidepressants
- Blood pressure medications
- Medications for urinary incontinence

Dry mouth is also a common side effect of cancer treatment. Nerve damage to the face, neck, and head; endocrine disorders; stress; and nutritional deficiencies can also cause dry mouth.

Treating dry mouth can be difficult. If a medication is the cause, talk to your doctor about possibly substituting another medication for your condition. Your doctor may have a sample to try first, that way you don't have to pay for another prescription that very well could carry the same side effects.

Try drinking more water — most people don't drink enough water anyway. As you age, the thirst sensation and the brain's response to thirst are sluggish and sometimes absent. Sucking on certain candies can help, but you can eat only so much candy.

weakening of the jaw bone, which holds your teeth. Eventually the bone will weaken to a point where gaps are created around the teeth and can accumulate and accelerate the effects of gum disease and tooth loss.

✔ **Avoid carbonated drinks as much as possible.** The carbonation, sugar, and acid in the soda attract bacteria and form damaging levels of acid that can eat away at the enamel of your teeth and contribute to tooth decay.

Cutting out the sodas is a great idea, but if you do drink them, researchers in Germany found that if you wait more than 30 minutes to brush your teeth after soda ingestion you can preserve enamel.

Taking care of dentures

Having dentures doesn't mean your dentist visits are over. Dentures needs to be periodically checked for proper fitting, and dentures can cause problems with your gums if they don't fit well or when you're first adjusting to them. Poor fitting dentures can be painful, causing rubbing and wear against your gums. Anytime you get skin abrasions, you increase your chances of infection; this is especially true in your mouth, which is full of germs. Because you need your dentures to talk, eat, and maintain a facial structure, taking them out while your gums heal is a difficult option. And dentures must be clean, or they can be an addi-

Bad breath: A sign of a deeper problem?

Halitosis is the medical term for bad breath — clinical, chemical, offensive odor. For most people, bad breath is situational and the result of something in their mouths. But if a mint or mouthwash doesn't do the trick, your dragon breath may be indicative of a health concern. Bad breath is often correctable with minimal effort — if you know you have it. Hopefully you're one of the lucky ones whose friends are honest enough to tell you or you figure it out on your own.

If you've determined the problem isn't from coffee, chips, a gyro, or something equally breathtaking, then check your teeth and gums. Halitosis is often a symptom of food caught between teeth, an infected tooth, or gum disease. In these cases, try the following remedies:

✔ Don't skip brushing and flossing. And don't do it just once a day, either — try to brush every time you eat something significant (this approach may cut down on your snacking, too!). Yes, it's a chore — especially in the middle of the day — to brush and floss, but nothing else is as effective in removing those evil bacteria that can cause disease and bad breath. (And it also ensures that you don't walk around with a piece of broccoli stuck between your teeth!) You may want to consider using a water pick, which can remove stubborn, stuck foods from hard to reach places in your mouth.

✔ Do a pain assessment on your mouth. If your teeth are painful or sensitive to hot and cold, you may have an infected tooth. If you have a painful lump on your gum, you could have an infection there. Any mouth infection can also cause bad breath — and you may have a bad taste in your mouth if the area is leaking pus. Call your dentist for an appointment.

- Take a look at your sinuses. If you have chronic pain over your eyes, frequent headaches, or pain over your cheekbones, you may have a chronic sinus infection, which can lead to bad breath.

- Drink something. Dry mouth can cause bad breath, so make sure that you drink plenty of water, and talk to your doctor if you feel that your mouth is abnormally dry.

If you're up-to-date on your dental visits and you floss regularly but still have issues with bad breath, look further down the pipes. The next common causes of halitosis are problems with your stomach, lungs, kidneys, or liver:

- Stomach problems that lead to chronic heartburn or reflux can cause bad breath.

- If you're having coughing fits, fevers, or shortness of breath, a lung infection can cause changes in your breath. See your doctor as soon as possible.

- Kidney disease can give your breath an ammonia smell, so see your doctor if you experience this odor.

- Liver disease can cause your breath to smell fishy. We strongly suggest you visit your doctor immediately if you suffer from this.

tional source of bacteria introduced into your mouth.

The following pointers are important for denture maintenance:

- **Dental checkups:** You may need new plastic added to the inside of the existing denture to fill the expanding space between the denture and gums due to the receding bone that can occur with aging and wear.

- ✔ **Cleaning:** This helps prevent bacteria from growing on your dentures. Rinsing thoroughly also keeps foreign particles that can accumulate on the dentures from irritating the gums. Don't use harsh abrasives; use products made especially for dentures. Keep your mouth and gums clean, too, by brushing with a soft toothbrush and toothpaste. And make sure that you use any rinse recommended by your dentist.

- ✔ **Replacement:** Dentures aren't forever. A denture worn too long can damage the facial appearance and the gums and cause a host of other complications. For example, muscles for chewing and talking begin to shorten to accommodate the decreasing space caused by the receding bone between the nose and chin. The longer a person waits to replace dentures, the more difficult the facial structure is to restore; this results in a sad or aged appearance. If you're doing routine denture maintenance, but your dentures aren't fitting well, it's time to get a brand-new shiny set of the pearly whites.

Can You Say "Eh?" Cleaning Out Your Ears

Have you noticed that the "volume" knob on your TV isn't working all that well these days? For some reason, you need to keep turning it up — and up. And everyone around you is mumbling — can't they just speak up? When these things start happening — guess what? It's probably you who has the problem, not everybody else!

When people talk about aging, many can't finish the conversation without talking about hearing loss. The development of hearing deficits can really impact your life or the lives of people around you. Often, loved ones are the main catalysts to having your ears checked out, because they can't take the high volume of the television, having to repeat themselves, and always needing to yell. Most people are in denial about the situation. When someone forces them to go to the doctor or convinces them that the hearing loss is affecting their job or social life, they finally realize that they should have it evaluated. Why do people wait? Mostly because they're afraid of the end result . . . hearing aids. Nobody wants to deal with the daily hassles of hearing aids.

Currently, over 20 million Americans suffer from hearing loss. It's the third most common chronic disabling condition, behind arthritis and high blood pressure. About 250 million people have disabling hearing impairment, and half of these cases are preventable.

A closer look at the causes of hearing loss

There are two types of hearing loss. One occurs when something is blocking the transmission of the sounds such as wax, while the other is a result of damage to the inner ear or the nerves that transmit sound signals to the brain. Age-related hearing loss (presbycusis) is a type of *sensorineural hearing loss.* It occurs when you have a problem with the transmission of the sounds from parts of the inner ear to your brain's auditory cortex. *Conductive hearing loss* occurs when the sound can't reach the inner ear. Whenever you suffer from hearing loss you may need specialized hearing tests and other diagnostic tools to ultimately know what type of hearing loss you have and what's causing it.

Common causes of conductive hearing loss include

- ✔ Wax (cerumen) buildup (the most common)
- ✔ External and middle ear infections (middle ear infections, or otitis media, are more common in children but can occur in adults)
- ✔ Perforated ear drum
- ✔ A tumor that lies directly behind the eardrum (this is rare)

Causes of sensorineural hearing loss include

- ✔ Age-related hearing loss (presbycusis)
- ✔ Noise induced hearing loss
- ✔ Tumor (acoustic neuroma)
- ✔ Autoimmune disorders
- ✔ Genetic disorders
- ✔ Meniere's disease, a middle ear disease that causes dizziness and hearing loss

Presbycusis, also known as nerve deafness, begins around age 40 and gets progressively worse as you age. Through the years of constant work, the little hairs in the middle ear are damaged or destroyed, and sound waves aren't processed well. Presbycusis does tend to run in families, so you may want to listen to see whether older family members have hearing difficulties and ask them (loudly!) at what age it started.

Noise induced hearing loss is the most preventable cause of hearing loss. Loud noises, such as explosions, gunfire, loud music, and other repeated occupational noise exposures (jackhammer, flight lines, factories), are the primary cause. That's one reason why being a rock musician isn't all that it's cracked up to be. More than 10 million people in the U.S. have noise induced hearing loss. Will the current craze of having music blasting directly into your ears 24/7 increase hearing loss in the future? It's a possibility — turn down the volume while you can still hear it!

Preventing hearing loss

Some causes of sensorineural hearing loss aren't preventable, and the one cause that can be prevented is only getting worse. The damage that occurs with all the causes of sensorineural hearing loss is permanent without any real effective cure. Although some hearing loss may be inevitable, you don't have to make it worse than it may already be.

Follow these tips for maintaining healthy and functioning ears:

- ✔ To prevent conductive loss

    - Do not — and we really mean never — stick anything smaller than your elbow in your ear canal. That means no cotton swabs. Often they just pack the wax in the canal like arming a musket with a ramrod.
    - Let soapy water run in and out of your ears in the shower to keep the wax out.
    - Schedule regular ear cleanings with your doctor if you have recurring problems with wax buildup and aren't able to clear it on your own.

- ✔ To prevent sensorineural loss

    - The main prevention for noise and age-related hearing loss is a no-brainer . . . ear protectors.

Use them in the form of earplugs or earmuffs. If you love to share your music with the cars next to you or with the people three machines over in the gym, you may want to turn the volume down a few notches. Save your own ears and everyone else's too!

Can you hear me now? Treating hearing loss

If you have hearing loss, see your healthcare professional to find the cause. If you have decreased hearing along with fever or with accompanied pain, you could have an inner ear infection or wax buildup, which needs to be evaluated by a medical doctor and treated.

Conductive hearing loss may be as easy to fix as having your doctor clean your ears. If it ends up being earwax, you can do a few things to keep the wax from building up in the ear canals. For example:

- Rinse your ears out with warm water and hydrogen peroxide.

- If ear wax is really packed, see your doctor for ear irrigation. You can buy kits over the counter that can be effective; just make sure you use the ear wax drops for a few days before trying to irrigate.

If you don't have wax and your doctor diagnosed you with sensorineural hearing loss, don't get too discouraged. Fortunately, there's a way to manage hearing loss through the use of hearing aids. Unfortunately, many people don't like them, and to make matters worse, they're not cheap and often not covered by insurance. They're often difficult to keep in the ear and static free; still, they can be helpful and

Considering LASIK

Getting rid of your glasses or contacts would certainly be nice, wouldn't it? No more searching the house or wearing a chain around your neck; no more expensive new prescriptions at ever increasing intervals. Yes, it would be nice — and thousands of people each year choose to have LASIK surgery. Do your homework first to increase your odds of having a positive — and healthy — experience with LASIK surgery. Having realistic expectations increases your chances of having a positive experience.

LASIK surgery involves surgically changing the contour of your cornea, the clear covering over the front of your eye, by using a laser. LASIK can't be done if your cornea isn't thick enough to be surgically altered. LASIK also can't repair every type of refraction error. If you have severe myopia, hyperopia, or astigmatism, LASIK may not work for you. And although most people have excellent results from LASIK, some have recurrent vision problems or problems with glare or halos around objects.

LASIK only corrects presbyopia — normal age changes in the eye — if a technique known as monovision is used. With monovision, one eye is corrected for distance vision and the other eye isn't.

As with any surgery, and especially one that's done on an irreplaceable organ, do considerable research on doctors in your area. Don't choose by price — in fact, price should be your last consideration. Choose a center that has a proven track record. Ask about success rates, infection rates, and complication rates. Ask your primary doctor who she would have operate on her own family. If you know an ophthalmologist, ask for a recommendation.

allow for better quality of life.

There's no cure for this type of hearing loss, so hearing aids don't correct the underlying problem; they just allow you to hear with assistance. Several companies and models of hearing aids are out there, so shop around before you buy. Find a company that will spend the time to teach you how to use the hearing aid and get the best possible results. Many supply free batteries with your purchase, too.

Examining and Preventing Age-Related Eye Conditions

Vision changes are inevitable as you age, and there's no real cure, just tools to compensate. In truth, most people have normal age-related vision changes; others have vision changes associated with diseases, such as diabetes. Some people retain good vision well into their 70s and 80s, but most people can expect some visual impairment. The number of people with vision impairment will increase in 2011 as the baby boomers turn 65 and double by 2030 as they continue to age.

Normal age-related vision loss is called presbyopia. *Presbyopia* is caused by hardening of the lens of the eye and usually begins after age 40. Presbyopia isn't a disease but rather a natural aging process, and it can be diagnosed by a simple eye examination.

Presbyopia is the inability to focus on near objects but is different then being farsighted (hyperopia), which is also associated with difficulty seeing close objects. With presbyopia, you may start to have difficulty reading, using the computer, or performing other day-to-day activities that involve things nearby. People with presbyopia often hold reading material at arm's length, trying to bring the words into focus. You may also complain of a headache from straining while reading or at work.

If your vision has never been corrected before, you may be able to get away with using drugstore reading glasses for some time — maybe even forever. But the most common treatment of presbyopia is prescription contact lenses or glasses. Eventually, you may need bifocals or trifocals, which incorporate reading glasses along with vision corrective lenses. You may also consider surgical options for correction, such as LASIK (laser-assisted in-situ keratomileusis) and lens implants. Consult your doctor to evaluate the best option for you.

Although presbyopia is a naturally occurring process rather than a disease, a number of diseases do cause vision changes that have different symptoms and treatments. Never assume that all vision loss in inevitable and unpreventable until seen by a medical doctor. A number of these diseases can be treated and the damage to your vision can be stopped or diminished. If vision changes come on suddenly, see an ophthalmologist (a medical doctor who specializes in treatment of the eye).

Seeing an eye doctor at regular intervals can help you recognize eye problems early and decrease further damage. Don't assume that it's just "normal vision loss" if you start to notice poor night vision, blurry vision, or floaters. The American Academy of Ophthalmology suggests the following exam schedule for people who have no visual problems:

✔ Every 5 to 10 years under age 40

✔ Every 2 to 4 years between ages 40 and 64

✔ Every 1 to 2 years beginning at age 65

If you have diabetes or other medical ailments that can affect your eyesight, make sure that they're treated correctly and strictly. Eye examinations under these conditions need to be done more frequently, usually at least yearly unless recommended differently by your doctor. Report any sudden change in your vision to your doctor immediately.

Clouding eyes — cataracts

When clouding on areas of the lens in your eye keeps light from passing through, you end up with cataracts. You may be developing cataracts if you have blurred or double vision and sensitivity to light, including glares from headlights, difficulty with night vision, and problems making out colors. If you have to change your prescription lenses more frequently than you once did, see a doctor, because this too could be a sign of cataracts. Cataracts may be worse in one eye than in the other.

 If vision changes start to interfere with your daily life, consider cataract surgery. The damaged lens is removed in a same-day surgery procedure and replaced with a synthetic lens made of plastic, silicone, or acrylic. If surgery isn't an option, wearing contact lenses or using strong magnifying glasses may help.

Leaking retinas: Diabetic retinopathy

Diabetic retinopathy is a major cause of vision loss for both type 1 and type 2 diabetics. Diabetes damages the blood vessels in the retina, causing them to leak fluid. Virtually everyone who has diabetes for 30 years or more has some degree of diabetic retinopathy. About 80 percent of people with diabetes has some retinopathy after 15 years.

If you have diabetic retinopathy, you may notice that your night vision is poor, or you may have floaters or blurry vision. See a retinal specialist as often as your doctor suggests to keep diabetic retinopathy from worsening as much as possible.

Diabetic retinopathy can be treated with a laser in the specialist's office. Early diabetic retinopathy is called non-proliferative; proliferative diabetic retinopathy is a later and more severe stage.

 The best thing you can do to prevent diabetic retinopathy is to try to keep from developing diabetes in the first place. Eat a healthy diet, keep your weight at a normal limit, and have yearly blood tests. If you do develop diabetes, keep your blood sugars under control and see your specialists frequently. Not smoking and maintaining normal blood pressure are also vital.

The pressure's up with glaucoma

Glaucoma results from increased fluid pressure (intraocular pressure, or IOP) in the eye, which damages the optic nerve. There are two types of glaucoma: open angle and angle closure. Open angle is by far the more common. If treated early, glaucoma can be controlled, but if left untreated, it can lead to loss of vision or blindness. Glaucoma is diagnosed by having the pressure measured by a special instrument called a *tonometer,* which measures the pressure in your eye. Your doctor also examines your optic nerve after dilating your eye with drops.

Glaucoma is treated by different types of daily eyedrops, which lower the pressure in the eye. You need regular checkups to make sure the pressure stays low, because glaucoma is usually painless.

Risk factors for developing glaucoma include race (glaucoma is the leading cause of blindness among African Americans), family history, previous eye injury, diabetes, high blood pressure, and extreme nearsightedness.

A decreasing ability to see straight (literally): Macular degeneration

The macula is located in the center of the retina, which is found at the back of your eye. Age-related macular degeneration (AMD) impairs central vision and can make driving and other common daily tasks difficult. The two forms of macular degeneration are

- ✔ **Dry:** A gradual breakdown of the cells of the macula

- ✔ **Wet:** From the formation of new, abnormal blood vessels grown under the center of the retina

The dry type is much more common — and the wet type has much more severe vision loss.

Only 10 percent of all cases of dry macular degeneration progress to wet. Risk factors for developing macular degeneration include family history, smoking, light-colored eyes, and eyes exposed to the sun over long periods of time. People developing macular degeneration may have blind spots in their central vision or blurriness or waviness in both the close and distant vision.

AMD has no known cure and there's no treatment for dry AMD, although your doctor may prescribe a type of multivitamin based on a study called the Aging Related Eye-Disease Study (AREDS) to slow macular degeneration. You can find these supplements, which should contain Vitamin C, Vitamin E, Vitamin A, Zinc, and Copper oxide, over the counter under a variety of name brands.

People with antioxidant deficiencies may suffer from macular degeneration due to the free radical destruction of the retina. Implementing antioxidants may improve these situations and also slow down other causes of AMD.

Other treatment options include intraocular injections

and laser procedures for the wet type of macular degeneration; although these may slow progression, at this time, neither is a cure.

Recognizing retinal detachment

Retinal detachment occurs when the inner and outer layers of the retina separate. The most common sign of retinal detachment is the sudden increase of the amount of floaters in the eye. Some people have halos around lights or bright flashes of lights, especially in the peripheral vision. You have no pain with a retinal detachment.

Retinal detachment needs to be treated with surgical procedures, either laser treatments or cryoplexy, which freezes the retina near the retinal tear, creating a scar that secures the retina. These procedures may be done in the office by an ophthalmologist who specializes in the retina or in the hospital as same-day surgery. If retinal detachments are left untreated, the retina may detach completely, causing blindness in the eye.

Chapter 5

Loving the Skin You're In

Your skin is the first line of defense against the outside world, and it takes a beating. Skin gets overheated, dried out, slathered with lotions and potions, scraped up, wrinkled, and wind burned, and the effects of the abuse you heap on your skin becomes more evident as you age.

In this chapter, we look at your skin with a magnifying glass, identifying the effects on your skin of too much sun, too little moisture, smoking, and an inadequate diet, among other things. We load you up with skin-care tips to help you avoid skin cancer and wrinkles. Although we can't guarantee that you'll keep the baby soft skin you came into the world with for your whole life, we can guarantee that taking proper care of your skin keeps it — and you — looking younger for longer.

A Primer on Your Body's Shell

Although you've probably heard the saying that beauty is only skin deep, it's obvious that society in general doesn't believe it. Most of the skin-care products on the market stress one thing — how it makes your skin *look.*

But there's much more to skin than its outward appearance. Skin covers your body for a reason — and although attracting a potential partner may be one of the reasons, it isn't the most important. The following sections educate you on the importance of the skin you're in, and why you can't live without it.

Your skin's all-important roles

Your skin is an *organ* (a body structure containing two or more different types of tissue that work together) — the largest organ of your body, in fact. Although your skin looks all of a piece from the outside, it's actually made up of three different layers, each with its own function. Your skin protects your insides from getting out and the outside world from getting in. More specifically, skin

- ✔ Serves as a waterproof barrier, keeping necessary moisture in your body where it belongs without allowing your insides to be flooded every time you get in the shower

- ✔ Keeps harmful bacteria, viruses, and other toxic elements from entering the body

- ✔ Regulates body temperature by releasing water and other toxins in the form of perspiration when you're hot and contracting tiny muscles (goose bumps) around hair follicles when you're cold

- ✔ Acts as a sensory receptor, allowing you to feel pain (a warning that something harmful is touching the skin) so that you pull away, pleasure (no pulling away there), and temperature changes so you protect your skin from damage from excessive cold or heat

 Your skin weighs about 8 to 11 pounds, and stretched out, it would cover 12 to 20 square feet! It's made up of 70 percent water, about 25 percent protein, and 3 to 5 percent fat. Dead skin makes up a majority of the dust in your house.

Your skin's anatomy and how it functions

Skin is more complicated than it looks on the outside. The three layers of the skin — the epidermis, dermis, and subcutaneous — each are further broken down into different layers. As you age, changes in your skin can make it more susceptible to damage — some visible, some not. Understanding what goes on "beneath the surface" can help you keep your skin from showing its age.

The three skin layers (and their sub-layers) each have a separate function:

- ✔ **Epidermis:** The epidermis is made up of five sub-layers. The top, very thin layer, called the stratum corneum, protects the body from the environment and consists of hard, flattened dead cells. In a process called *exfoliation,* your skin cells shed, at a rate of about 30,000 per minute, to reveal the newer cells that are produced in the bottom layers of the epidermis and pushed up through the middle layers until they reach the stratus corneum.

Over a two to four week period, new cells die, shed, and are replaced by newer cells.

Beneath the stratum corneum, the remaining layers consist mostly of two types of cells: squamous cells and basal cells. Squamous cells produce keratin, a protein that makes up a large part of skin, hair, and nails. Basal cells are found in the bottom layer of the epidermis, where new cells are continually produced. Both squamous cells and basal cells can become cancerous; most skin cancers, 70 to 80 percent, arise in basal cells.

Melanocytes are cells that produce skin pigment, or melanin. These cells can also become cancerous.

The skin on your eyelids is only 0.05 millimeters (mm) thick; on your palms and the soles of your feet, it's 1.5 mm thick.

✔ **Dermis:** The middle layer, the dermis, is the thickest, making up about 90 percent of your skin. The main role of the dermis is to regulate temperature and supply the epidermis with nutrient-rich blood. The dermis contains nerve fibers, fat cells, blood vessels, sweat and oil glands, and hair follicles. Sweat glands keep you from becoming overheated and help keep you at a constant 98.6 degrees (although everyone's internal temperature is a little different). The dermis also contains *collagen* and *elastin,* two proteins responsible for the structure and elasticity of the skin.

- **Collagen:** Between 75 and 80 percent of your skin is made up of collagen, a protein manufactured in the dermis by cells called fibroblasts. Collagen is one of the strongest proteins in your body, and it gives skin its strength and durability.

- **Elastin:** Another protein manufactured in the dermis, elastin gives skin its elasticity, allowing it to stretch out and then bounce back in shape.

- **Subcutaneous:** This layer is composed primarily of subcutaneous fat and connective tissue. A certain number of fat cells are essential; they provide energy, serve as heat insulators for the body, and act as a shock absorber to protect underlying tissue and organs from injury. However, too much subcutaneous fat, or adipose fat, makes you — well, fat! Sweat glands originate in this layer and excrete waste matter through perspiration.

Although normal skin cells rejuvenate constantly, you can't actually grow new skin over a large cut or injury like you can grow new bone when you break one (refer to Chapter 7 for more info on bone growth). A large cut or skin injury is covered with scar tissue instead of normal skin. Scar tissue, made up mostly of fibrous tissue, grows in an area where the underlying layers of the skin have been damaged or destroyed and can no longer perform their normal functions. Your body compensates by creating new tissue, which, while strong and durable, doesn't contain the blood vessels, glands, hair follicles, or nerve endings of the original skin.

How skin ages

Your skin is as subject to aging as any other organ in your body. If you've put extra stress on your skin — by spending too much time in the sun, smoking, yo-yo dieting, or eating poorly — the natural effects of aging are magnified.

When you're young, your skin's turnover rate is about every 15 to 18 days, which is why you have that youthful glow — a new layer of cells appears every few weeks. When you start approaching your mid-30s, the cell turnover process slows down to about every month. By age 70, the cell regeneration rate can be as long as several months.

Skin is damaged in two ways — by intrinsic factors and by extrinsic factors. *Intrinsic* factors are directly related to aging; an example is a slowdown in cell regeneration. *Extrinsic* factors are outside factors, like sun and pollutant exposure. According to the National Institute of Health, 90 percent of visible skin damage is from ultra-violet sources. That means that a great deal of the damage done to your skin may be preventable, or at least modifiable. The younger you start, the better!

Looking at intrinsic (age-related) aging factors

Because everyone inherits different genetic characteristics, keeping skin lovely as you age is, in part, a matter of inheriting good genes. For most people, though, the same intrinsic changes occur over the years. All these changes working together add up to wrinkles, fine lines, sagging skin, dry skin, flaky skin, and easily damaged skin. Here's what happens:

- ✔ The epidermis layer of the skin becomes thinner.

- ✔ Cell turnover slows.

- ✔ Collagen begins to break down, the subcutaneous layer thins, and the skin's elastin is less able to "spring back" (think of an overstretched rubber band). The results are wrinkles and saggy, baggy skin.

- ✔ Oil production from the sebaceous glands decreases.

- ✔ Melanin production slows, increasing your susceptibility to sun damage and also causing you to appear paler.

✔ Pores enlarge and become clogged.

✔ Capillaries and broken blood vessels become more visible, as well as more frequent, due to the fragility of the blood vessels as you age.

Intrinsic effects don't occur in a vacuum; they're affected for better or worse throughout your life by extrinsic effects. The skin damage you see as you age isn't a result of just one factor, but a number of factors working together to produce the results you'd rather not see in the mirror.

Examining extrinsic aging factors

You can't control what type of skin you inherit, but you can control the damage you inflict on your skin yourself. Extrinsic factors are factors not related to normal aging or genetics; effects from sun, smoking, and pollution are all examples of extrinsic damage. The extrinsic factor that causes the most skin damage over the years is — you guessed it — sun exposure. But any or all of these factors contribute to premature aging of your skin:

✔ Ultraviolet (UV) rays from the sun damage the DNA in epidermal cells, often resulting in mutations that can cause cancer.

✔ UV radiation accelerates the breakdown of collagen in the dermis.

✔ UV radiation increases the accumulation of abnormal elastin, which leads to increased wrinkling.

✔ Cigarette smoke constricts blood vessels in the skin and reduces the amount of oxygen and nutrients that reach facial tissues, resulting in increased wrinkling and loss of elasticity.

Fleeing the Free Radicals: Recognizing and Preventing Extrinsic Skin Damage

Free radicals are a hot topic these days, and although they sound like an alternative rock group, free radicals are actually a complicated molecular phenomenon. Free radicals are the result of unpaired electrons; electrons don't like to be alone, so they look to correct this imbalance. Free radicals try to take an electron from some other cell to pair up with, leaving the donor cell missing part of its structure.

The effect of free radical molecules on skin — taking electrons from healthy cells and leaving the donor cell dysfunctional in the process — creates visible damage (think wrinkles, thinning skin, and diminished muscles) and advances the aging process. The sun, pollution, smoking, alcohol, poor nutrition, and harsh skin products can all damage the skin at the cellular level by increasing free radical formation.

We start with the most damaging skin toxin — the sun's powerful damaging rays — and then we look at a few of the other free-radical-forming skin irritants, the way they damage the skin, and some ways that you may be able to protect against them.

Unfortunately, extrinsic factors can't be avoided entirely, and intrinsic factors can't be avoided at all. Both, however, can be modified or reduced. In the next sections, we describe the most common causes of skin damage and what you can do to minimize their effects.

The scorching sun: Putting a block between you and the rays

The number one cause of wrinkles is sun damage — not old age. No matter what your age, lifestyle, or geographic location, your skin is exposed to the sun's ultraviolet rays (UVA and UVB radiation), which can cause irreversible damage to your skin by decreasing its ability to *synthesize* (manufacture) collagen and elastin. Sun damage can result from long-term or cumulative exposure over the years, or it can show up years after severe sunburn. Sun damage can cause the following:

- ✔ Worsening wrinkles

- ✔ Tough, leathery, wrinkled, blotchy skin

- ✔ Precancerous growths called actinic keratoses, which are dark, flaky, hardened areas of skin

- ✔ Basal or squamous cell carcinoma (in layman's terms, skin cancer)

- ✔ Melanoma, a form of skin cancer that can show up years after severe sunburn

Sun exposure is one of the easiest skin damages to avoid, if you're willing to take a few extra minutes every day to slather on some sunscreen. This may seem foreign to you if you spent the first 20 years of your life slathering on baby oil to perfect your tan! But, as people become more conscious of protecting their skin from sun damage, you see a shift from the deep tan look to the smooth, creamy skin look. Some of the new sunscreen products are spray-on lotions that are easier to apply and reduce missed spots. A couple of minutes is all you need to get a thorough application — and the result can be life saving.

UV rays aren't all equal; different types have different effects. To oversimplify a bit, UVA rays = aging changes; UVB rays = sunburn. Sun Protection Factor (or SPF; see the nearby sidebar "Conundrum! Choosing a sunscreen" for more info) measures your degree of protection only against the sun's burning *UVB* rays. So, what about the most harmful *UVA* rays? Good question. If your sunscreen provides only UVB protection and you stay in the sun for three and a half hours, you expose your unprotected skin to the most damaging of the sun's rays and don't even feel it. After all, UVA rays don't burn you. They do, however, damage your skin.

UVA rays aren't blocked by glass, like UVB rays are, so you can acquire skin damage by riding in the car or sitting in a bright sunny window. Having your windows tinted with a UVA blocking tint can prevent this damage; consider having your windows tinted especially if you have very sensitive skin or live in an area where the sun rays are stronger. Check out Table 5-1 for additional comparisons of UVA and UVB rays.

Table 5-1	Comparing UVA and UVB Rays	
Factor	*UVA Rays*	*UVB Rays*
Wavelength	320–400 nanometers	290–320 nanometers
Skin effects	Skin aging and damage	Sunburning
Cancer risks	Melanoma	High (basal cell, squamous cell, and melanoma)
Prevalence	All day, year-round	10 a.m. to 3 p.m.; mostly in the summer months

 Protecting your skin from damaging UV radiation is possible; we recommend the following tactics to keep the sun's damage to a minimum:

- Make sure that your sunscreen is effective against both UVA and UVB rays.

- Apply a liberal amount of a double-duty sunscreen with SPF 15 daily; low dose daily sunscreen is more effective in preventing damage than occasional use of a higher SPF.

- Look for makeup that has sunscreen in it so that when you put on your face, you also apply your daily dose of sunscreen on your most delicate area.

- Completely cover your skin with a thin layer of sunscreen; most people don't put enough on.

- Don't wait until the last minute; sunscreen takes 20 to 30 minutes to soak into the skin to be effective, so don't just slap your sunscreen on right before you head out the door.

- If you use topical retinoid products on your skin for exfoliation or any other reason, you're more likely to have sun damage, due to the loss of some of your body's first layer of defense. Use a higher SPF and apply diligently.

- If you're going to have continual sun exposure, reapply sunscreen 30 minutes after exposure begins and then every 2 to 3 hours, and after activities that may wash away the coverage (swimming and sweating).

- Don't be afraid to wear a hat. Many hats are very effective at blocking sun from the head and face.

 If bugs bother you and you use sunscreen and insect repellent together, use a higher SPF sunscreen. Insect repellent decreases the effectiveness of sunscreen by one third.

Conundrum! Choosing a sunscreen

As you look at the array of sunscreens available, you may be unsure of whether to buy one with a 15, 30, or even 50 Sun Protection Factor (SPF). According to the Federal Drug Administration, a product's SPF number tells you how long you can stay in the sun before getting burned. An SPF 15 product lets you stay in the sun 15 times longer than you would normally be able to without getting burned. If you normally stay in the sun for 15 minutes before you start turning pink, use an SPF 15 to get 225 minutes (15 × 15), or approximately 3 and a half hours of sun exposure before you start burning. If you begin turning pink after 10 minutes, an SPF 15 lets you stay in the sun approximately 2 and a half hours, or 10 minutes times 15.

In addition to telling you how much longer you can stay outside, the following SPFs block a certain percentage of the sun's UVB rays:

- SPF 2 blocks about 50 percent of UVB rays
- SPF 10 blocks about 85 percent of UVB rays
- SPF 15 blocks about 95 percent of UVB rays
- SPF 30 blocks about 97 percent of UVB rays

Note: An SPF over 30 doesn't increase the amount of blockage; it just increases the length of time you can stay in the sun without burning

Consider the UV index (strength of the sun's ultraviolet rays), skin type, how frequently you're reapplying, and whether you're in water when choosing a proper SPF. All these factors may make a higher SPF more appropriate for you. Visit www.webMD.com and www.americancancersociety.com for information on choosing and applying sunscreens.

Sunscreen ingredients (17 are approved for use in sunscreen) fall into one of two categories: absorbers and blockers, also called reflectors. Absorbing ingredients absorb UV rays before they can penetrate your skin, and blockers are physical barriers to absorption. Octyl methoxycinnamate (OMC) or oxybenzone are examples of chemicals in sunscreens that absorb UV rays. Zinc, a thick white paste, is an example of a blocker — remember seeing pictures of people with white noses at the beach?

Your sunscreen should contain both blockers and absorbers, and should include ingredients that block UVA rays as well as UVB.

For UVA protection, your sunscreen label should list one of the following active ingredients:

- Zinc oxide, a blocker

- Titanium dioxide, a blocker

- Avobenzone or butyl methoxydibenzoylmethane (Parsol 1789, Eusolex 9020, Escalol 517, and others), which block both UVA and UVB

- Ecamsule (Mexoryl), which absorbs UVA rays

 We highly recommend applying and reapplying sunscreen, but we know that it isn't always easy or convenient. Take these additional preventative measures to protect your skin against the damaging effects of the sun's radiation:

- Remember that sun exposure is more intense at higher altitudes and close to the equator; in both cases the sun's rays have to travel less distance through the atmosphere. For every 1,000 feet you rise in altitude, your sun exposure increases 2 percent. Grass, sand, snow, ice, and water all

Scary skin stats

Skin cancer is the most common form of cancer in the United States. Does that surprise you? Here's even more startling news:

- ✔ Globally between 2 and 3 million non-melanoma skin cancers and 132,000 melanoma skin cancers occur each year.

- ✔ According to the American Cancer Society, about 7,800 adults in the U.S. die of skin cancer each year.

- ✔ Melanoma, the most serious form of skin cancer, can spread to other parts of the body quickly.

- ✔ Melanoma is the leading cause of cancer death among women ages 25 to 29.

- ✔ Melanoma is second only to lung cancer as the leading cause of cancer in women ages 30 to 34.

The good news, though, is that you can largely prevent skin cancer by practicing consistent skincare protection from UV ray exposure (see the nearby section "The scorching sun: Putting a block between you and the rays" for more on this topic).

increase sun exposure as well, as much as 20 to 30 percent in the case of sand.

- ✔ Avoid sun exposure between 10 a.m. and 3 p.m.

- ✔ Wear protective clothing and a wide-brimmed hat when you're outside (UVA rays are present even on cloudy days).

Toxic smoke (that is, all smoke): Snuffing out its effects

Smoking damages skin by releasing free radicals and also by the repetitive muscle contractions that accompany each puff. Secondhand smoke can be a culprit, too, because it stirs up free radicals. Free radicals initiated by smoking reduce the delivery of needed oxygen and nutrients by their effects on the blood vessels. The smoke also increases certain proteins that break down collagen. Collagen is already decreasing with age, so speeding up this process isn't doing your skin any favors.

Cellular damage from free radicals isn't the only problem you can pin on smoke. It also leaves a nasty residue on the surface of your skin, much like the stains on a smoker's fingertips or the grime on the walls of a smoky bar. You've likely seen the classic "smoker's face," identified by the number of wrinkles all around the mouth from drawing in on a cigarette, and lines around the eyes from squinting through smoke irritation.

Obviously the way to prevent or reverse the skin damage that smoking causes is to stop smoking. If you quit smoking, but wrinkles and skin damage from past smoking have already occurred, the following tips help reduce already present wrinkles:

- Exercise to increase oxygen to the skin thereby increasing blood flow.

- Drink plenty of water to improve skin integrity (smoking can dehydrate the skin).

- Take extra vitamin A and vitamin C to help overcome previous damage. These vitamins help protect the skin, but they aren't well absorbed in smokers.

Aggressive skin treatments, such as chemical peels and laser resurfacing, can be costly and often are only temporary. Botox can help paralyze the muscles that cause the wrinkling around the mouth and eyes, and cosmetic fillers can fill the fine crevices in the skin for a better cosmetic appearance.

Other ways to fight for your skin

If you don't smoke, and if you do protect your skin from the sun, you're off to a great start at protecting your skin. Unfortunately, a few other elements can have damaging effects to the skin. These problems aren't hard to avoid if you remember a few important points:

- **Fight free radicals with good nutrition.** A good diet, high in antioxidants, can help fight damage from free radicals. Antioxidants can bind with free radicals to stop their damaging effects.

  Foods high in antioxidants aren't difficult to find; food high in beta carotene, selenium, vitamins C and E, and zinc all fall into the category of antioxidants. (We talk in detail about nutrition and the benefits of antioxidants in Chapter 7, but a diet high in green and yellow vegetables, fruits, fish oils, eggs, legumes, and whole grains will help you fight off the free radicals.)

- **Modify your alcohol intake.** Light alcohol intake has some beneficial aspects, particularly in regard to cholesterol levels and the heart. The problem is that drinking too much alcohol puts your entire detox system into overdrive because the liver and kidneys have to filter out a huge amount of additional toxins, and so does your skin (remember, that's one of its jobs). Alcohol also depletes your body of nutrients for healthy hair and skin and accelerates the aging process in your skin (as well as other organs). Specifically, it depletes your body of vitamin A, a very important antioxidant. Drinking alcohol in excess also leads to a nutrition deficiency of vitamin B complex, a vital group of nutrients that can fight against skin damage, as well as diarrhea and depression.

To minimize the damage from alcohol, limit the amount of alcoholic drinks to no more than one to two per day for men and no more than one per day for women.

✔ **Decrease your pollution exposure.** Pollution is so prevalent that you can't completely avoid it; car exhaust, chemically infested water, and toxic air have you covered. It's in your hair, on your skin, in your nose, under your nails, and between your toes. You ingest it when you eat your food and drink your water (even bottled!). Pollution doesn't allow your skin to breathe and function properly, so it promotes and accelerates the aging process.

To combat the effects of pollution, we recommend that you stick to a daily cleansing routine to get rid of as much toxic buildup as possible (see the later section "Aging Beautifully: A How-To Guide for Interested Folks" for specifics) and be sure to eat foods rich in antioxidants and keep your body hydrated.

✔ **Avoid harsh weather conditions and other things that strip moisture from your skin; on the contrary, make sure you stay well hydrated.** Dry skin is a nearly universal problem, but certain factors make you more likely to develop tightness, flakiness, and fine lines. These factors include

- **Your age:** Skin tends to become drier as you age because your oil-producing glands become less active. The lack of oil also causes cells to clump together in flakes or scales. At the same time, the skin-cell regeneration process slows down, and the skin's ability to hold on to moisture diminishes. Your complexion can appear rough and dull.
- **Your gender:** Everyone's skin changes with age. Women usually experience an increase in dry skin during and after menopause. Men have minimal changes in the moisture of their skin as they age, unless of course they have other damaging risk factors such as smoking.

Extreme weather conditions like temperature and moisture level extremes, biting wind, and stinging cold all wreak havoc on your skin. In the winter, your skin may become dry, red, and flaky. In the summer, it may be sweaty, burned, and oily. Even though your skin is designed to handle just about anything you throw its way, it still needs time to adjust to these changes. The increased cold or dryness actually affects your skin most when it first occurs; after a few months, your skin has adjusted to the change.

You can control some things. The following activities affect your skin:

- Central air and heating, wood-burning stoves, space heaters, and fireplaces all reduce humidity and dry your skin in the winter months. (And if you live in an older home that has radiator heating, your cells are even more parched.)
- Frequent showering or bathing, especially if you like hot water and long baths, can break down

the lipid barriers in your skin.

- Frequent swimming, particularly in heavily chlorinated pools can have the same effect.
- If you're subject to dry skin, limit activities that involve submersion of your skin in water for long periods of time. Some people with severe dry skin may need to consider taking only showers — and not every day. You may be able to enjoy the water if you can find a good moisturizer.

If you have dry skin, dry off quickly after getting out of the water, and quickly apply a moisturizing lotion. This combination often manages dry skin and can give you more freedom to partake in a nice warm bath from time to time.

Because you can't change the weather, you should provide your skin with some protection from the harsh effects and subsequent reactions. Prepare and protect your skin from moisture loss by using moisturizers, covering your face in harsh wind and cold, and shielding your face with a hat in excessively dry climates.

Recognizing and Managing Skin-Damaging Diseases

Many diseases are directly reflected in your skin. Some diseases primarily target the skin, like rosacea; others (like systemic lupus erythematosus, or SLE) are *systemic* (affecting your whole body) diseases that can target several organs, but often have the presence of skin manifestations.

Many of the following conditions are quite common; psoriasis alone is estimated to affect 125 million people worldwide. We start with the conditions that predominantly affect the skin first and finish with the ones that are systemic:

194

- **Eczema:** Eczema is dry skin; the problem with dry skin is that it becomes more susceptible to bacterial, fungal, and viral infections that cause the manifestations called "eczema." Moisturizers, gentle cleaners, and topical steroids for flare-ups can help control eczema, which can be found on any part of the skin.

- **Rosacea:** Rosacea is a skin disease characterized by enlarged blood vessels resulting in red, bumpy, blotchy skin. The cause is unknown, but the effects are quite visible. Found initially on the face, rosacea may be dismissed as merely adult "pimples" when it first appears. In addition to affecting the skin, rosacea can cause your eyes to become dry, red, and irritated. Antibiotic creams can help keep rosacea under control. Using sunscreen regularly and keeping a list of what seems to trigger flare-ups can also help.

- **Psoriasis:** This autoimmune disease is marked by a rapid buildup of rough, dry, dead skin cells that form thick scales. Skin cells in psoriasis are replaced every few days rather than every few weeks, resulting in patches called plaques. Cold, dry weather, stress, skin abrasions, and injuries can cause flare-ups.

  This is another disease that affects the skin but can affect other body systems as well. Psoriatic arthritis (joint inflammation) affects between 10 and 30 percent of psoriasis cases. The treatment for mild cases includes using a topical salicylic acid (aspirin), vitamin D_3, or steroid cream. Severe cases, whether they affect skin only or a combination of skin and joint involvement, may need systemic medications such as steroids, methotrexate, remicade, and enbrel. Another option for severe skin disease is using a

UVB light source regularly for a set time. You can purchase home units that provide excellent results. Some of the medications for psoriasis are very strong and can have serious side effects, so discuss treatment options with your doctor.

✔ **SLE:** SLE is a systemic disease that affects nearly every organ in the body, including your skin. SLE may first come to your attention because of the characteristic "lupus rash," which goes across the cheeks (the wings) and bridge of the nose (the body), resembling a butterfly. SLE may require systemic treatment with steroids to decrease flare-ups — if you think you may have it, consult your doctor for evaluation and you may be referred to a rheumatologist or dermatologist for further care.

✔ **Hypothyroidism:** This condition occurs when your thyroid produces too little thyroid hormones. It reduces the activity of your sweat and oil glands, leading to swollen, dry, waxy skin. Some people may have a yellowish color to the skin due to poor vitamin A absorption and can often suffer from hair loss. This condition can be diagnosed with blood tests, but may need further evaluation of the thyroid gland itself if the gland is enlarged. Thyroid disease can be treated with thyroid hormone replacement and is easy to control with proper monitoring. Your primary care doctor or an endocrinologist will direct your management.

Inspecting Your Skin for Cancer

 In addition to prevention, assess your skin monthly for strange looking spots or textures. Once a month, check your whole body. Don't limit this check to the obvious places that you can easily see — you also need to check places like your back, scalp, and the bottoms of your feet. Ask a loved one to help you, or use a hand mirror to check the places yourself. Women often find melanoma on their legs, an area that many people don't think to check. Men frequently find melanoma on the trunk of the body. But melanoma can strike anywhere, so make sure that you do a thorough check.

Closely examine your moles during these monthly checks. Your moles are good indicators of change and can be early warning signs of skin cancer. Use the *ABCDE* rule to evaluate moles; look for the following signs:

- ✔ **A for asymmetry:** A mole that doesn't look the same on the left and right or on the top and bottom

- ✔ **B for border:** A mole with edges or a border that's blurry or jagged

- ✔ **C for color:** A mole that darkens or loses color, or whose color spreads or otherwise changes. Look for the appearance of multiple colors like blue, red, white, pink, purple, or gray

- ✔ **D for diameter:** A mole larger than 1/4 inch in diameter (about the size of a pencil eraser)

- ✔ **E for elevation:** A mole that's raised above the skin and has a rough surface

In addition the *ABCDE* test, watch for the following changes in moles:

- ✔ A mole that bleeds

- ✔ A mole that grows quickly with notable changes within a few weeks to 6 months

197

    A mole that itches

Moles aren't the only type of lesion that can be cancerous; just watching your moles may mean missing another type of skin cancer. Basal cell and squamous cell cancers don't grow as quickly as melanomas, so you may not notice their growth unless you're doing a systematic monthly skin check. Look for the following:

    A scaly or crusted growth on the skin that isn't the result of your latest rollerblading stunt

    A sore that doesn't heal

    A place on your skin that feels rough, like sandpaper

Tell your doctor immediately if you experience any of the changes in this section or find that a lesion fits any of the descriptors in the ABCDE. Early diagnosis and treatment of cancer is extremely important.

Aging Beautifully: A How-To Guide for Interested Folks

Although preventing skin damage is extremely important as you age, you may be interested in going a step further — not only preventing damage but also pampering your skin. Aren't you worth it? Sure you are! Men, don't think that this section doesn't apply to you; great looking skin is for everyone!

Maintaining a healthy cleansing regimen

Skin-care people tend to fall into a few different categories — the "buy every product on the market" group, the "I never touch the stuff" group, and the vast majority group — the group that buys products and forgets to use them. Certainly, you can find an incredible number of promising skin-care products — maybe too many, if you unknowingly use everything you can to clog your pores, age your face, and eventually require a putty knife and a bottle of vodka to remove it all. But the best place to start good skin care is with a regular, complete cleansing routine.

Wash your face twice a day; once in the morning and again at night before bed. When you do, follow these steps:

1. **Cleanse your skin.**

   Choose a gentle cleanser that leaves your skin feeling clean, not tight and dry. It should be close to your skin's pH, which is slightly acidic, around 4.5 to 5.5, with some alpha and beta hydroxies to open pores, dissolve oil, and slough off some dead skin.

   Facial cleanser doesn't have to be expensive to be good and effective, so keep it simple. This is one area where you can skip the high price name brands for a cheaper brand. It isn't on your skin long; save your money for your moisturizer. Skip the fancy fragrance, harsh detergents (they can irritate your skin), and soap — especially the same soap you use on the rest of your body. Soap can dry your skin, and can irritate it if too alkaline; most bar soaps have a pH around 9 (a pH of 7 is neutral; a lower number is acidic, a higher number alkaline).

   Don't go to bed with makeup on your face. That residue clogs your pores and doesn't allow dead skin cells to be shed. In addition, your skin can't regulate its temperature, breathe properly, or release toxins.

2. Use a toner to remove excess dirt and oil.

Do you really need a toner? It depends on who you ask (even beauty experts don't always agree), what type of skin you have, and the type of toner you choose. Even a good cleanser doesn't remove all the dirt and oil from your skin, so a toner wipes up what a cleanser leaves behind. Toner also tightens pores, hydrates your skin, restores proper pH, and increases circulation. However, toners that contain alcohol can dry skin excessively.

Choose a non-alcohol based astringent (alcohol can irritate your skin). Most toners indicate whether they're for oily, dry, or even acne-prone skin; read labels before buying the product nearest you on the shelf! Toners, like cleansers, don't need to be expensive. The ingredients in toners are inexpensive, so you may be paying a high price for a pretty label or a brand name.

3. Exfoliate to stimulate cell turnover.

To *exfoliate* doesn't mean to rub your face with stones or wire brushes until the skin's raw. It simply means to remove *dead* skin cells, and many dermatologists believe that it would be hard to over-exfoliate. Exfoliating that outer layer helps nutrients in the topical products you apply (serums and moisturizers) to get down to the live skin cells. This step also opens up clogged pores, keeping under-the-skin bumps and blackheads from becoming a nuisance. Exfoliating needs to be done only a few times a week.

A quality exfoliating product is essential. Unfortunately, the labels and claims for exfoliating products can be a bit confusing, with many products over-promising and under-delivering. See the

"Distinguishing between promising products and bogus beauty claims" sidebar later in this chapter for guidance.

Choose an exfoliant for *faces only* if you're exfoliating your face. Select other exfoliating products for other parts of your body that get rough and dry (feet, hands, and elbows). Follow these guidelines:

- A good daily facial exfoliant has an 8- to 10-percent-strength glycolic acid pad to slough off dead skin cells. (Any weaker strength can't achieve exfoliating results.)
- Using Alpha Hydroxy Acid (AHA) and Beta Hydroxy Acid (BHA) facial peels a couple times a week is a fantastic way to exfoliate without overdoing it. But unless you have free access to an *esthetician* (a qualified skin care specialist), you may be spending more on your face than you bargained for.
- Weekly *microdermabrasion* (an exfoliation treatment where the skin is "sandblasted" to remove dead skin cells) scrubs with very fine granules are magnificent but pricey. Over-the-counter microdermabrasion creams are good once a week to polish your face.

The best judge of whether the product is working or not is your own reflection in the mirror. Is your skin softer, less blotchy, free of acne? Sounds like you've found the right combination of skin-care products! Want to make sure you keep getting good results? Write down products that really work well for you so that you remember them the next time you're at the store.

4. **Moisturize to keep your skin supple.**
   Your skin is coated with *sebum,* a natural
   moisturizing oil that you shower away with harsh
   soaps and expose to environmental assaults. Sebum
   also rubs off on your clothes and wipes off when you
   sweat. So whether you live in Arizona, Idaho, or near
   the Tropic of Cancer; whether you have oily skin, dry
   skin, or a combination; whether you're a man or
   woman; you still need a moisturizer to

   - Help replenish your skin with the vital nutrients
     and hydration it needs to stay healthy
   - Replace oils and nutrients you strip away during
     cleansing
   - Help minimize the appearance of fine lines

   Invest in a quality product. Just make sure that
   you're paying for the quality and not just the label.
   Look for these ingredients:

   - *Oil-free* for oily skin and *cream* for normal to dry
     skin
   - An SPF of 30 (If you don't want a product that
     includes an SPF, be sure that you also apply a
     broad spectrum sunscreen; see the earlier
     section, "The scorching sun: Putting a block
     between you and the rays," for more on SPF.)

   Skip the mineral oil because it can clog pores and
   trap perspiration. It doesn't get absorbed into the
   skin because the molecules it contains are too big.
   Apply moisturizer twice a day after cleaning,
   toning, or exfoliating.

Keeping your skin well hydrated

Keeping the skin moist from the inside out is important regardless of your age or gender, because dry skin looks flaky and dull and feels itchy. The stores contain a plethora of moisturizing creams, liquids, and lotions. Don't forget that you have skin that could use moisturizing in places besides your face! Moisturize your legs and other potentially dry areas, like elbows and knees. Moisturizing products come in several types:

- ✔ **Oil-based creams:** These creams retain moisture and serve as a barrier by blocking the release of water from the skin. As you age, oil-based creams aren't very effective because your skin loses its ability to attract moisture in the first place. Oil-based creams can retain moisture only if your skin has moisture to begin with. Oil-based creams may work for some dry skin.

- ✔ **Water-based lotions:** A good remedy for aging skin is a natural moisturizer that attracts and retains water. Water-based lotions are also a good choice if you have oily skin.

- ✔ **Gels:** More solid than creams, gels are good for oily faces.

Toning muscles for a face-lifting effect

Remember Mom telling you that if you made funny faces, your face would freeze that way? Actually, the opposite may be true; not working your facial muscles and exercising them regularly can result in wrinkles, lines, and furrows that can become permanent.

Exercise is good for you — *all* of you! Exercising the muscles in your face and neck can help keep the skin firm and relax muscles you may tense without even realizing it. The good thing about face and neck exercises is that you can do

Essentials to look for in skin-care products

The number of skin-care ingredients on the market are virtually as limitless as a chemist's imagination. But you don't have to be a chemist to figure out what to use on your face; this list includes the most essential skin-care ingredients, many of which can limit or reverse the effects of aging or damage to skin:

- **Alpha Hydroxy Acid (AHA):** This ingredient has been around since the 1980s as a chemical peel to exfoliate dead skin cells and give a noticeable improvement to the skin's appearance. Benefits include the disappearance of fine lines and wrinkles, and a fresher looking skin tone. Hydroxies also act as a stimulator of collagen production and cell growth.

    The percentage of AHA concentration depends on where you get it and who applies it. You can apply over-the-counter AHAs, which have glycolic acid in a solution up to 10 percent. An esthetician or licensed cosmetologist can use up to 30 percent AHA; these facial peels are similar to microdermabrasion, and erase fine lines and smooth the skin's texture. Finally, a dermatologist can use a 50- to 70-percent AHA solution; after you get past the pain, redness, and oozing for up to four weeks, your results can last two to five years.

- **Beta Hydroxy Acid (BHA):** This ingredient, commonly known as *salicylic acid,* is also an exfoliant. It's oil-based, while AHA is water-based. As a result, BHAs are better at penetrating and unclogging pores where those nasty little blackheads and whiteheads get stuck. Most products geared toward oily or acne-prone skin contain this product.

- **Alpha-Lipoic Acid:** This acid is an antioxidant with many skin-rejuvenating benefits, including an inhibiting effect on wrinkles. Lipoic acid also has moderate anti-inflammatory benefits (thus reducing inflammation that can cause red, blotchy skin) and is capable of removing several toxic metals from the body.

- ✔ **Dimethylaminoethanol (DMAE):** One of the major skin problems of advanced aging is loss of elasticity due to the tissue destruction of collagen and elastin. DMAE is a topical agent that functions as a cell-membrane stabilizer to produce a firming effect on the skin.

- ✔ **Vitamin A (tretinoin):** This vitamin switches on receptors that tell the skin to grow new cells, synthesize elastin and collagen, and produce sebum. Indirectly, it stops the enzyme that breaks down collagen and elastin. As your skin ages, this breakdown process speeds up.

  Research confirms that tretinoin reduces fine wrinkles and skin roughness, increases middle-layer skin thickness, and stimulates collagen production. Retin-A, developed to treat acne, is the most recognizable form of tretinoin. It's available by prescription only.

- ✔ **Vitamin C:** This is one of the most widely used ingredients in skin-care products for wrinkle reduction and skin rejuvenation. Vitamin C is also essential for collagen synthesis, and it contains antioxidant properties that help fight free-radical damage. Vitamin C undergoes oxidation when exposed to air and can lose its effectiveness. New derivatives of vitamin C that are more stable and less likely to break down upon exposure to air are being developed. Look for a colorless product with a 10-percent concentration of vitamin C.

Distinguishing between promising products and bogus beauty claims

You've seen all the brightly colored bottles and packages of skin-care products, watched infomercials with celebrities, and seen the ads with models who have ravishing bodies and pristine skin — all flaunting the latest breakthroughs in skin-care technology. Everything looks so promising, so you keep pulling out your wallet faster than they can take your money. You try the products again and again — but the results are disappointing. Another $120 for 1 ounce of snake oil down the toilet.

So are any of these products for real? How can those companies make those claims if they aren't true? Both valid questions. The short answer to the first one is, "Yes, many products are real and do provide real benefits to your skin." The short answer to the second question has to do with regulations in the cosmetics industry.

Just like labels on food, household cleaners, and clothing, you need to read the labels on skin-care products. The labels list ingredients by their chemical or scientific name from highest to lowest content. (Most people aren't familiar with these chemicals, so a copy of a paperback cosmetic-ingredients dictionary is nice to have. Never heard of such a book? Type the words "cosmetic ingredients dictionary" into the search engine at Amazon.com or BarnesandNoble.com and choose from any one of a dozen options.)

Here's the tricky part. Say you want to buy a face-firming cream with DMAE because you've heard that it's great for firming skin. Great choice! The department store has two choices — both with DMAE and both promising to firm your skin — but one is twice as expensive. Which one do you buy? Of course, the one that contains the highest, safest, and most effective amount of the active ingredient DMAE. But the label doesn't tell you that (and the clerk probably doesn't know!).

The law (Food, Drug and Cosmetic Act) only requires the ingredient to be in the product. Manufacturers don't have to disclose how much or at what percentage. So both products can *claim* to have the same benefits even if one product has only a *dusting* (just a pinch) of DMAE and can't begin to deliver on the promise. And yes, it still costs a premium.

In order to be a smart and knowledgeable consumer, your best bet is to

✔ Understand the most familiar terms in skin-care products.

✔ Check out some of the manufacturers and their products as well as smaller companies and doctor brands that disclose this kind of information on their labels.

Note: Not all companies are bad or out to get you. Many great products are available from several companies. But if you rely solely on fancy boxes and marketing promises for your educational research, you'll likely *not* get what you paid for.

them anytime and anywhere — in the car, right before you go to sleep, or to scare off strangers on the street!

Neck and throat

If you want to firm up or avoid saggy skin, double chins, and loose skin on your neck, these quick exercises can help:

1. **Sit up straight, tilt your head back to look at the ceiling, and keep your lips closed.**

2. **Start a chewing movement.**
   Repeat 20 times.

3. **Gently turn your head to the right for 20 big**

chews, and then turn to the left for 20 big
chews.

4. **Look at the ceiling, and pucker up.**
That's right — try to kiss the ceiling. Stretch and
hold your kiss for ten counts and then relax.
Repeat this step five times. You should really feel
the stretch in your neck and under your chin.

5. **Sit in your chair, look up at the ceiling, tilt your
head back, and open your lips.**

6. **Stick out your tongue and try to touch your
chin; try to keep your tongue in this position for
ten counts.**

7. **Relax and tuck your tongue back in your mouth
where it belongs.**
Repeat Steps 5 to 7 ten times.

Lips and cheeks

Do these exercise steps to help erase lip lines and to prevent
saggy cheeks:

1. **Sit comfortably, close your lips, and keep your
teeth together.**

2. **Smile as wide as you can without opening your
lips.**
Hold for five seconds.

3. **Move immediately into a big puckered kiss;
hold it for a count of five, and then relax.**
Repeat Steps 2 and 3 ten times.

4. **Relax your smile with your lips closed.**

5. **Suck your cheeks in toward and onto your
teeth.**

Hold this pose for ten counts, and then relax.
Repeat Steps 4 and 5 ten times.

Eyes and forehead

To decrease frown lines and forehead furrows, and to keep eye crinkle lines at bay, try these steps:

1. **Sit up and look straight ahead with your eyes open.**

2. **Look up, and then look down, moving just your eyes.**
   Repeat ten times.

3. **Look left, and then look right, moving just your eyes.**
   Repeat ten times.

4. **Make a really big frown.**
   Try to bring your eyebrows over your eyes while pulling your eyebrows toward one another.

5. **Lift your eyebrows as far as possible while opening your eyes as far as possible.**
   Repeat Steps 4 and 5 five times.

Chapter 6

Building Bones and Preserving Joints

. . . .

In This Chapter

▶ Understanding bone matters
▶ Staying ahead of bone problems
▶ Taking the ache out of aging bones
▶ Managing joint and arthritis pain
▶ Working out your back kinks

. . . .

Bone and joint problems, such as arthritis, bum knees, bad hips, back problems, and brittle bones, used to be philosophically accepted as the price to be paid for getting older. But today you can find better-than-ever ways to treat and even prevent some of the problems that result from a lifetime of wear and tear. In this chapter, we give you a primer on bone growth and aging. We also explain the best ways to preserve your mainframe by slowing the aging process, and we offer suggestions for dealing with bone and joint damage that can occur after a lifetime of hard use.

Examining Your Bones' Biggest Role

If you were asked to associate one word with the word bone, you may choose "calcium." Your bones contain 99 percent of the calcium in your body, and you have more of this mineral in your body than any other. Calcium together with phosphorus is responsible for the strength of your bones and teeth. Calcium and phosphorus keep your bones strong; their levels are kept in a constant balance in your body. As blood calcium levels increase, phosphorus levels decrease. Maintaining constant concentrations of calcium and phosphorus in blood requires your body to make frequent adjustments. Your body relies on a system of checks and balances, described in the following sections.

Vitally important vitamins and minerals

Almost all of the body's calcium is stored in the bones (99 percent). Getting enough calcium in the diet is essential starting at a young age because the body needs that to help prevent bone loss in the future. Next to calcium, phosphorus is the most abundant mineral in the body. The problem is that some minerals need help to maintain a healthy balance in the body and be available for important functions. Calcium and phosphorus are like stranded hitchhikers without Vitamin D to help transport them to the bones from the intestines and also help reabsorb calcium in the kidneys before excretion. There's a sensitive balance between phosphorus and calcium and these minerals' teamwork is important in building strong bones and teeth. Take a closer look at these vitamins and minerals:

✔ **Calcium:** Healthy bones need calcium, but calcium is also essential for other vital functions in your body, like regulating your heartbeat, blood clotting,

Two bones in one

Your bones, like your skin, are made up of layers:

✔ **Cortical (compact) bone:** Cortical bone forms the outer layer or protective "shell" of your bone and accounts for 80 percent of the weight of the skeleton.

✔ **Trabecular (cancellous) bone:** This spongy part is located inside the bone, where the bone marrow and blood vessels are. This area of bone is light and porous and makes up the remaining 20 percent of the skeleton weight.

All the bones in your body are a combination of both cortical and trabecular bone. The mix of the two bone types determines the bone's strength.

muscle contractions, and nerve function. Blood calcium levels (between 2.2 and 2.6 millimoles per liter or mmol/L) need to remain stable for your body to work normally; both too much calcium and too little calcium can be harmful. Too much calcium and too little are described in the following terms:

- **Hypocalcemia:** A condition that refers to low levels of blood calcium. Signs of low calcium include involuntary muscle spasms, muscle cramps, heart irregularities, and stomach cramps and pains.

 If you don't have enough calcium in your blood, your body takes it from the bones. Calcium taken from your bones has to be replaced by dietary calcium, found particularly in dairy products, green vegetables, and eggs.

- **Hypercalcemia:** A condition in which you have abnormally high amounts of calcium in your blood. Too much calcium and phosphate in blood and extra cellular fluid can cause widespread organ dysfunction and damage.

  Very large doses (over 2,500 milligrams) of calcium may cause blood calcium levels to rise and lead to calcium deposits in soft tissue, such as the heart and kidneys (kidney stones). Large calcium intakes may reduce zinc and iron absorption and impair vitamin K metabolism. Very high blood levels of calcium can cause heart or lung failure.

✔ **Phosphorus:** Phosphorus, like calcium, is also used in other parts of the body to contract muscles, build and repair bones and teeth, and help nerves function. Most of your body's phosphorus (about 85 percent) is found in your bones. The rest of it is stored in tissues throughout your body. High dietary sources of phosphate include dairy products, nuts, and meat. Your kidneys help control the amount of phosphorus in your blood. Extra phosphorus is filtered by the kidneys and passes out of the body in the urine. A high level of phosphate in the blood is usually caused by a kidney problem. The amount of phosphorus in the blood affects the level of calcium in the blood. The normal level of phosphate in the blood is 0.8 to 1.4 mmol/L.

✔ **Vitamin D:** Vitamin D helps you absorb calcium and phosphorus in your small intestine. A little vitamin D is absorbed from food, but most is made in the skin, in a process that occurs when your skin is exposed to sunlight. After that, vitamin D has to be converted to an active form in your kidneys.

Vitamin D, PTH, and calcitonin (see "Hormones that lend a helping hand in maintaining calcium balance" later in this chapter) help control the total amount of calcium in your body. They also regulate the amount of calcium absorbed from food and the amount removed from your body by the kidneys.

Organs and hormones that maintain the body's calcium balance

Three parts of the body participate in supplying calcium to blood and removing it from blood when necessary. These parts don't make these decisions on their own, but instead need to be signaled to absorb, excrete, or trigger bone mineralization or resorption to maintain calcium levels. Those signal callers are called hormones. Take a closer look at the players in calcium balance:

- **Small intestine:** The small intestine absorbs dietary calcium in different places depending on the dietary intake. Active absorption takes place in the duodenum when dietary calcium is low. Passive (movement across membranes without using energy) absorption occurs in the jejunum and the ileum when dietary calcium is higher. The small intestine absorbs about 40 percent of the total calcium.

- **Bone:** The bone is the major storage bin of calcium. Calcium and phosphate are stored in your bones and can be released from your bones into your blood as well as deposited back into your bones as needed.

- **Kidneys:** Your kidneys play a vital role in calcium homeostasis (keeping levels in balance). Normally, almost all the calcium that enters the kidneys for the formation of urine is reabsorbed back into your blood, which preserves blood calcium at a fairly constant level. However, if blood calcium levels become too high, the excess calcium is excreted in your urine.

Hormones also play an integral part of bone development, maintenance, and unfortunately bone destruction. Hormones are the key to controlling the sensitive balance of calcium, vitamin D, and phosphorus that your bones need in order to stay strong and healthy. Some of the major hormones that affect bone health are as follows:

- **Parathyroid hormone (PTH):** Parathyroid hormone helps regulate blood calcium levels. PTH is produced in the parathyroid glands (behind the thyroid gland in your neck). If your blood calcium levels are too low, the parathyroid gland releases PTH, which results in bone resorption and the release of calcium from the bones into the blood. If the calcium level in the blood rises above normal, PTH secretion falls, and the level of calcium in the blood falls back to normal. PTH also increases the production of vitamin D, which helps increase the absorption of calcium in the small intestine.

- **Calcitonin:** This hormone functions to reduce blood calcium levels and therefore can slow further bone loss. Calcitonin is secreted in response to *hypercalcemia* (too much calcium) and increases the excretion of calcium into urine and the release of calcium from the bone through the inhibition of bone resorption. Calcitonin can help with some of the pain that can occur with osteoporosis.

- **Estrogen:** This hormone inhibits the removal of

calcium from the bones by activity on the *osteoblasts* (see the previous section). It also helps keep the osteoblasts alive and active.

- ✔ **Calcitriol:** Calcitriol is the active form of vitamin D and is actually a hormone. In response to dropping blood levels of calcium or phosphorus, calcitriol increases the absorption of calcium and phosphate from the gastrointestinal tract and increases the bone's absorption of calcium. Calcitriol also inhibits the release of PTH.

Zooming in on the bones' role in calcium delivery and balance

Human bones thrive on a personal recycling program called the *bone remodeling cycle.* This cycle of remodeling is a continuous process of removing old bone and creating new. The bones become lighter, less dense, and more porous — like a sponge or limestone rock.

Here's how it works:

1. **The osteoclasts secrete an acid that dissolves enough old bone to create a tiny cavity.**
   Osteoclasts are bone cells responsible for demolition; it usually takes these cells a few weeks to create a tiny cavity.

2. **Calcium and other minerals are released from the dissolved bone into the bloodstream.**
   When your body needs extra calcium, it signals the osteoclasts to dissolve more bone. Most of this material is recycled later in the remodeling process.

3. **Osteoblasts line the cavity that the osteoclasts left with *collagen* (the soft, sticky stuff that**

forms the main frame for bone).

4. **The osteoblasts pull in calcium and other minerals (like phosphorus and magnesium) from the blood, forming crystals on the collagen to lengthen and thicken the bone.**

5. **The collagen and minerals harden or *calcify* into bone tissue.**

6. **When the osteoblasts are done working, they transform into mature bone cells, called *osteocytes*, and become part of the new bone.**

    The osteocytes no longer participate in bone remodeling, but they do help maintain the bone and also help balance the calcium and phosphorus concentrations.

At the end of the remodeling cycle, the cavity has been re-filled with new bone. The whole process takes three to six months, which explains why developing osteoporosis can take a long time. This is also why taking early measures can prevent osteoporosis.

The Big Dilemma: How Your Bones Change Over Time

Your bones continue to grow in length and mass from birth until about the age of 25 to 35 when they hit their peak mass. This age varies from person to person and can be influenced by physical activity, gender, and lifestyle choices. After you reach your peak bone mass, it's all downhill from there, though your outer bone can continue to thicken with certain exercises. From the climax on, you start to lose bone faster than you can form new bone. During your younger years, you have excellent bone building ability and good calcium absorption capacity to build up the bones as much as possible; then as you age you move to maintain your bone mineral density through a calcium-rich diet and strength training. You have some control over how fast and how much bone you lose, so read on for more information on how and why bone loss occurs and what you can do to slow it down.

Decline in calcium absorption

As you move past age 30, your rate of calcium absorption goes down slowly and steadily until about the age of 50. After 50, bone loss accelerates more quickly due to the normal decline in hormone levels for men and women and the onset of menopause for women. Go ahead and add another aging loss to the list — your hair, your eyesight, your waistline, and now your bone mass. But, despite the fact that bone loss is another part of the aging process, you aren't doomed to the life of a glass menagerie. You do have some control in delaying the onset. The thicker your bones are, the longer it takes to develop bone loss.

Calcium absorption slowly decreases from 75 percent in childhood to 25 percent by adulthood and even decreases further as you age. Because calcium absorption declines with age, dietary needs of calcium are higher for adults ages 50 and over. Here are some reasons why absorption goes down as age goes up:

- ✔ **Vitamin D:** As your body ages, skin becomes less effective at making vitamin D, which aids in calcium absorption.

- ✔ **Gastrointestinal changes:** As you age, the amount of stomach acid production goes down, especially in women. If your stomach isn't producing enough stomach acid (hydrochloric acid), the calcium remains in a form that isn't readily absorbed by the intestines.

- **Medications:** Several medications can either reduce calcium absorption or cause increased calcium loss from bones. Some examples are antacids, blood pressure medications, cholesterol-lowering medications, thyroid hormone, certain diuretics, seizure medications, and corticosteroids. Corticosteroids are great medications for inflammatory conditions such as asthma and arthritis, but long term steroid use can decrease the formation of new bone and increase the breakdown of old bone.

- **Interfering foods, drinks, and other lifestyle choices:** Caffeine can increase the amount of calcium lost in the urine, as can excess sodium. Soda has been looked at in several studies as a culprit in disturbing calcium balance. It may be replacing the intake of calcium-rich fluids, and the phosphorus in the soda interferes with calcium metabolism. Smoking is associated with poor bone health, but it isn't clear whether it's the multiple health issues related to the smoking or the tobacco itself that weakens the bones. Alcohol intake can also disrupt bone health by effects on the parathyroid hormone (PTH) and the environment in the stomach.

Bone degeneration and loss

Both men and women start having age-related bone loss at about age 50, but bone loss can be accelerated in individuals who didn't develop maximum peak bone mass. There are two levels of bone loss that can occur and are associated with an increased risk for fractures:

- **Osteopenia:** Osteopenia, which is loss of bone mineral density (BMD), is the warning siren that the bones are thinning. This phase begins when existing bone breaks down faster than the body can replace it. Preventing transition into osteoporosis takes the combination of exercise, calcium, and possibly some medications prescribed by your doctor.

- **Osteoporosis:** Osteoporosis — Latin for *porous bone* — takes years to develop as bones slowly lose minerals, density, and structure, which makes them weaker. If left untreated, osteoporosis can lead to stooped posture, loss of height, and broken bones. See Figure 6-1 to compare a bone with osteoporosis with a healthy bone.

  The good news is that not everyone ends up with osteoporosis and there are tests to determine how dense your bones are. The news may not be that bad if you've made lifestyle choices that help and not hinder bone strength. Making good choices still can't guarantee that you won't develop osteoporosis, but it significantly helps your odds. After you've been diagnosed with osteoporosis, you still have options to maintain bone density, but prevention is your best bet for preserving bone.

All bones aren't created equal. Women's bones are smaller and less dense than men's, and women are four times more likely than men to suffer from osteoporosis. This is because men in their 50s don't experience the rapid loss of bone mass that women do in the years following menopause. By age 65 or 70, however, men and women are losing bone mass at the same rate, and the absorption of calcium decreases in both sexes. Excessive bone loss causes bone to become fragile and more likely to fracture.

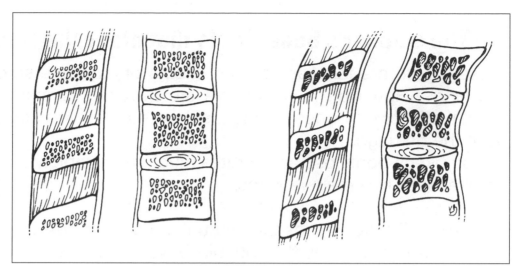

Figure 6-1: The differences between a healthy bone and one with osteoporosis.

Maintaining Healthy Bones

Face it: You take your bones for granted. Many folks haven't had a broken bone and don't realize how important preserving that statistic is. Imagine having to use crutches or a wheel chair for weeks due to a broken hip or leg. Fractures of the spine, secondary to osteoporosis, affect more than 20 percent of post-menopausal women and account for pain and interference with activities of daily living. Mobility is important at any age, and supporting good bone health as you age is one way to keep you on your feet.

An ounce of prevention: Live a healthy lifestyle

It's never too late to start thinking about bone loss, but the earlier the better. Whether you're 20-something and still have time to build up your bones or 60-something and want to preserve what you have, keep reading to find out the best ways to keep your bone bank balance on the plus

The smoker's bone: Facts that clear the smoke

Most people are familiar with the effects of cigarette smoking on the lungs. However, fewer people are aware of smoking's detrimental effects on bones — and just how early bones start to ache from the damage.

A smoker's bone loss accelerates much more rapidly than a nonsmoker's for two main reasons:

✔ Smoking decreases the amount of calcium absorbed from food and the way that vitamin D works to manage calcium.

✔ Smoking inhibits the production of bone cells.

✔ Smoking lowers estrogen in men and women. Estrogen is important because it helps hold calcium in the bones.

The combination of these effects puts smokers at a much higher risk for developing osteoporosis.

Substantial research shows that after surgeries or broken bones, the healing time for smokers is almost double that of nonsmokers.

In addition, female smokers have a 50 percent greater risk of developing osteoporosis than nonsmokers. Smoking causes a decrease in the production of estrogen, so menopausal symptoms begin earlier than in nonsmokers therefore increasing their risk for osteoporosis from early estrogen deficiency.

side for as long as possible. Just like an early investment of money, your early investment in bone health can pay the biggest dividends when you're older.

The formula for maintaining healthy bones isn't a secret, but it does take a heavy dose of practice and good common sense in the following areas:

✔ **Exercise regularly.** The effects of exercise on the bones are continuously researched, but it's quite clear that certain exercises cause stress on the bones, which stimulates the bones to hold on to calcium. The reason weight-bearing exercise helps keep bones strong is that pulling the muscles against the bone creates a force that stresses the bone. That kind of stress drives calcium back into your bones, reinforcing their strength. See Chapter 10 for specific ways to increase bone density through weight training.

If you have osteoporosis, there are a few exercises that you should avoid. High-impact exercises — such as jumping rope or jogging — or exercises that make you bend or twist can place too much stress on the bones and can increase your risk of fractures. Talk to your doctor about an appropriate exercise regimen that's good for your health condition.

✔ **Consume good nutrition and supplements.** Your body has two primary ways to feed your bones a balanced meal: the foods you eat and the supplements you take. Of course, getting the daily recommended nutrients through fresh whole foods is your best bet because they're in natural form — your body is made to digest them. In addition to the obvious calcium benefit of dairy foods and calcium-fortified beverages, you can get calcium from eggs, canned fish (sardines, salmon with bones), soybeans and other soy products (soy-based beverages, soy yogurt, tempeh), some other dried beans, and some leafy greens (collard and turnip greens, kale, bok choy, and broccoli).

Your body can't absorb more than 600 to 700 milligrams of calcium at a time. Eat small meals and snacks rich in calcium throughout the day to ensure that you're absorbing adequate calcium.

Getting regular bone-density screenings

As you age, the list of tests you should have done as a baseline reading just keeps growing. Testing for osteoporosis is one more test that you should add to the list. Exactly when you should have your first evaluation depends on several factors. Here are some guidelines to go by.

We recommend screening if you have any of the following risk factors:

- ✔ You've gone through early menopause

- ✔ You're 60 to 65 years old

- ✔ You're over the age of 50, post menopausal, and have at least one other risk factor for osteoporosis

- ✔ You have other diseases that effect bone loss, such as diabetes, kidney disease, or hyperparathyroidism (excess release of parathyroid hormone)

- ✔ You're taking medications, such as steroids or anticonvulsants, that affect bone mineralization and resorption. Bone mineral density tests (BMD) measure how saturated your bones are with minerals such as calcium. By using X-rays, CT scans, or ultrasound technology, your doctor can review the results and advise you of your bone strength.

You have a few options for a professional measurement of your bone density:

- ✔ **Ultrasound:** Your doctor may use ultrasound as the first test to see whether your bone density is low. The test is usually performed on your heel rather than the bones most likely to break from osteoporosis (like your hip or spine). If the results are positive, your doctor schedules DEXA (see the next bullet) to confirm the results.

✔ **Dual-energy X-ray absorptiometry (DEXA):** This fast test uses very low doses of radiation and is the most accurate method for measuring BMD (it can measure as little as a 2-percent bone loss per year). DEXA uses two X-ray beams to estimate bone density in your spine and hip. The amounts of each X-ray beam that are blocked by bone and soft tissue are compared to each other. Bones with higher mineral density allow less of the X-ray beam to pass through.

A regular X-ray can't detect bone loss until the loss is greater than 25 percent.

✔ **Quantitative computed tomography (QCT):** This test measures the density of a bone in your spine. QCT isn't usually recommended because it's expensive, uses higher radiation doses, and is less accurate than DEXA.

BMD is described in terms of standard deviations (SD) from two different norms. The T score compares your bone density to that of a typical 30 year old, and the Z score compares you to others of your age. Being one standard deviation below normal on either test is considered normal. Lower than –1, the breakdown is as follows:

–1 to –2.5 SD = osteopenia
–2.5 or more = osteoporosis

–1 SD is equal to a bone loss of 10 to 12 percent on most tests.

Treating Osteoporosis

Osteoporosis can be detected early and treated effectively with diet, exercise, and medication. It can't be cured, but the main risk of osteoporosis — fractures — can be reduced. After proper screening and evaluation, your doctor can help you decide on the best treatment options based on your test results and any other contributing medical factors. Women are the main candidates for osteoporosis, and estrogen is essential for healthy bone density. When the production of estrogen is reduced (primarily due to menopause in women), bones become brittle and break easily. One of the options for treatment of osteoporosis, therefore, is hormone therapy (HT), also called hormone replacement therapy (HRT).

HT was once the mainstay of treatment for osteoporosis because it treated the slowing of the bone resorption that occurs with estrogen deficiency. After some major studies done by the Women's Health Initiative (WHI) found concerning conclusions about hormone therapy and cardiovascular and breast cancer risks, management with this therapy changed. Women at risk for certain forms of cancer (endometrial and breast cancer) as well as some clotting disorders are cautioned against HT. Also, estrogen replacement therapy (ERT) increases the risk for heart attack, stroke, breast cancer, and blood clots. Discuss the various options with your doctor to determine which may be best for you.

Hormone replacement therapy (HRT) has been used much more conservatively in recent years in light of its potential risks. HRT is now primarily used in lower doses for shorter periods of time as a temporary treatment for the worst menopausal symptoms, but only in women who don't have heart disease or a strong family history of breast cancer or cardiovascular disease. In such cases, HRT gives women relief from menopausal symptoms, and it slows down the resorption of bone that occurs with estrogen decrease during menopause.

If your doctor determines that HRT isn't for you, and lifestyle changes don't help control your osteoporosis, prescription drugs can help slow bone loss and may even increase bone density over time. These medications include the following:

- **Calcitonin** (Miacalcin) is a naturally occurring substance found in the body that works to balance the bone production and breakdown process. This product is available as a nasal spray.

- **Alendronate** (Fosamax) and **Risedronate** (Actonel) represent a class of medicines called bisphosphonates that treat osteoporosis. They serve as an alternative to hormone replacement therapy and are available in convenient once-a-week dosage forms. Studies have shown significant improvement of bone mineral density following treatment. You need to be able to remain upright for 30 minutes after taking bisphosphonates to avoid damage to your esophagus. These medications may also cause osteonecrosis of the jaw, which is a deterioration of the jawbone, in some patients. Make sure to discuss the possible risks with your doctor before taking these medications.

- **Ibandronate sodium** (Boniva) is a once-a-month bisphosphonate for postmenopausal osteoporosis. It not only maintains bone density, but also builds bones with just one tablet a month. As with other bisphosphonates, remain upright for at least 30 to 60 minutes after taking your dose. Cases of osteonecrosis have also been reported in patients taking Boniva, so discuss all options with your doctor.

- ✔ **Raloxifene** (Evista) is a selective estrogen modulator. In other words, it offers the beneficial effects of estrogen on the bone but doesn't have the detrimental effects of estrogen on *endometrial* (the tissue that lines the uterus) and breast tissue.

- ✔ **Teriparatide** (Forteo) helps to reverse bone loss. It's a natural bone-building hormone that doubles the normal rate of bone formation and stimulates new bone growth by increasing the number and action of bone-forming cells.

Discuss medical treatment options with your doctor before taking any medications. As with many prescriptions, certain risks and side effects may be associated with each drug, and you also need to watch out for interactions that may occur if you're taking other meds.

Maintaining the Parts that Join Your Bones

As you age, your joints start to show the wear and tear from years of stooping, bending, jumping, running, and twisting in the form of osteoarthritis or degenerative joint disease. You may be able to not only feel the effect of joint disease, but also hear it — this kind of grinding noise when your joints rub against each other is called *crepitus.*

Just because you can hear the effects of joint wear doesn't mean that it's worse. Some people may have no audible crepitus and have much more severe pain and disease. You may develop pains in your joints and realize that other members of your family suffered from similar symptoms. There are a few hereditary forms of joint disease that can cause symptoms at an early age and can be much more severe than the age-related arthritis. Check out the joints themselves for a better understanding of how arthritis works.

The components of joints and how they age

To get a better understanding of how your joints work, here's a breakdown of the components involved and the specific roles each one plays.

- ✔ **Synovial fluid:** To limit wear and tear in your joints, the cartilage is filled with *synovial* fluid (a substance with a sticky consistency like a raw egg). The joints can then move without friction.

- ✔ **Ligaments:** A ligament is a short band of tough fibrous connective tissue composed mainly of long, stringy collagen fibers. Ligaments connect bones to other bones to form a joint.

- ✔ **Tendons:** Tendons join muscle to bone and are very elastic in nature. Tendons are tough and fibrous tissue. They're often long and straight and act as shock absorbers in your body. They help you walk, jump, skip, and hop because when you contract your muscle, the tendon moves the bone.

- ✔ **Cartilage:** All bones have a lining of cartilage to cushion the ends of the bones, preventing them from rubbing against each other when they move. Cartilage is a type of dense connective tissue. It's composed of fibers of collagen and elastin. If you've ever looked at the end of a chicken bone, you may have noticed how white it is — cartilage doesn't contain blood vessels. You have cartilage in many places other than just your ear and nose — like your joints, rib cage, bronchial tubes, and between intervertebral discs. Your tendons are also made of cartilage.

Cartilage is one of the first body parts you start to lose as you age. Because cartilage no longer provides a cushion between your bones to keep them from rubbing together, that old knee injury you suffered on the ski slopes in your 20s is now bugging you in your 40s.

Think of it this way: When a spring-coiled seat cushion that was once as comfy as a cloud starts to age, the padding wears away, the fabric becomes threadbare, and the coils begin to poke the sitter painfully in the posterior! Similarly, the cartilage that provides cushioning between the bones begins to break down with age or excessive wear and tear (or both!). The friction of two uncushioned bones rubbing together causes painful joint inflammation, better known as *arthritis.* Ouch!

Keeping your joints flexible (or making them that way)

Although arthritis isn't preventable, you can take steps to reduce your risk of developing the disease:

- **Keeping off the pounds:** Excess weight puts an extra strain on joints, which can lead to arthritis.

- **Eating right:** Consuming foods rich in calcium and vitamin D helps with weight control and strengthens bones and muscles.

- **Maintaining reasonable physical activity and fitness levels:** Exercise helps develop strong muscles, which can protect and support joints. In particular, strengthening the core muscles of the body (abs, back, and stabilizer muscles) can enhance

Self-induced snap, crackle, and pop

Your joints can make all types of sounds when you stretch them, but have you ever wondered why your knuckles "pop" when you crack them? All the joints in your body are surrounded by synovial fluid that acts as a lubricant. This fluid contains gases such as, nitrogen, oxygen, and carbon dioxide. When you stretch your fingers to crack the knuckles, you cause the bones of the joint to pull apart causing the pressure in the capsule to drop so low that gas is rapidly released forming bubbles, which then burst . . . and "crack."

And old wives' tale associates this self-induced joint cracking to arthritis. This cracking hasn't been found to be associated with any future risk of arthritis.

flexibility and improve balance.

✔ **Stretching:** Stretching the joints of the extremities can maintain joint health by increasing range of motion and maintaining strength of the muscles that support the joints. See *Stretching For Dummies* (Wiley) by LaReine Chabut for more information.

In addition, some of the most effective ways to prevent joint pain may not make you happy if you're a smoker, professional athlete, or body builder, or if you have a family history of related illnesses. If none of the aforementioned factors describes you, then you have a much better chance of preventing joint pain.

If your joints are stiff and achy but you're afraid that moving them will hurt worse, think again. Movement is the best recommendation to loosen and limber up stiff, achy joints. The longer your joints are immobilized, the more they ache and the stiffer they become because the ligaments contract, leaving you feeling like the tin man left out in the rain. If you already have arthritis, read on to find out what you can do to feel better.

Coping with Joint Pain and Arthritis

The pain and deformity of arthritis have plagued human beings for as long they've walked the earth. It shows up in the bones of cavemen and the mummies of Egyptian pharaohs. For just as long, people have searched for medications, herbs, and other concoctions to assuage achy joints — but a cure for arthritis has proved elusive. As a result, sufferers are willing targets for both effective therapies *and* snake oil.

Understanding arthritis

Arthritis is a single term that covers a wide range of joint disorders: *Arth* means *joint* and *itis* means *inflamed.* More than 100 different types of arthritis are known, and each type can have different symptoms. Most types of arthritis show signs of joint inflammation like swelling and stiffness. Three of the most common types of arthritis are

- ✔ **Osteoarthritis:** This is a degenerative joint disease in which the joint's cartilage breaks down faster than your body is capable of rebuilding it. After the cartilage wears down the ends of the bones, they start to rub together, which causes inflammation and is painful. Figure 6-2 compares a healthy joint to a joint with osteoarthritis.

- ✔ **Rheumatoid arthritis (RA):** This is actually an autoimmune disorder. It causes chronic inflammation in which your own immune system attacks your joints. It's a disabling and painful inflammatory condition, rendering a person

232

immobile and in pain due to joint destruction. RA is a systemic disease, often affecting tissues throughout the body, including the skin, blood vessels, heart, lungs, and muscles.

✔ **Gout arthritis:** This common type of arthritis (also called metabolic arthritis) is caused by the chemical uric acid, a byproduct of protein breakdown. In this condition, uric acid crystals are deposited on the articular cartilage of joints, tendons, and surrounding tissues when too much uric acid is in the bloodstream. These crystals create inflamed tissue. Gout usually attacks the big toe (approximately 75 percent of first attacks), but it can also affect other joints, such as the ankle, heel, knee, wrist, elbow, fingers, and spine.

Osteoarthritis isn't just for the elderly. Younger people can get it too. Many athletes suffer from osteoarthritis after years of repetitive motion and excessive wear and tear on their joints. People who work in repetitive or heavy-lifting jobs should use joint-protecting devices and techniques to ensure proper lifting and posture to help avoid injury, which can lead to the development of arthritis.

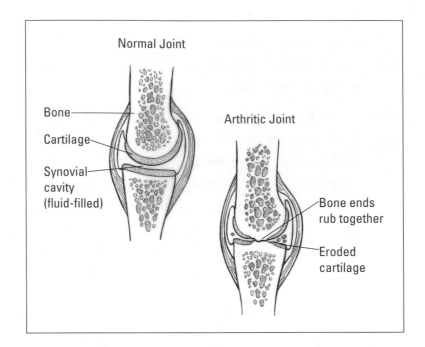

Figure 6-2:
A healthy joint and a joint with osteoarthritis.

Formulating a medical treatment plan for arthritis

If you're experiencing joint pain and don't know whether it's an acute injury or arthritis, see your doctor. Together you can formulate an inclusive plan for your health that may include medication, nutrition, and exercise. If you have a joint injury, you can be causing more damage by waiting. If you have osteoarthritis, you're only delaying your options for relief and treatment.

 Regardless of the type of joint pain you experience, treatment options are available. The following list provides examples of herbals and pharmaceuticals:

- ✔ **Supplements:** Glucosamine and chondroitin are large proteins naturally present in joint tissue; glucosomine is used to build and repair cartilage, and chondroitin gives cartilage its elasticity.

Glucosamine is derived from shellfish shells (if you're allergic to it, talk to your doctor about alternatives) and chondroitin from cow cartilage. Study results are often more anecdotal than scientifically based, and the most comprehensive study conducted by the NIH found no benefit to using the supplements over a placebo. The two supplements are sometimes sold in a combination pill.

- **Nonsteroidal anti-inflammatory drugs (NSAIDs):** Drugs like Aleve and Advil or ibuprofen are available over the counter for joint pain. Talk to your doctor before taking NSAIDs on a regular basis. The COX2 inhibitors like Mobic and Celebrex are good NSAIDs, although they need to be used with caution. Some have been pulled from the market due to their risks and associations with adverse cardiac events (like Vioxx).

- **Steroidals:** Often steroids are injected right into the joint. If you have an inflamed or swollen joint, or if you have pain or inflammation near a joint, your doctor may inject a steroid preparation into the affected area. The mildest is hydrocortisone; prednisolone, methylprednisolone, and triamcinolone are stronger. The stronger steroid preparations tend to be less soluble, and therefore remain in the joint longer. Benefit from the stronger drugs is associated with a slightly increased risk of local side effects.

Fighting arthritis in other ways

In addition to combating arthritis with medication, you have some natural options for relieving the pain. Get relief from making these changes:

- ✔ **Weight loss:** Maintaining a healthy weight goes a long way as a natural and healthy remedy to arthritis and joint pain. Experts say that every extra 10 pounds of weight you carry feels like 30 pounds on your knees. Eliminating excess weight lightens the load for your body, freeing you to move more easily and comfortably.

  Keep in mind that you can't eat your way out of arthritis or joint pain. In fact, overeating, or more specifically, being overweight is the most controllable factor you have in alleviating joint pain.

- ✔ **Exercise:** Low impact exercise, such as swimming, bicycling, or an elliptical machine may be right up your alley if you've sustained a joint injury but still want to lose weight through exercise. You may also consider these exercises if your arthritis pain prevents you from engaging in more invigorating activity. The point is to keep moving. You need to maintain muscle tone for joint stability. Yoga is another option for opening up your range of movement, which is important if you have arthritis.

- ✔ **Getting up in the morning:** Arthritis is most painful in the morning when you first wake up because you've been at rest all night. Your first step is to get out of bed, but do so slowly and carefully. You'll find the most benefit to relieving your stiffness and achiness if you continue to move and stretch for 20 to 30 minutes first thing in the morning. Try going for a walk or doing some yoga, but get up and move to lubricate your joints. Oh, and don't forget to breathe!

- **Nutrition and dietary supplements:** The information is mixed on what type of diet is most helpful if you have osteoarthritis. Some studies suggest that antioxidants such as those found in cherries may reduce osteoarthritis. One Duke University study showed that diets high in carotenoids, the chemicals that give some fruits and veggies their orange and yellow colors, helped decrease the inflammation of osteoarthritis, while another Duke study (done on animals rather than people) showed that high doses of vitamin C can increase the inflammation of osteoarthritis.

  Also, the *bromelain* (a mixture of protein-digesting enzymes) in fresh pineapples may have an anti-inflammatory effect.

  What's the best bet for now? Eat a healthy diet with a variety of fruits and veggies and make note of what makes your osteoarthritis worse. Different people may react differently to certain foods, and a food diary may help you pinpoint what's good — and not so good — for you.

- **RICE method for an aching joint:** The RICE method is a popular and widely used method for treating joint pain, as well as minor injuries:

  1. **Rest:** Reduce or stop using the injured area for 48 hours. If you have a leg or foot injury, you may need to stay off it completely.

  2. **Ice:** Put an ice pack on the injured area for 20 minutes at a time, four to eight times per day. Use a cold pack, ice bag, or a plastic bag filled with crushed ice that's been wrapped in a towel.

  3. **Compression:** Compression of an injured ankle, knee, or wrist may help reduce the

swelling. These compresses include bandages, such as elastic wraps, special boots, air casts, and splints. Ask your doctor which one is best.

4. **Elevation:** Keep the injured area elevated above the level of the heart. Use a pillow to help elevate an injured limb.

Combating an Aching Back

If you're like 80 percent of Americans, you've had back or neck pain at some time in your life. Back-related complaints are the number one reason for work related disability claims, and one of the most common reasons for people to see their family doctor — not to mention the chiropractor or the orthopedist. Why do so many people have bad backs? Most of them aren't spending all day outside planting crops or doing back breaking labor.

Backs can hurt for a number of reasons. Sometimes the reason is obvious, such as muscle strain after a day of shoveling snow or raking leaves. Other times there seems to be no cause at all — you get up in the morning, feel a sharp twinge in the lower part of your back, and fall back onto the bed. Oh, your aching back!

Back pain is considered chronic if it lasts for three months. Back pain can be caused by any number of things; among the most common are

✔ **Sprain or strain:** Doing an activity you aren't used to, like shoveling, can strain or sprain muscles or ligaments. Work up to new activities slowly, and remember that you won't immediately feel pain from a sprain (a ligament injury) or strain (a muscle injury); it may take up to 24 hours for the pain to grab hold of you. Symptoms are usually short lived (less than one month) and easily treated by rest, icing, NSAIDs, and time.

✔ **Disc problems:** The discs in your back act as cushioning shock absorbers, but as you get older, the discs dry out and become brittle (disc degeneration). If a disc ruptures and the thick inner jelly-like substance leaks out and pushes on the spinal canal, this can cause pressure on the nerves resulting in pain, weakness, or numbness. Surgery to remove the disc and fuse the vertebra above and below may be necessary if conservative measures don't have any effect after three months.

✔ **Sciatica:** Sciatica pain results when the sciatic nerve, which runs down your buttocks and the back of your leg, is "pinched" by bulging discs or excess bone or soft tissues. Surgery is necessary only if conservative measures fail and you have dysfunction of the affected area, such as foot drop or numbness. Surgery called laminectomy or lamintomy removes or goes through the *lamina,* the roof of the spinal canal, to remove the disc causing the problem.

✔ **Spinal stenosis:** This condition is most often associated with aging and disc degeneration; the spinal canal narrows, putting pressure on the spinal nerves, causing an achy or electrical pain down an arm or leg. Spinal stenosis progresses over time and may require surgery if conservative measures like rest, exercise, anti-inflammatories, or spine support don't work.

If you're having any symptoms such as weakness, numbness, or severe pain in your arms or legs you should see your medical doctor. You may need to have further testing done to see if there is severe damage to your discs. You don't want to start any therapy or exercise prior to having these tests done. If tests are normal, you can proceed to try other modalities, such as chiropractic or massage therapy.

Part III

Using Nutrition to Extend Your Expiration Date

The 5th Wave   By Rich Tennant

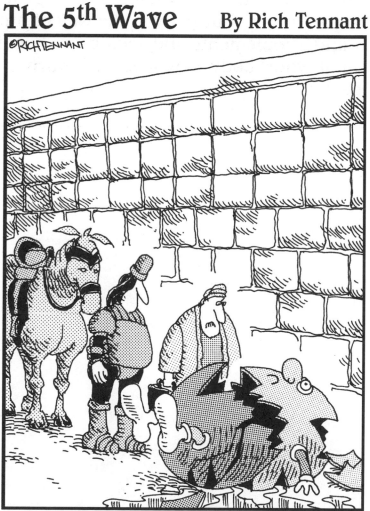

"The way I see it, if the fall off the wall didn't get him, the protein imbalance in his system would have sooner or later."

In this part . . .

It's no secret that good nutrition can help you live a longer, healthier life. Understanding what makes food good for you — the nutrients, phytochemicals, vitamins, and minerals — can help you make wiser choices about what you eat.

This part gets you started on improving what you put in your body in the way of nutrition and supplements and seeing the benefits of what your body can give in return . . . longevity.

Chapter 7

You Are What You Eat: Nutrition 101

● ●

In This Chapter

▶ Knowing the importance of nutrition as you age
▶ Checking out different kinds of food that are good for your body
▶ Living a healthy life and making healthy habits
▶ Reading labels on your food

● ●

The phrase "Garbage in, garbage out" is just as true for your body as it is for your computer. If your diet lacks nutrients, or if you eat too much or too little, the results show up as health problems and feeling ill, especially as you age. Although you may think of nutrition issues primarily in terms of your weight, the effects of a poor diet are far more than skin deep; serious health problems such as diabetes, heart disease, high blood pressure, cancer, and osteoporosis can stem from poor nutrition and can reduce your chances of living a long and healthier life.

In this chapter, we look at the importance of good nutrition (and we define it) and how your body's nutritional needs may change as you age. We also offer info on reading

243

nutritional labels (the ones you need your glasses to read!), and then we recommend some diets for healthy, nutrition-smart aging.

The Importance of Nutrition — and Why You Should Care

All food isn't equal when it comes to keeping you healthy as you get older. Case in point: Although a plate of brown rice and a candy bar have about the same number of calories, the brown rice is much healthier. But given a choice between the rice and the candy bar, most people would choose the candy bar. In this section, we plan to educate you about food — what's in it, why some foods are much better for you than others, and why getting the proper nutrition helps you age well. Our goal is to increase your motivation to put down the candy bar and pick up something that's good for you . . . at least most of the time.

How the good foods work for you . . .

A healthy diet helps you age well, but what constitutes a healthy diet? The answer is, a diet that delivers the nutrients you need after the food's broken down and absorbed by your digestive system.

Most everything you put in your mouth has some nutrients, but some foods have more *macronutrients* — nutrients that your body uses in larger amounts, which comprise proteins, carbs, and fats — and micronutrients — nutrients that your body requires in smaller amounts, such as vitamins and minerals — than others. In addition, some foods have additional properties that promote extra health benefits and help boost your immune system, which weakens as you age. These additional components may include the following:

- **Antioxidants:** These compounds help fight free radicals that result from oxidation. *Oxidation* is the loss of electrons in atoms; free radicals can damage cells and cause disease or deterioration in your body. Oxidation appears to increase as you age, making antioxidants a valuable player on the anti-aging field.

  Foods that contain vitamins A, C, and E, beta carotene, selenium, and lycopene (found in tomatoes) are rich with antioxidants. Most brightly colored fruits and vegetables contain essential antioxidants too, which are more beneficial when consumed in food than taken in supplement form. Antioxidants also help keep your immune system strong.

- **Bioflavanoids:** Bioflavanoids are the brightly colored pigments found in fruits, red wine, and vegetables; they're a class of antioxidants (see preceding bullet) necessary for vitamin C absorption. They also strengthen blood vessels and have anti-inflammatory properties.

- **Omega-3 and -6 fatty acids:** These essential oils are found in some fish, meats, eggs, walnuts, corn, safflower, and oils such as canola and flaxseed. Studies show that they may protect against heart disease by lowering triglyceride blood levels as well as possibly decreasing rheumatoid arthritis, depression, macular degeneration, and asthma. These fatty acids are best utilized by the body when obtained from food instead of supplements.

- **Phytosterols:** Phytosterols are found in plants; they work to lower LDL (low density lipoproteins, the "bad" cholesterol) blood levels. There are two types of phytosterols: sterols and stanols. Both are found in fruits, legumes, nuts, seeds, vegetables, and vegetable oils. Some food products are fortified by phytosterols. These foods include orange juice, some cereals, salad dressing, and lowfat milk.

✔ **Probiotics:** Probiotics are living microorganisms that positively benefit you. They improve the health and functioning of your gastrointestinal tract (GI) and may help boost your immune system. Probiotics such as bacteria and yeast help balance the flora (microorganisms) found in your intestinal tract, killing off the bad bacteria and allowing the good bacteria to flourish.

You never knew there was such a thing as good bacteria? Yes, indeed. One example is one many women are familiar with — the development of a yeast infection after taking antibiotics. This infection happens because bacteria, not being too choosy, kill off the good bacteria that normally keep yeast proliferation under control. Without them, yeast runs rampant and you have a yeast infection. Probiotics are found in some yogurts and dairy products, as well as supplements.

✔ **Prebiotics:** Prebiotics are found in whole grains, bananas, honey, onions, artichokes, and fortified food products. They also help balance flora in the GI tract and may aid in calcium absorption.

. . . and how the bad foods work against you

Sooner or later, bad nutrition shows up in your health. While you may be able to eat poorly for a few months (or even a few years) without getting sick, sooner or later the sustained effects of poor eating habits appear in various forms, the most dangerous being serious disease.

The following diseases can be brought about or worsened by poor food choices:

- ✔ **Heart disease:** Heart disease is the nation's leading killer for both men and women and is caused by a number of factors including heredity, high blood pressure, high cholesterol, diabetes, obesity, and inactivity. Factors like heredity can't be modified (you can't ever really fire your relatives), so watching what you eat is one way to try to prevent heart disease.

- ✔ **Diabetes:** Type 2 diabetes can be mostly attributed to controllable factors including excess weight, lack of exercise, and poor nutrition. Although the genes you inherit may influence the development of type 2 diabetes, they pale in comparison to your behavioral and lifestyle factors.

  The Diabetes Prevention Program (DPP), a landmark study sponsored by the National Institutes of Health, found that people with an increased risk for diabetes can prevent or delay the onset of the disease by losing 5 to 7 percent of their body weight through a lowfat, low-calorie eating plan and by getting 30 minutes of physical activity five days a week.

- ✔ **High blood pressure:** Uncontrolled high blood pressure can lead to stroke, heart attack, heart failure, or kidney failure. Saturated fat can increase your blood pressure as well as your cholesterol. Saturated fat increases the level of low density lipoproteins (LDL), which tend to stick to the sides of the arterial wall. This deposit, called *atherosclerosis,* begins with the accumulation of fatty streaks on the inner arterial walls. When this fatty buildup enlarges and becomes hardened with minerals, such as calcium, it forms plaque. Plaque stiffens the arteries and narrows the passages through them. As a result, blood pressure rises.

Increasing the amount of vegetables and fruits and reducing the amount of fat and cholesterol not only reduces blood pressure but also helps with weight loss, which also lowers blood pressure.

Sugar may be as big a villain in raising blood pressures as salt, according to research, because consumption of sugar induces salt and water retention. A diet high in processed foods and sugar caused study blood lipid levels to rise significantly.

- **High cholesterol:** Cholesterol is necessary for the formation of cell membranes, some hormones, and vitamin D. LDL carry cholesterol through the bloodstream from the liver to the rest of the body. Excess LDL can be deposited on the walls of blood vessels, causing heart disease. High density lipoproteins (HDL) carry cholesterol back to the liver, so a high level of HDL in your blood removes excess cholesterol from the bloodstream so it doesn't get deposited on the blood vessel walls.

    Fats are also an essential part of your diet; they carry cholesterol to and from your liver. But saturated and trans fats are bad for you because they can raise blood cholesterol levels, which can lead to increased risk for heart disease. Saturated fats are found mostly in animal fats and dairy products, while trans fats are found in commercially prepared baked goods, snack foods, and just about anything that tastes really good but that you know is bad for you. Saturated fats raise both good cholesterol (HDL) and bad cholesterol (LDL), with a negative effect overall, while trans fats go one bad step further, lowering HDL and raising LDL.

- ✔ **Osteoporosis:** Bones need calcium to stay strong, especially as you get older. As many as one half of women over 50 and one quarter of men (yes, men get osteoporosis too) have osteoporosis. Calcium can be obtained from dairy products and leafy green vegetables.

    You can take calcium supplements but you need to take your daily dose in divided doses, because only around 500 mg of calcium can be absorbed into your bloodstream at one time.

- ✔ **Cancer:** Changes in your diet and regular exercise are critical components to prevent cancer. Up to 30 percent of cancers in developed countries like the United States may be linked to poor nutrition, obesity, and lack of exercise, according to the American Cancer Society. For example, a high-fat diet is linked to an increase in colorectal cancer. Obesity in general is an independent cancer risk, according to some studies, linked to colon cancer and postmenopausal breast cancer in particular, as well as cancers of the endometrium, pancreas, prostate, and kidney.

How Nutritional Needs Change As You Age

As you age, changes occur in your body that can affect your nutritional needs. The aging process affects the body's absorption of many nutrients. For example, you're less able to absorb nutrients such as calcium. This change occurs because as you age your stomach secretes less hydrochloric acid, which may reduce the amount of calcium absorbed. Your body also excretes, or eliminates, more nutrients. For example, hormonal changes may result in more calcium being excreted through the kidneys. So with these examples in mind, you need to take in more nutrients to absorb the same amount, or you may become deficient in that vitamin or mineral.

As you age, focus on increasing the levels of the following nutrients:

- ✔ **Calcium:** Hormonal changes may decrease calcium absorption as it increases loss of calcium through the kidneys. In addition, you may become *lactose intolerant* (lose some of your ability to digest lactose, the sugar in milk). Because of this condition, some people decrease their intake of dairy products, which are good sources of calcium. But you still need to get the calcium from somewhere. Most people don't eat enough dairy products or veggies to get adequate calcium from their diet and should consider supplementation. The amount of calcium can vary with age or medical conditions, but in general adults should have about 1,000 mg a day, and if you're over the age of 50 increase the dose to 1,200 mg daily.

- ✔ **Iron:** Iron is necessary to carry oxygen to your cells, but it's difficult to get all you need because most foods contain only a little iron. The best source of iron is in red meat, but you can also get iron from poultry, fish, whole grain or enriched breads and cereals, dry beans, and some fruits and vegetables. Women over age 50 should get 50 mg of iron a day where as men only need 10 mg.

  Vitamin C helps you absorb more iron from foods, so be sure you include foods with vitamin C (such as citrus fruits, greens, and tomatoes) in the same meal as foods with iron.

  Taking too many iron supplements can be lethal. Talk to your doctor before taking iron supplements. A less common, but very serious problem, more often found in men, is caused by excessive absorption and storage of iron. This condition is known as *haemochromatosis.* Over time, iron builds up in body tissues and because the normal body can't increase iron excretion, the absorbed iron accumulates in the body. This excess iron can damage organs like the liver and heart, and may contribute to heart disease.

Figuring Out Which Types of Foods You Need

Sure, you've seen the food pyramid — colored horizontal lines with bottles of milk and smiling vegetables plastered on it, telling you what percentage of which nutrients you need each day. Ho hum. And out of date, besides. Welcome to the interactive age, and the *new* improved food pyramid (see Figure 7-1), which is all about personal nutrition — *you* and your individual needs. (And the bars on the pyramid are now vertical instead of horizontal, making it look more like a pyramid and less like a squashed layer cake).

MyPyramid was unveiled by the USDA in April 2005. Its purpose is two-fold:

✔ To convey the USDA and Department of Health and Human Services dietary guidelines (there's a noble, but somewhat boring sounding goal)

✔ To make Americans aware of the vital health benefits of simple and modest improvements in nutrition, physical activity, and lifestyle behavior (in other words, how small changes in nutrition and activity can make you a much better *you*)

We know you're just dying to know what kinds of foods

make up the new and improved pyramid. You can visit the Web site at www.mypyramid.gov, but here are the general guidelines:

- ✔ **Grains:** Grains, which include bread, rice, cereal, and wheat, are big — very big — on the new food pyramid. Daily recommendations are five to eight ounces (a serving is about an ounce). A half cup of cooked rice or grains such as couscous or a slice of bread also count as a serving (if you're not big on ounces). Three servings should be whole grain foods.

- ✔ **Veggies:** The USDA wants you to eat your veggies — two to five servings each day. Vegetables are divided into five different categories: leafy green, orange, starchy, dry beans and peas, and other, which includes such odd fellows like lettuce, onions, tomatoes, and brussel sprouts.

- ✔ **Fruits:** The new food pyramid suggests two cups of fruit a day in most cases, depending on your age and sex. One fruit generally counts as a cup. Check out the Web site for a chart with individual fruits.

- ✔ **Oils:** You can have between five to seven teaspoons of oil daily. That doesn't sound terribly appetizing straight, so you can use oil to prepare foods, or you can also take your oils in nuts or fish, which are also in this category.

- ✔ **Milk:** Just about everyone needs three cups a day from the milk group, which includes cottage cheese, yogurt, and pudding.

- ✔ **Meat and beans:** You need around five to six ounces of protein, which includes meat, eggs, peanut butter, chicken, and fish. This category also includes dry beans.

- **Discretionary calories:** Your government realizes that you're only human and are probably going to eat some things each day that aren't part of any recognizable food group, like Pop-Tarts. You're therefore allowed between 200 and 500 calories to squander any way you wish, but the pyramid suggests you eat something from one of the recognizable food groups.

- **Exercise:** Get off the couch and *do* something every day — for at least 30 minutes. Walking through the discount chain store does *not* count as a moderate or vigorous activity, so plan to walk briskly, run, play golf (no cart allowed!), play basketball, or climb rocks, if your heart desires.

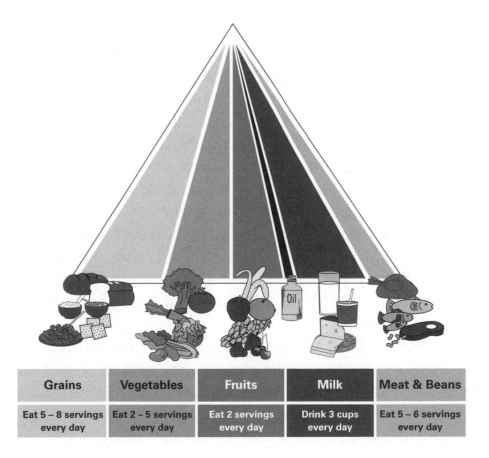

Grains	Vegetables	Fruits	Milk	Meat & Beans
Eat 5 – 8 servings every day	Eat 2 – 5 servings every day	Eat 2 servings every day	Drink 3 cups every day	Eat 5 – 6 servings every day

Figure 7-1: *The USDA food pyramid.*

To get your *individual* recommendations, use the online tool that helps you know the amount of each food group you need daily. Go to www.mypyramid.gov/mypyramid/index.aspx and enter your age, sex, weight, height, and amount of physical activity to find out and receive a customized food guide. Who said your government never did anything nice for you?

Counting Calories and Determining Your Daily Need

It's common for people to say they're "counting their calories" or "watching their calories", but in reality, calories aren't something you can get your hands around. A *calorie* is the amount of energy, or heat, that it takes to raise the temperature of 1 gram of water 1 degree Celsius (1.8 degrees Fahrenheit). To lose one pound of fat, you need to burn 3,500 calories.

To further complicate the terminology, what we refer to as a calorie isn't really a calorie at all; it's a kilocalorie, which equals 1000 calories. Who decided to drop the "kilo" when counting calories in foods? Probably someone who got tired of writing the word *kilocalories!*

For better or for worse, however, the term calorie is used in general conversation to describe food energy. You need a certain number of calories each day based on the amount of energy you burn. And the amount of energy you burn is determined by your metabolism, your weight, and your activity levels.

Regardless of your diet, if you take in more calories than you need, you gain weight. In fact, if you consume 3,500 more calories per week than you need, you gain one pound. If you want to lose one pound, the reverse is also true — you need to consume 3,500 fewer calories per week or burn

3,500 more calories (although keep in mind that your body requires a minimum amount of calories everyday to function, so cut back on calories slowly). If you reduce your daily calories by 500 each day (the max you should eliminate from your daily intake), in one week you can lose one pound.

If you eat all the recommended servings of each food group, no more, no less, you can get your recommended amounts of nutrients without consuming too many calories. Monitoring your portion sizes is also important to make sure you get just the right amounts (see the nearby sidebar, "Portion sizes made simple" for help understanding appropriate portion sizes).

To figure out how many calories you need to consume each day, check out the following sections.

Calculating daily calories burned just by being alive

Your *basal metabolic rate* (BMR) is the basic number of calories you need every day to keep your body up and running and to maintain your breathing, heartbeat, and body temperature. Everyone's BMR is different.

About 60 to 70 percent of your body's energy goes into pure maintenance. The other 30 to 40 percent is used for your daily activities. The more you do physically each day, the higher number of calories (energy) you need.

A common BMR calculator is the *Harris-Benedict* formula (if you're really bad at math or have problems using the formula you can use an online BMR calculator).

- **Adult male:** 66 + (6.3 × body weight in lbs.) + (12.9 × height in inches) – (6.8 × age in years)

- **Adult female:** 655 + (4.3 × weight in lbs.) + (4.7 × height in inches) – (4.7 × age in years)

Gauging daily calories burned through activity

Calculate how many calories you expend per day with physical activity.

This formula is a bit more complicated. It uses an activity multiplier (a number that adjusts the calculation for activity levels) and your BMR (see preceding section). Be honest about your activity level (some people aren't) when figuring out how much you can eat each day.

You expend the following calories, depending on your lifestyle:

- ✔ Sedentary = BMR × 1.2 (little or no exercise, desk job)

- ✔ Lightly active = BMR × 1.375 (light exercise/sports 1–3 days per week)

- ✔ Moderately active = BMR × 1.55 (moderate exercise/sports 3–5 days per week)

- ✔ Very active = BMR × 1.725 (hard exercise/sports 6–7 days per week)

- ✔ Extremely active = BMR × 1.9 (hard daily exercise/sports and physical job or training twice daily for marathons, contests, and so on)

Figuring out total calories your body needs to function well

After you know how many calories your body needs for basic functions and what your body is going to use based on your activity level (see preceding two sections), you can calculate your daily total caloric need or Total Daily Energy

Portion sizes made simple

Because you can't always take measuring cups or a scale with you when you dine, here are some fun ways to eyeball your food portions using your hands or some other household object:

- ✔ 1 teaspoon of butter or peanut butter is about the size of the tip of your thumb.

- ✔ 1 ounce of cheese is about as thick as two dominoes.

- ✔ 1 ounce of nuts can fit in the palm of your hand.

- ✔ A 3-ounce serving of meat is about the size and thickness of a deck of playing cards.

- ✔ 1/2 cup of ice cream is about the size of a tennis ball.

- ✔ 1/2 cup of fruit or vegetables can fit in the palm of your hand.

- ✔ 1 cup of cooked mashed potatoes is about the size of your fist.

- ✔ 1 cup of broccoli is about the size of a light bulb.

- ✔ A medium apple or orange is about the size of a tennis ball.

Expenditure (TDEE). This is the amount of calories your body expends in 24 hours. All you need to do to get that number is multiply your BMR times your activity level.

For example, if your BMR is 1339 calories per day. Your activity level is moderately active (work out 3–4 times per week). Your activity factor is 1.55 (see preceding section). Your TDEE = 1.55 × 1339 = 2075 calories/day.

Picking the Right Macronutrients (Protein, Carbs, and Fats)

The changes in recommendations on what type of macronutrients are best for you from year to year may have you feeling a bit like Alice in Wonderland — which foods make you healthy, which ones make you sick? They may also leave you feeling like, "What's the use? The recommendations are going to all change next year anyway." One year butter's out, the next year it's margarine. Fish is good, but watch out for mercury. Beef is bad — no, it's good, at least some types are.

If you read the food-pyramid section earlier in this chapter and discovered your daily needs online, you know how many servings of each food type you should have — now you just need to refine your choices. In the next section, we help you figure out how to pick the best macronutrients out of the bewildering number of choices available.

Consuming complete proteins, no matter your lifestyle

Protein is a dietary essential, even for vegans, who don't eat animal protein in any way, shape, or form. Proteins are made up of tissue building blocks called *amino acids,* and proteins that contain all the *essential amino acids* (amino acids that the body can't make and therefore must be obtained in foods) are called "complete." Animal protein is a good example of a complete protein, while the proteins found in grains, nuts, and vegetables are incomplete, and you must carefully balance them to obtain all the essential amino acids in your diet.

Although protein isn't a high source of energy, your body uses proteins to grow and to build hormones, antibodies, and the enzymes that regulate the chemical reactions within the body. Proteins are essential for healthy aging because they maintain healthy tissues and sustain growth. Because protein can't be stored in the body, you need a new supply every day to keep tissues from breaking down.

Getting just enough

The U.S. Department of Agriculture (USDA) says that to be healthy, 20 percent of your total daily calories should come from protein. So if your optimal daily caloric intake is 1,800 calories (more on counting calories earlier in this chapter), 360 of them should be in the form of protein.

Can you eat too much protein? It depends. A large study indicated that women who ate over 95 grams of protein per day were 20 percent more likely to suffer a wrist fracture over a 12-year period. The same study, however, showed that women who ate the most protein (up to 110 grams a day) were 25 percent less likely to have a heart attack or stroke compared to women who ate less protein (68 grams a day). The safest bet is to take in around 70 grams of protein each day.

On the other hand, too little protein has serious health consequences, leading to muscle loss, failure to grow properly, and a weakened immune system.

Considering the source

Red meat is a good source of complete protein, but some red meat also contains a large amount of saturated fat, which can raise your cholesterol levels and contribute to heart disease. So poultry and fish, which contain less saturated fat, provide a better source of protein. And if you're vegetarian, you don't have to worry about the high levels of saturated fats in meat — dry beans and nuts are excellent sources of protein. Most servings of protein supply around 24 grams of protein.

A calorie-estimating tool for the mathematically challenged

You can estimate your daily calorie needs by using this easier formula:

- ✔ For sedentary people: Weight × 14 = estimated cal/day

- ✔ For moderately active people: Weight × 17 = estimated cal/day

- ✔ For active people: Weight × 20 = estimated cal/day

Your protein needs depend on your activity level, age, and if you're dieting. Use the following equation to calculate your protein needs:

Weight x 0.6 grams of protein per pound

For example: 170 pounds × 0.6 = 102 grams of protein per day. Remember that this formula is an approximation. Check with your doctor, too.

You can break down your protein choices like this:

- ✔ **Complete proteins:** These contain all essential amino acids. Examples include the following:

  - **Beef:** Lean beef contains less than 10 percent fat, but be careful — this doesn't apply to ground beef, which, in some states, doesn't even have to display the exact fat content on the label. Mix ground turkey with regular ground beef to cut the fat.
  - **Poultry (chicken, turkey, and duck):** Some people eat so much poultry that they really

should cluck. And that's a good thing, because the white meat in poultry is high in protein, low in fat, and low in cholesterol. Remember to remove the skin (that's where most of the fat is) and stick to white meat, which has less fat than dark meat. Poultry contains about 0.5 grams of saturated fat and delivers a walloping 30 plus grams of protein per serving.

- **Fish:** Some fish is very low in saturated fats; most types of fish have less than 1 gram of saturated fat per serving. A few have 2 grams — salmon and tuna among them. Fish is a good source of protein as long as you don't fry it in saturated fat. Fish is also a good source of omega-3 fatty acids. The fish that's best for these fatty acids include salmon, tuna, trout, mackerel, and whitefish. Fish contains around 20 grams of protein per serving.

  Farm raised fish don't have the same amounts of omega-3 fatty acids and can have high levels of mercury.

- **Pork:** Pork has about the same amount of saturated fat (2 grams per serving) as lean beef, even when you trim the fat before eating. Although the pork industry is promoting it as the "other white meat," pork is higher in saturated fat than poultry and shouldn't be a nightly dinner choice. Pork has around 25 grams of protein per serving.

- **Lamb:** Lamb is also high in fat compared to poultry; in fact, it's slightly higher (3 grams per serving) than pork in saturated fat.

- **Eggs:** Eggs contain about 6.25 grams of protein and are only 75 calories. The egg white is only 17 calories. They have 3.5 grams of saturated fat, which is mostly contained in the yolk, but the yolk contains most of the amino acids and 40 percent of the protein.

✔ **Incomplete proteins:** These don't contain all essential amino acids. Incomplete proteins include

- **Dry beans:** Dry beans and lentils are excellent sources of protein, although you may not think of them as such. Beans contain around 7 grams of protein and lentils about 9 grams of protein per half cup and less than one gram of saturated fat. To obtain all the essential amino acids, you need to combine them with other sources of protein that contain the rest of the essential amino acids.

- **Nuts:** Nuts are a good source of protein, around 5 grams per serving, but are also high in saturated fats; a serving contains anywhere from 4 grams (almonds) to 16 grams (brazil nuts). Macadamia nuts are also high in saturated fats, about 12 grams per serving. Nuts are also an incomplete source of protein.

The added benefits of soy protein

What about soy? Soy products are everywhere, and you may have heard that soy is superior to animal protein and can lower cholesterol and reduce the risk of heart disease. Recent studies by the American Heart Association show that taking in 50 grams of soy protein a day (over half your daily requirement of protein) reduced LDL only about three percent, not a large amount but worth considering if you're fighting high cholesterol.

Choosing good carbs

Carbohydrates are an important part of your diet because they help supply the energy that your body needs to function. They are so important that the USDA recommends that half of your daily calorie intake should come from carbs. Carbohydrates fall into two categories:

- ✔ Simple, which contain refined sugars, with minimal fiber, vitamins, and minerals

- ✔ Complex, which contain more fiber, vitamins, and minerals

All carbohydrates are broken down and used for energy. The goal when choosing carbs is to chose complex carbs that increase energy storage at a slow, steady pace, to help control blood sugar levels. Sugars (simple carbs) are broken down most easily and cause a quick infusion of glucose (blood sugar) into your blood. This surge gives an immediate boost of energy, but it also causes blood sugar to drop rapidly and can leave you feeling weak.

Separating healthy carbs and unhealthy carbs: The glycemic index

Today, there's an increased emphasis on the glycemic index (GI) of foods. The glycemic index categorizes foods by how quickly they're broken down and enter the bloodstream and how high your blood sugar rises after eating them compared to pure glucose. Foods with a low glycemic index are considered most healthy. They're rated on a scale from 0-100, with the lower numbers being healthiest.

Sugars have a high glycemic index, while starches such as whole grains have a lower glycemic index and stabilize your blood sugar because they take longer to break down.

(Fibers can't be broken down in the body and pass through unchanged.) So starches like whole grains and vegetables with a low glycemic index are your best choice for carbohydrates. Processed foods like white bread are stripped of much of the fiber, vitamins, and minerals, and they have a higher glycemic index, making less processed food like whole grain bread a much healthier choice.

Assessing a food's carbohydrate makeup: Glycemic load

Just to complicate things, carbohydrates are further categorized by their *glycemic load* (GL), which takes into consideration the amount of carbohydrates consumed. Two items might be similar on the GI but your blood sugars and insulin response are affected differently if you eat a greater amount of one than the other, which is the GL. You determine the glycemic load by taking the GI, dividing by 100, then multiplying by the carbohydrate count in the food. For example:

1. **A cup of cooked spaghetti has a GI of 42.**
   42 ÷ by 100 = .42.

2. **A cup of cooked spaghetti contains 38 carbs (subtract fiber, if any, from the total carb count since it isn't digested).**
   .42 × 38 = 16. So 16 is the GL for a cup of cooked spaghetti.

For a list of common foods and their glycemic loads, see Table 7-1. The table helps you pick carbs with the lowest glycemic load per serving, anything below 10 is considered low, anything over 20 is considered high.

Table 7-1		The Glycemic Load of Common Foods		
Food Source	Glycemic Index	Serving Size	Carbs	Glycemic Load
Apples	38	1 medium	21	8
Bananas	51	1 large	26.5	14
Brown rice	55	1 cup boiled	42	18
Carrots	47	1 large	6	3
Grapefruit	25	1/2 large	11	3
Ice cream	61	1 cup	16	10
Lowfat yogurt	33	1 cup	47	16
Oatmeal	58	1 cup cooked	21	12
Oranges	48	1 medium	12	6
Peanuts	14	4 oz	15	2
Pizza	30	2 slices	42	13
Popcorn	72	2 cups popped	10	7
Potato chips	54	4 oz	55	30
Raisins	64	1 small box	32	20
Spaghetti	61	1 cup boiled	45	27
Watermelon	72	1 cup	11	8
White bread	70	1 slice	14	10
White rice	64	1 cup boiled	40	26

Fighting off the bad fats and getting enough of the good ones

You may be conditioned to think of fat as something bad to eat, but you need "good" fat in your diet for your body to function properly. You need fat to help with absorption of fat soluble vitamins, to regulate cholesterol metabolism, and to keep your skin soft and healthy.

Eating fat doesn't make you fat. Excess body fat comes from consuming too many calories (of any kind) that aren't used as energy but are stored away in the body as fat reserves.

Fat is either saturated or unsaturated:

✔ Saturated fat can be included in your diet, but should be limited due to the risks of elevated cholesterol.

✔ Unsaturated fat is good for you, lowering your LDL and raising your HDL.

High cholesterol can be related to heredity. Seventy-five percent of the cholesterol in your blood is manufactured in your liver; only 25 percent comes from what you eat. Reducing cholesterol rich foods can play a small part in reducing your cholesterol levels. Total cholesterol levels are optimal if under 200 milligram per deciliter; LDL should be less than 100 mg/dl, and HDL should be greater than 40 mg/dl.

Gathering near the good fats

Most people don't realize that fat plays a necessary role in their diet. The important thing is to make sure you have the right balance of good and bad fats. Healthy fats such as polyunsaturated and monounsaturated fats are beneficial to your body, but they need to be consumed in moderation.

You need healthy fats in your diet for the following vital reasons:

- ✔ To develop and maintain gray matter in your brain
- ✔ To achieve optimal growth
- ✔ To maintain the health and structure of cell membranes
- ✔ To keep skin healthy
- ✔ To maintain proper visual development
- ✔ To maintain a healthy nervous system
- ✔ To regulate blood pressure, blood clotting, and your body's inflammatory response

Experts don't always agree on exactly what percentage of your daily calories should come from fat. According to the World Health Organization (WHO) people should restrict dietary fat intake to 30 percent of daily calories, and according to the USDA, you *need* 30 percent of your daily calories from fats. The American Heart Association suggests 20 to 30 percent, while some experts believe that people may only need as little as 10 percent of calories in the form of fat.

You don't need to add a lot of extra fat to your diet; just make healthy food and cooking choices to get enough of the nutrients from the healthy fats you need.

Omega-3 fatty acids are one type of "good fat." There are many supplements that provide these fatty acids, because most people don't consume enough of the foods that contain omega-3s. Good sources of the omega-3 fatty acids are found in the following foods:

✔ Cold-water fish like mackerel, salmon, sardines, anchovies, and herring. The oils of wild-caught fish contain a significantly higher proportion of omega-3 than the oils of farm-raised fish.

✔ Nuts, such as walnuts, Brazil nuts, and almonds along with pumpkin, sunflower, and flax seeds

Saying no to the bad fats

Many foods nowadays have been processed and reformulated to create a variation of the original (think chicken nuggets or peanut butter). The same is true with fat. On the one hand, polyunsaturated fat is an essential fatty acid that's good for you; but on the other hand, saturated fats and trans fatty acids clog your arteries, raise your bad cholesterol, lower your good cholesterol, and — unfortunately! — taste scrumptious in donuts.

Saturated fats and trans fats are bad for your health for the following reasons:

✔ **Saturated fats** are usually solid at room temperature, and they're a major dietary factor in raising cholesterol. The main sources of saturated fat in the typical American diet are foods from animals and some plants. These sources include whole milk, butter, cheese, ice cream, red meat and dark meat, milk chocolate, coconuts, coconut milk, and coconut oil.

✔ **Trans fats** should be avoided altogether because they can raise your total LDL (bad) cholesterol *and* lower HDL (good) cholesterol, putting you at risk for high blood pressure and heart disease. Examples of trans fat include most margarines, vegetable shortening, partially hydrogenated vegetable oil, deep-fried anything, many fast foods, and most commercially baked goods.

According to the USDA, no more than 10 percent of your daily calories should come from saturated fats. There's no official recommendation from the USDA for trans fats percentage, so we recommend that if you eat them at all, you share your 10-percent allotment between the two.

Make sure to read your food labels and ask about trans fat when you dine out. But generally, some foods to avoid with saturated and trans fats include

- Butter
- Cookies
- Crackers
- Doughnuts
- French fries
- Fried foods (like fried chicken)
- Ice cream
- Margarine

According to a recent study of some 80,000 women, for every 5 percent increase in the amount of saturated fat a woman consumes, her risk of heart disease increases by 17 percent. But just a 2 percent increase in trans fats increases her risk of heart disease by 93 percent!

Positive Nutritional Habits for Healthy Living

Nutrition isn't just about food. Nutrition is the foundation for a strong immune system, disease prevention, and a healthy body. Nutrition offers multiple opportunities to improve health without a lot of effort. Boost your nutritional intake by purchasing organic foods, avoiding unhealthy food additives, and reducing salt.

Put down the salt shaker

Sodium causes *vasoconstriction,* which is the narrowing of blood vessels which decreases the amount of space through which blood can travel (think water through a fire hose). This increased resistance makes it more difficult for the arteries to expand with each beat of the heart, causing the internal pressure to rise.

A high sodium intake can raise your blood pressure, so hiding the salt shaker and avoiding processed foods may help lower your blood pressure. High sodium foods include processed meats, salted snack foods, cheeses, and canned foods. Also, many frozen dinners and canned soups are loaded with sodium.

Start reading food labels to help lower your sodium intake. Your body gets all the sodium it needs from a balanced healthy diet. If you miss the flavor of salt, try fresh herbs, which are full of essential vitamins and bursting with flavor. These herbs include oregano, cilantro, and basil.

Restricting sodium intake to lower blood pressure appears to work better if accompanied by increasing your potassium intake. Good dietary sources of potassium include bananas, potatoes, avocados, tomato juice, grapefruit juice, and acorn squash.

Make mine organic?

Organic foods are grown using farming techniques designed to reduce pollution, decrease use of pesticides, and conserve soil and water resources. These types of food are all the rage these days — even your local grocery store may have an organic section. Organic foods don't *look* any different from foods throughout the rest of the grocery, but the price tag is surely different. So should you shell out the extra bucks for expensive organic foods? Is *USDA Organic* just another designer label? We give you the answers in this section.

Organic foods have less exposure to pesticides, antibiotics used for growth, and chemical fertilizers — all of which certainly sound like they should lead to healthier food. But is it that much more healthy than what you've been eating for years?

Researchers debate the importance of the organic label based on the lack of substantial evidence supporting differences in quality or safety, but some studies show that organic produce contains more nutrients than traditionally grown products. Organic products are definitely exposed to fewer pesticides, additives, and preservatives. If you can find them and afford them, organic products are probably healthier for you.

Organic foods can be labeled in several different ways, and they're increasingly government regulated, so anyone who sells more than $5,000 a year worth of organic foods must be certified. Foods marked with the USDA Organic seal meet one of the first two criteria listed below:

- ✔ **100 percent organic:** Must be completely organic or made of organic products. USDA Organic seal approved.

- ✓ **Organic:** Products that are 95 percent organic. USDA Organic seal approved.

- ✓ **Made with organic ingredients:** Must contain at least 70 percent organic ingredients

The USDA requires that all the organic foods must follow these standard guidelines regardless of having a USDA organic stamp:

- ✓ Prohibit the use of irradiation, sewage sludge, or genetically modified organisms in production

- ✓ Reflect National Organic Standards Board (NOSB) recommendations concerning items on the national list of allowed synthetic and prohibited natural substances

- ✓ Prohibit antibiotics in organic meat and poultry

- ✓ Require 100 percent organic feed for organic livestock

Foods that are less than 70 percent organic can't be labeled as organic. Also, foods labeled "free range," "hormone free," or "natural" aren't certified organic. Because meat has to be completely free of any antibiotic exposure at all to be called organic, it's difficult to find truly organic meat.

Wash all organic fruits and vegetables before you eat them, just like commercially grown produce. One concern about organic food is that it could be more susceptible to bacterial contamination, although studies haven't confirmed this to be a definite risk.

Make sure you get enough H$_2$O

What could be simpler than water? Second only to air, this element is essential to your survival. You can go for almost two months without food but only a few days without water. In this section, we discuss why your body needs water, why you need more as your body ages, and how water can reduce health complications and stress on your body when you consume enough of it daily.

Consider these facts:

✔ More than two-thirds of the weight of the human body is water.

✔ The brain is 95 percent water.

✔ Your blood is 82 percent water.

✔ Your lungs are 90 percent water.

✔ Your muscles tissue contains 73 percent water.

Water is essential to regulate body temperature and transport oxygen to your cells as well as nutrients to your organs. Water also removes waste and protects your joints and organs. If you take in less or lose more fluid than you need, the end result is *dehydration,* the excessive loss of water from the body.

You need water to maintain the following:

✔ To replenish what's lost via perspiration and respiration (breathing)

✔ To flush toxins

✔ To keep your body's core temperature balanced

✔ To help keep blood circulating

You can, of course, be dehydrated if you've spent a long time in the heat, are running a fever, have severe diarrhea or vomiting, have exercised strenuously, or haven't been drinking at all. Serious effects of dehydration include hypotension (low blood pressure), heatstroke, urinary tract infections, nausea, dryness of the mouth and skin, vomiting, constipation, and reccurring headaches. Recent studies have also linked the lack of water to arthritis, kidney stones, and heartburn.

Most likely, if you're drinking 6 to 8 glasses of water a day, you're getting plenty of hydration. As you age, however, you may experience the following, which can lead to an increased need to stay hydrated:

- **The diminished thirst mechanism:** As you age you experience a reduction in your sensitivity to changes in fluid status in your body. Your brain doesn't tell you that you're thirsty. This factor significantly impairs your ability to maintain water level balance and increases your risk for dehydration.

- **Medications with a *diuretic* (a substance that increases the discharge of urine water):** As many people get older, they need medications that have a diuretic side effect. If you're on a medication like this, you may need to increase your fluid intake. Make sure to talk to your doctor before making any changes.

- **Changes in renal physiology and anatomy:** Due to a decreased size in kidneys, blood flow to the kidneys is restricted and the kidneys function more slowly.

So you don't necessarily need more water as you get older — you may just need to be more conscious of getting enough.

Deciding what to drink

Although water is the best source of replenishing your body's fluids, there are a variety of fluids you can drink that can still provide you with hydration to replace your body's daily fluid loss. There are several electrolyte drinks or drink mixes that work, but realize that they have more calories and can contain artificial sweeteners and other additives.

Common sense, though, says that taking in 64 ounces of a soft drink every day isn't going to do anything for your nutrition besides add a bunch of "empty" calories to your daily intake.

Staying well hydrated without wasting calories — or money — is pretty straightforward:

✔ Drink tap water, if yours is safe from bacteria and pollutants.

✔ Skip regular and diet sodas, which have no nutrition whatsoever. Regular soda is nothing but sugar and diet sodas contain artificial sweeteners.

✔ Substitute sugar laden 10 percent "real juice" types with real 100 percent fruit and vegetable juices.

✔ Eat more fruits and veggies, which have natural high-fluid content.

✔ Drink lowfat or skim milk and get your calcium and calories without the fat.

Avoid the unpronounceable: Chemical additives

If the labels on the food you eat have you shaking your head over the long list of unpronounceable ingredients, you're not alone! There are over 14,000 man-made chemicals added to the food supply today.

Food additives are *not* natural nutrition. Additives are used to preserve food's shelf life, add flavor, or make food look "pretty" by adding or enhancing color. They may also keep products like mayonnaise from separating, increase bulk, add a nice smell, or control acidity or alkalinity of certain foods.

Most additives aren't known to be harmful, but some such as food dyes and sulfites, are known allergens. Some additives, such as artificial sweeteners, have been linked to increasing the cravings for simple carbs and are commonly consumed by people over their ideal weight. A few of the most common additives and their possible effects are listed below:

- **Acesulfame K:** This additive, where the K stands for potassium, is one of three sugar substitutes (the other two are aspartame and saccharin) sold in packet or tablet form. It's used to sweeten chewing gum, baked goods, dry mixes for beverages, instant coffee and tea, gelatin desserts, puddings and non-dairy creamers, among other things. The drug is excreted without being absorbed.

- **Aspartame:** Equal, NutraSweet, and Canderel are just a few of the names that aspartame is marketed under. Aspartame is found in products worldwide and the list of foods is enormous. Some of the common products that you find it in are diet soft drinks, chewing gum, and as a packaged sweetener.

    Aspartame has been under public scrutiny for some time due to the suspicion of harmful side effects. In 1995, over 90 symptoms of health concerns were reported by medical professionals or consumers thought to be attached to aspartame.

Some studies have concluded adverse effects and some have not. With the emergence of other sweeteners like sucrolose and stevia, many folks just avoid aspartame, although the debate goes on.

✔ **Artificial coloring:** Coloring is found in everything from Cheetos to Popsicles. Artificial coloring (there are nine FDA certified color dyes) serves no purpose except to enhance the appearance of food. They're also blamed for an increase in hyperactivity in children and allergic reactions. But is the blame deserved?

Researchers at Columbia University and Harvard reviewed 15 previous studies and came to the conclusion that the claims of increased hyperactivity were inconclusive. On the other hand, occasional hives have been reported after exposure to Red 40 and Yellow 5 dyes. As with all artificial food products, limiting exposure is the best policy. It's not like most of the food colored with them have much, if any, nutritional value.

✔ **Caffeine:** This stimulant is found naturally in tea, coffee, and cocoa. It's also added to many soft drinks. It is one of the few drugs — a stimulant — added to foods. Caffeine promotes stomach-acid secretion, temporarily raises blood pressure, and dilates some blood vessels while constricting others. Caffeine is mildly addictive, which is why some people experience headaches when they stop drinking it. If you have high blood pressure or are at risk for heart disease, skip the caffeine.

✔ **Monosodium Glutamate (MSG):** MSG is used as a flavor enhancer in many foods, despite the fact that it has no flavor of its own. It may work by stimulating certain receptors in the tongue.

A *small* number of people may have a sensitivity reaction called MSG symptom complex after consuming 0.5 to 2.5 mg of MSG, especially on an empty stomach (a typical serving of MSG in food is less than 0.5 mg). A *small* percentage of asthmatics also experienced worsening asthma symptoms after the same dose. MSG symptom complex symptoms include headache, chest tightness, fast heartbeat, tingling, and burning and numbness of the face and upper extremities. If you're asthmatic or you've had an MSG reaction, avoiding MSG is probably a good idea. MSG is found in many foods and dishes, (including many Chinese dishes) so read labels.

✔ **Sodium nitrite and sodium nitrate:** These two closely related chemicals have been used for centuries to preserve meat and keep it from changing color when heated.

- *Sodium nitrite* provides some protection against botulism. The main concern with nitrites is that they can form a known animal carcinogen called nitrosomine when combined with gastric juices or during the process of frying. For this reason, ascorbic acid, which inhibits formation of nitrosomines, is added to processed meats. Our recommendation? Limit processed meats to one or two servings a week; they contain a lot of "bad" fat anyway. Nitrites have also been found to be triggers of migraines; migraine sufferers are often coached to stay away from processed meats for this reason.

- *Sodium nitrate* is used to preserve meat. When it's used, the bacteria converts the sodium nitrate into nitrite, which has the preserving benefits stated above. Sodium nitrate isn't often used and is replaced with sodium nitrite.

Most meat processors have stopped using sodium nitrate over concerns about its safety and have decreased the amount of nitrites used to cure meat over the last twenty years.

- **Saccharin:** This additive is 350 times sweeter than sugar and is used in tiny amounts in dietetic foods or as a tabletop sugar substitute. An epidemiology study done by the National Cancer Institute in the early 1970s found that a high dose of artificial sweeteners (saccharin and cyclamate) in rats was associated with an increased risk of bladder cancer and was listed as a possible carcinogen in 1981. Subsequent studies didn't show a connection, and in 2000 saccharin was removed from the National Toxicology Program's report as a carcinogen.

  Occasional use of artificial sweeteners can help curb your sweet tooth, but in the long run, anything made out of chemicals shouldn't be part of your regular diet.

- **Sulfites:** These additives are used to prevent discoloration in fruits and veggies; they also keep bacterial growth and fermentation under control in wine and aid in food preservation. Some people — possibly as many as one in a hundred — are sensitive or allergic to sulfites and may have a reaction that can range from a mile headache to life threatening breathing problems. Allergies and serious reactions are more common in asthmatics. Sulfites are no longer allowed to be used on most fresh fruits and vegetables, but they're found in a number of processed foods, including beer, wine, dried fruits,

Curbing unhealthy cravings

Have you ever felt like you just HAD to have a chocolate bar or an order of salt and vinegar potato chips? You weren't really hungry, you were just craving a certain something. No? Lucky you! One survey showed that almost 100 percent of women and nearly 70 percent of men have had food cravings during the last year. A history of food craving is associated with excessive snacking and poor diet compliance.

A study done at the University of Pennsylvania showed that food cravings activate three regions of the brain associated with emotion, memory, and reward, so cravings may really be "all in your head." What this means is that cravings are related to your emotional state and your memories of how certain foods made you "feel" rather than to a need for a specific food or a dietary lack.

For most people, occasional cravings are harmless and won't wreck an otherwise nutritionally sound diet. But if your cravings are a daily (or hourly!) event, the following suggestions may help:

- **Eat something every few hours.** Letting yourself get hungry not only leads to eating "whatever's handy" but also allows you time to "think" about the foods you want, which can activate cravings for them.

- **Give in to your cravings once in a while.** Cravings don't go away when you're dieting (what a shocker, eh?) so plan to "give in" occasionally. Diet plans like Weight Watchers allow for this by giving you "anytime" points for when a craving hits or when you want to have a big meal or dessert.

- **Find better ways to handle stress.** According to a study done by University of California, San Francisco, food craving may be the body's way of calming chronic stress.

So other ways of combating stress, such as biofeedback, relaxation techniques, and journaling, will result in fewer pounds gained and healthier stress management techniques perfected.

✔ **Choose lower calorie substitutes that satisfy cravings without wrecking your diet plan.** Figuring out how to suppress food cravings is an important part of long-term weight loss success, so it's good to be prepared for cravings.

baked goods, and canned vegetables. Look on food labels for indications that the product contains sulfites: sulfur dioxide, potassium bisulfate, sodium bisulfate.

Reading Food Labels

Food labels have moved way outside the supermarket; everything from fast food to restaurant menus these days contains nutritional breakdowns of calorie count, percentages of protein, carbs and fat, calcium and iron recommended daily allowance (RDA) percentages, and much more in grams, milligrams, or percentages. There's no excuse today for not knowing what you're eating!

While food labels are a great source of info, and sometimes even more than you want to know, they do have some caveats. For one thing, the percentages of RDA are based on a 2,000 calorie a day diet, with 60 percent of calories coming from carbohydrates, ten percent from protein, and thirty percent from fat, based on the average nutritional needs of a 170 pound man. If you're not a 170 pound man, but a 100 pound woman, the RDA percentage of, say, fat, contained in a food may not be accurate for you. If a candy bar (just to use a bad example) contains 30 percentage of the "RDA" of fat, it may actually be more like 50 percent of *your* RDA of fat. If you're on a diet higher in protein, or lower in carbs, these percentages won't apply to you, either. So read labels with a grain of — dare we say? — salt when it comes to the exact percentage, unless, of course, you're a 170 pound man on a diet composed of 60 percent carbs.

By law, all food labels contain the following information:

- ✔ **Serving size:** The most important thing to remember is that the serving size may not be the whole box, bag, or container. This fact may be obvious when you're looking at a 20 ounce bag of chips and not so obvious with a two-ounce bag. But if you're eating the entire bag thinking you're taking in 200 calories, and then notice there are two servings in a bag, you've just eaten twice as many calories as you intended.

- ✔ **Servings per container or package:** This information states the number of servings in the package. Don't forget — check this info *before* you start eating!

- ✔ **Calories and Calories from Fat:** The calorie content is important because excess intake can lead to weight gain. And the calories-from-fat number is crucial to help you limit fat intake, especially saturated and trans fats. Ideally the calories from fat should equal no more than 30 percent of the total number of calories in a serving. For example 2 tablespoons of peanut butter has about 210 calories and 16 grams of fat. That means 69 percent of the calories come from fat.

- ✔ **% Daily Value:** This information compares the contents of the product to the RDA based on a 2,000-calorie diet. These numbers help you judge whether the food has enough or too much of the nutrients you need. For example, a box of macaroni and cheese (prepared) has 48 grams of carbohydrates, which is 16 percent of the RDA.

- ✔ **Total Fat, Carbohydrates, Protein; Cholesterol, Sodium:** This part of the label lists several important numbers. The label identifies the specific types of fat in the product (unsaturated, saturated, and trans fat) and their amounts. No more than 10 percent of your total 30 percent daily allowance of fat should come from saturated fats or trans fats. This label also helps if you're trying to track your carb and protein intake, your daily sodium intake, or if you're trying to cut down on cholesterol.

- ✔ **Vitamins and Minerals:** Percentages of RDA will also be listed on the food label, although it may be way too small for you to read without a magnifying glass!

Chapter 8

Supplementing Your Daily Diet

In This Chapter

▶ Choosing vitamins and minerals for your needs
▶ Understanding the forms and delivery systems of supplements
▶ Considering the importance of *probiotics*
▶ Checking out the natural values of herbs

As you get older, you may think that you need to take some vitamins or supplements. You may have heard that some supplements help with memory loss, or others give you the stamina of a 20 year old. But do you really need to take dietary supplements to get the vitamins, minerals, and other nutrients that you need? The answer is possibly, especially if your diet, like many people's, is heavy on the processed and fast foods and light on fruits and vegetables, or if you just want to make sure you're getting all the nutrients you need, especially as you get older.

In this chapter, we explain why nutrient supplements may be vital to your health, and how to find the best ones, because all supplements aren't created equal. We also look at the side effects of some supplements, their interactions with certain medications, and why it's not a good idea to take supplements without discussing them with your doctor first. We also probe the preventative properties of *probiotics,* the good bacteria, and how you can incorporate them into your diet.

Nutritional supplements can *never* take the place of food and should never be used as a replacement for a healthy diet. Use supplements as just that — a supplement to an already healthy diet and notify your physician any time you begin taking a new supplement.

Knowing Which Vitamins and Minerals You Need (and How Much)

Vitamins and minerals are both micronutrients (substances that the body requires only in small quantities), found in many of the foods you eat, but these small nutritional powerhouses are important for many essential reactions in the body. You need vitamins and minerals for growth and development, particularly with vision, muscles, blood cells, teeth, and bones. Vitamins and minerals sound pretty similar, but they're very different; in this section, we look at vitamins first.

Vitamins

Vitamins are *organic,* which means that they come from plants and animals; they're found in food but can also be obtained from supplements. Vitamins fall into two categories:

✔ **Water soluble:** With these vitamins, excess amounts are washed out in your body fluids. You need to take in adequate amounts of water-soluble vitamins every day because your body doesn't store them.

- **Fat soluble:** These vitamins are stored in the body's fat tissue and liver for a few days to several months to be used when needed.

Be careful not to overdo fat-soluble vitamins, because large amounts can be harmful if they build up in your tissues, leading to *hypervitaminosis* (excess vitamins in the body with potentially dangerous toxicity). There's no definitive level of vitamin intake that will absolutely lead to toxic levels, so it's very important to stick to the recommended guidelines for fat-soluble vitamin intake.

You don't need to read the tiny print on the multivitamin bottle to know what the daily dosages of different vitamins should be. To make it easy, the FDA has created a handy table of the recommended daily allowance (RDA) of the most common vitamins — see Table 8-1.

Table 8-1	Daily Vitamin Needs		
Vitamin	*Category*	*Amount Needed*	*Benefit(s)*
Vitamin A	Fat soluble	10,000 IU	Helps regulate immune system; protects vision; helps maintain skin
Vitamin B1 (thiamine)	Water soluble	50 mg	Helps regulate nervous system; helps glucose metabolism
Vitamin B2 (riboflavin)	Water soluble	50 mg	Helps maintain skin; helps process proteins, carbs, and fats

Vitamin	Category	Amount Needed	Benefit(s)
Vitamin B3 (niacin, niacinamide)	Water soluble	100 mg	Helps maintain skin, and nervous system, digestion; helps process protein, carbs, and fats
Vitamin B5 (pantothenic acid)	Water soluble	100 mg	Helps make red blood cells
Vitamin B6 (pyridoxine)	Water soluble	50 mg	Helps make red blood cells; helps maintain immune and nervous systems
Vitamin B12	Water soluble	300 mcg	Helps maintain red blood cells and nerve cells; helps make DNA
Biotin (part of B complex)	Water soluble	300 mcg	Helps synthesize amino acids and fatty acids
Folic acid	Water soluble	800 mcg	Protects from neural tube defects
Vitamin C with mineral ascorbates	Water soluble	3,000 mg	Helps regulate immune system; helps form connective tissue

Vitamin	Category	Amount Needed	Benefit(s)
Vitamin D	Fat soluble	400 IU	Helps absorb calcium and phosphorus; essential for bones
Vitamin E	Fat soluble	600 IU	Helps with immune function and DNA repair
Vitamin K	Fat soluble	100 mcg	Helps make blood-clotting factors

IU = international unit; mg = milligram; mcg = microgram

Minerals

Minerals differ from vitamins in that, unlike vitamins, the body can't make any minerals. Your body relies completely on external sources, like food and supplements, for your minerals. In addition, minerals are *inorganic,* which means that they come from the soil and water that animals and plants ingest. (Or absorb, in the case of plants.) Some minerals are routinely added to certain foods; the iodine added to salt is one example. See Table 8-2 for your daily mineral needs.

Not all minerals are beneficial. Some minerals, like lead, are contaminant minerals and not nutrients; they can cause harm by disrupting rather than helping normal body functions.

Table 8-2	Daily Mineral Needs	
Mineral	*Amount Needed*	*Benefit(s)*
Calcium	1,500 mg	Essential for building strong bones and teeth
Chromium (GTF)	150 mcg	Regulates the breakdown of sugar and carbohydrates
Cobalt	3 to 25 mcg	Helps with red blood cell formation
Copper	3 mg	Help forms hemoglobin, the oxygen-carrying component of a red blood cell
Fluoride	1.5 mg	Strengthens teeth and bones
Iodine (kelp is a good source)	225 mcg	Regulates the thyroid
Iron	18 mg	Stimulates a healthy immune system
Magnesium	750–1,000 mg	Helps facilitate muscle and nerve function and has a role in regulating your heart beat
Manganese	10 mg	Fights cancer cells
Molybdenum	30 mcg	Synthesizes protein for a healthy nervous system
Potassium	99 mg	Helps maintain a normal fluid balance between cells and body fluids
Selenium	200 mcg	Destroys free radicals with vitamin E

Mineral	Amount Needed	Benefit(s)
Sulfur	There's no RDA, but 850 mg is thought to be the basic need and is obtained mostly in the amino acids methionine, taurine, cystine, and cysteine	Possesses antibiotic capabilities and immune system support
Zinc	50 mg	Helps heal wounds by producing white blood cells

mg = milligram; mcg = microgram

Deciding Whether You Need to Supplement Your Diet

If you're looking to get the best nutritional bang for your buck, get your vitamins and minerals from food rather than pills, because more nutrients are absorbed from food than from supplements. From a nutritional standpoint, if you eat a well-balanced, healthy diet, you won't need much, if anything, in the area of supplements (see Chapter 7 for more information on a healthy diet). Supplements should never be used as meal replacement and need only be used if your diet is deficient.

At certain times in your life, supplementation is a good idea — some medical conditions can benefit from adding vitamin and mineral supplements. Folic acid for women who are pregnant or thinking of pregnancy has been shown to reduce neural tube defects (a birth defect involving the brain and/or spinal cord). Vegetarians should consider taking vitamin B12, vitamin D, calcium, and iron, which are found predominantly in meat and dairy products. In the next sections, we look at factors that can help you decide whether or not to supplement your diet.

Taking stock of your lifestyle

If you have the food pyramid shellacked onto the front of your refrigerator and follow it religiously every day, you probably get all the essential nutrients you need. People who grow their own vegetables, buy all their fruit at a local stand, raise their own free-range chickens, and have never been inside a fast food restaurant probably don't need to take vitamin supplements. However, this doesn't apply to most people today; research shows that people in the industrialized world eat fast food twice a week and that one-third of American children may eat fast food daily.

The problem with fast foods (including the frozen kind, the shelved kind, and the drive-up kind) is that most of them have been processed in some way in order to preserve them for longer shelf life, or to make them taste better. True, processing is good in some ways: It allows food to be kept longer without spoiling, kills dangerous bacteria like salmonella, and lets you eat fruits and vegetables out of season. Food processing additives also make food taste better by adding salt and flavor enhancers. The caveat? The price you pay for stronger flavors includes more salt and unhealthy fats, not to mention that processing strips food of essential nutrients. Even cooking is considered a form of food processing that can disturb the balance of nutrients because exposure to high temperatures, light, and oxygen causes the greatest amount of nutrient loss.

One way to avoid processed food is to eat more raw foods. It would be wonderful, nutritionally speaking, if more people jumped on this bandwagon, but many folks

Vitamins and minerals in the news

Some vitamins and minerals get more press than others. Here are a few related to aging that have been in the news recently and the latest findings about their use:

- ✔ **Vitamin E:** Vitamin E has drawn some bad press lately. Long touted as an antioxidant that boosted the immune system and protected against cardiac disease, vitamin E took a hit when a recent research project done at Johns Hopkins University showed that people who took vitamin E in amounts larger than 400 IU daily were more likely to die of any cause than people who didn't. With this new information, vitamin E supplements are no longer recommended.

- ✔ **Vitamin D:** Recently, a number of reports say that people who live in climates where sun exposure is limited for a good part of the year have serious vitamin D deficiencies. If you live in a cold climate, vitamin D supplementation should be part of your daily intake, especially as you get older; vitamin D is essential for strong bones and aids in calcium absorption.

- ✔ **Vitamin A:** Vitamin A has been in the news lately for two reasons; some studies have shown that one form of vitamin A, retinol, may increase the risk of osteoporosis in high doses (over 5,000 IU). You should look for a multivitamin where the dose of vitamin A is less than 2,500 IU, or one where half of the vitamin A present comes from the second form of vitamin A, beta carotene.

  However, beta carotene also has risk factors. Some studies have indicated that beta carotene may increase the chance of developing lung cancer in smokers and should be avoided. If you smoke, choose a vitamin with less than 2,500 IU of retinol and no beta carotene.

✔ **Calcium:** Your body contains more calcium than any other mineral, and 99 percent of your calcium is found in your teeth and bones. Calcium is essential for good bone density. It's impossible to get enough calcium from a daily multivitamin; you need between 1,000–1,200 mg daily, and a multivitamin containing that much calcium would be too big to swallow. Your body also can absorb only about 500 mg of calcium at one time, so you need to take supplements preferably three times a day, with food, to get maximum absorption.

✔ **Iron:** After age 50, you should take a supplement that doesn't contain any iron, because after menopause, women are no longer losing blood on a monthly basis (which can lower your iron count), and most men get enough iron from their diet. Too much iron can be harmful because the body doesn't excrete much iron; toxic levels can occur when iron accumulates. Take iron only if your physician prescribes it; iron supplements should be kept out of the reach of children because death can occur with small ingestions.

✔ **AREDs vitamin preparations:** Age-related eye disease (ARED) vitamin preparations are recommended for people with age-related macular degeneration (AMD) or those with a family history of the disease. Studies found that the ARED preparations reduced the incidence of developing AMD by around 25 percent.

There are two ARED formulas: one contains beta carotene, the other doesn't. Smokers should take the formulary without beta carotene. Other ingredients in the ARED formulas are zinc, vitamin E, vitamin A, and copper.

don't care for raw vegetables unadorned with butter or salt and don't want to take the time to wash and peel fresh fruits and veggies. Many have chosen to replace the nutrient loss with vitamin and mineral supplements, which we strongly advise against. The *best* source of vitamins and minerals is still from foods; however, getting vitamins indirectly is still better than not getting them at all.

So what's a person to do? Our suggestion is to adhere to a healthy diet and take supplemental vitamins or minerals only if you really need them. The bottom line is that if you're eating a well-balanced diet and have no medical conditions that may be affecting your nutritional balance, you can save some money by not taking extra vitamins that your body doesn't need. However, if you eat mainly processed foods or absolutely can't eat the recommended intake of fresh fruits and vegetables (see Chapter 7), and if you do have medical conditions that affect your body's ability to absorb nutrients, you may want to take nutritional supplements. Also consider your habits; if you smoke or consume alcohol, you may want to take supplements, because tobacco and alcohol have been found to affect nutrient absorption of vitamin C, B1, zinc, and iron. Talk to your doctor if you feel that a supplement may be the right choice for you.

Getting your doctor involved

Sometimes, supplementation isn't beneficial and could be harmful, particularly if you have existing medical conditions or are taking prescription or over-the-counter medications. (Vitamins can interfere with some medications and can have toxic effects if taken in too-large of quantities; too much chromium piccolinate, for example, can result in kidney failure, according to some reports.) Therefore, you should always discuss your interest in supplements with your doctor to make sure that nothing in your medical history makes taking certain supplements unwise for you.

Many supplements are available on the market and new ones always pop up on the horizon, but most people simply look for a quality daily vitamin. A well-balanced multivitamin is a sensible choice when you're not sure exactly what your body needs — it may not be sufficient, though, if you have specific deficiencies. Some multivitamins contain some vitamins with higher strengths. Some supplements are manufactured and marketed for specific groups categorized by age, gender, and medical conditions. Your doctor should help guide you toward supplements that may benefit any medical conditions you have or be appropriate for your age and gender. Basically, a 25-year-old male needs a different supplement list than a 55-year-old female with killer hot flashes!

Another important consideration is the brand and form (liquid, capsule, or pill) of supplement you'll take. You can choose from many brands of supplements, and not all are created equally; your doctor can help you navigate the vitamin-laden shelves.

The Absorption Factor: Comparing Supplements

What's in *your* waste treatment plant? It seems that one of the things that's "left behind", so to speak, is remnants of undigested pill casings, tablet fillers, and binders from the medications and supplements people ingest. So how much of your expensive supplement is actually ending up in the toilet? While it's a lot simpler to just grab the nearest inexpensive bottle of vitamins off the shelf or maybe the ones with the prettiest label, it's not the smartest way to choose your supplement. In the world of vitamins, marketing ploys

Poor soil quality, poor food (and nutrient) quality?

Depending on which journals or magazine articles you read, the soil food is grown in is becoming depleted. Despite persuasive arguments and studies on both sides, no certain proof exists that food today is less nutritious than what was grown 100 years ago, though some researchers claim otherwise.

Most plants grow by absorbing nutrients from the soil. Soil quality is important and is the foundation for the development of nutritious produce. Depending on where in the world the soil is located, fertile soil contains some combination of sand, silt, clay, and organic matter. The consistency of a soil (soil texture) and its acidity (pH) determine the extent to which nutrients are available to plants.

Studies of forests in New England have shown a decrease in calcium and magnesium in the soil on the forest floor, most likely due to acid rain. Other potential culprits for soil depletion are the overuse of fertilizers and overfarming without letting the land recover between crops.

At this point, it's hard to say whether this problem is serious; many studies are being conducted to either verify or deny allegations that food isn't as nutritious today as it once was. Taking supplements may give you peace of mind about what your food may be missing.

of supplements promise to be the next big medical breakthrough, but make sure that you take time to become an educated consumer.

It may be helpful to know a few terms and basic components of supplement manufacturing before you start digging through the rows of bottles in the health food store. If you settle for a supplement that doesn't supply exactly what you need in the way you need it, not only will it fail to benefit your health, but it will also be a waste of money. Understanding the different ways that supplements are manufactured and designed to deliver the vitamins and minerals helps you make more educated decisions when looking to purchase.

The importance of supplement form

Clearly, you can't sit at home and receive all your nutritional needs from an IV hung overhead while watching your favorite TV show — at least, not yet! You need to choose between liquids, capsules, or tablets. Learning how supplements are made and what maximizes absorption can help you choose.

Vitamin supplements come in many forms. Fortunately, discovering new or improved methods of getting vitamins into your cells quickly is a vital goal of nutritional manufacturing companies, and those methods largely relate to form. The term for this characteristic is *bioavailability*, which is the rate at which a substance is absorbed and made available to your body. It's affected by how quickly a supplement dissolves and is absorbed in the gastrointestinal system (mostly the stomach and small intestine); substances that need to be broken down the least are absorbed fastest.

Here are some key factors to keep in mind regarding supplement forms:

- **Tablets:** This form is the most common one. According to the Physicians Desk Reference, only about 3 to 10 percent of the vitamins in pill or tablet form actually make it throughout your body and enter the bloodstream. Tablets have the slowest rate of bioavailability.

- **Capsules:** Capsules are coated with a substance that makes them easier to swallow than traditional tablets.

297

Gel-form capsules also digest more quickly than powder-form capsules, and in general, capsules have a better bioavailability than tablets but less than liquids.

✔ **Liquid:** Liquids are quickly absorbed into your bloodstream because they don't have to be broken down — and they're much easier to swallow! As such, they have the fastest rate of bioavailability of all the over-the-counter forms.

The differences among brands

Should you care which supplement you spend your money on? After all, tossing the closest supplement in your shopping cart is easier than reading the labels to make sure that you're getting your money's worth. And isn't the government looking after you by regulating all the supplements on the shelf?

If you aren't familiar with the actual regulations that control supplement production — and not too many people are — you can get to know them (see the nearby sidebar "The Dietary Supplement Health and Education Act of 1994 (DSHEA)" to find out what those regulations are). Supplements don't have to meet the same high standards that food and conventional medications do, although this regulation is changing and becoming more stringent.

Unfortunately, you'll rarely find a supplement that is simply the intended active ingredient without the addition of some inactive substances that help mold the supplement to the right size, shape, and color and aid in its dissolving. Some of the added substances can also negatively affect the way you digest and absorb the supplements. Consider the following:

✔ **Filler:** One area where supplements differ greatly is in the filler they use. Some filler is necessary to take up space, but fillers are nothing more for the supplement than volume. However, some fillers are better than others for absorption, and some companies use more filler than needed to give the appearance of a larger quantity.

- ✓ **Disintegrant:** Disintegrants help dissolve a tablet after you swallow it. Some of the popular disintegrants are gellan gum, crospovidone, and croscarmellose sodium.

- ✓ **Binder:** In tablets, binders are mixed with fillers to stick to the components of the tablet during compression. Some common binders are starch, cellulose, povidone, and xanthan gum.

- ✓ **Flavor:** Flavoring is added to add a pleasant taste — or to disguise a bad taste! A few other things you can do without are added sugar, salt, or starch — a vitamin isn't something you're having for lunch!

- ✓ **Colorant:** Colors are added to tablets to make telling them apart easier and so that they look more appealing. One thing you absolutely, positively have no use for in a multivitamin or supplement is artificial coloring. Vitamins don't need to be pretty to be effective.

To ensure that you're taking a supplement of the highest quality, look for a USP (United States Pharmacopoeia) or BP (British Pharmacopoeia) designation on the label.

To make things easier on you, Web sites such as www.consumerlab.com have tested supplements and can provide you with lists of the ones that don't contain the amounts of the ingredients that they claim to have or those that have too many fillers or binders to be beneficial.

Nutraceuticals: The future form of supplements?

The development of high-standard nutraceuticals is an exciting and evolving field focused on providing nutrients with proven medical benefits with better concentrations and absorption rates. But what are nutraceuticals?

According to the FDA, a nutraceutical is any substance that has additional medical or health benefits beyond general nutrition and can include vitamins, minerals, herbs, foods, and supplements. This broad definition leaves much room for interpretation and confusion, and many products may call themselves nutraceuticals, but they don't really fit the bill. Nutraceuticals can be pills, capsules, liquids, juice, or just about any form that combines a food product with a medical benefit. Many supplements are also nutraceuticals, but many are not. The key to nutraceuticals is that research-supported proof shows that they have medical benefit.

Nutraceuticals aim to counteract the effects of stress and free radicals by boosting your body's immune system and reducing specific health risks. Research has proven that you can slow down various components of early aging by using the right combination of vitamins, minerals, and antioxidants contained in nutraceuticals.

Furthermore, with insurance premiums continuing to rise, the uninsured population will increase, leaving a large portion of consumers looking for ways to improve health and decrease the potential for costly medical care. As the quest for good health continues, pharmaceutical-grade supplements are becoming more mainstream and highly popular because they provide people with what they're looking for — the right nutrients that the body can readily absorb and utilize quickly in a delivery system with minimal wasted product through poor digestion and absorption.

Currently, nutraceuticals aren't required to follow pharmaceutical-grade standards because of their dietary supplement classification. Nutraceutical manufacturers are required to adhere only to the regulations set forth under the Dietary Supplement Health and Education Act. Despite having few regulations, some of the nutraceutical companies are setting high standards for quality products. However, as a result of less stringent requirement practices of dietary supplement manufacturers, some nutraceutical manufacturers have made exaggerated or false claims (as always, if it sounds too good to be true, it probably is). However, there are reputable manufacturers of quality nutraceutical products available. Eniva Corporation is one of the companies setting the pace for standards and quality in the nutraceutical industry with a long line of products including their best seller, VIBE. Amerisciences is another company with a full range of products and, along with Eniva, uses manufacturing standards as high as many pharmaceutical companies in their product development and research. Other supplement companies will be looking to improve their standards and even major pharmaceutical companies have been looking to get into the arena of nutraceuticals due to consumer demand.

Warning: Nutraceuticals, like all supplements, need to be treated as medicine, because they could interact with some prescription medications, or even other nutraceutical products. Discuss with your doctor before you take any nutraceutical products.

Adding a Pinch of Good Bacteria: Probiotics

Bacteria aren't always a bad thing. Although you may associate bacteria with infections, your intestines play host to a number of bacteria considered to be "good" or even necessary. Probiotics (the name comes from a Greek word meaning *for life*) are good bacteria that help keep the body in proper balance. Good bacteria in the intestines carry out a number of functions:

- Assist in breaking down food so you can absorb the nutrients

- Help maintain proper pH levels in your body

- Create antibodies that help support your immune system

Problems occur when the bad bacteria start to take over, overwhelming the good bacteria. The resulting imbalance can cause symptoms such as intestinal distress (excessive gas, bloating, and constipation), urinary tract infections, or yeast infections for women.

The most common and well-known cause of bad bacteria overgrowth is the use of antibiotics; many women are familiar with the yeast infections that result when they take antibiotics. Diseases like Crohn's disease and diverticulosis, which slow muscular activity in the intestine, also allow bad bacteria to multiply.

It's also possible that parasites, mold, viruses, chlorinated drinking water, alcohol, and a high-sugar intake can contribute to bacterial overgrowth. One way to correct the problem is to get more good bacteria into your intestines by consuming probiotics.

The importance and function of probiotics

Clinical studies have shown that probiotic supplements improve your ability to fight off intestinal infections and also help you digest your food better. But those aren't the only positive effects probiotics can have. For example, probiotics

- **Aid in digestion and absorption:** Probiotics are necessary for manufacturing the B vitamins, biotin, and folic acid, which aid in food absorption, as well as antioxidants and iron from your diet. They remove the harmful toxins you ingest in your foods (like pesticides) and assist in the removal of digestive waste products.

✔ **Slow down the growth of bad bacteria that cause upset stomach:** When bad bacteria multiplies in the intestines, things get "backed up" causing gas, bloating, diarrhea, and constipation, and nutrient absorption is inhibited. Taking probiotics can help restore the balance of your intestinal tract and calm down "tummy troubles" and traveler's diarrhea.

✔ **Reduce food intolerance:** Probiotics can help you digest lactose or gluten if you're lactose or gluten intolerant.

✔ **Stimulate the immune system:** Probiotics produce natural antibiotics, which can help fight off harmful bacteria such as salmonella, E. coli, and shigella.

✔ **Support urinary tract health:** Women are more susceptible than men to contracting urinary tract infections (UTIs). Because a woman's urethra is much shorter than a man's, the bacteria has a much shorter distance to travel to cause an infection. A UTI or *cystitis* occurs when bacteria coming from normal intestinal flora makes its way into the bladder. Replenishing the intestines with probiotics helps restore the balance.

✔ **Support vaginal health:** The vagina and its normal, healthy microflora (*microbiota*) form a finely balanced ecosystem. Disruption of this ecosystem can lead to *bacterial vaginosis* (BV, an overgrowth of bacteria or yeast that causes unwanted symptoms,

Getting a personalized multivitamin

If you're looking for something designed for your specific needs, ask your doctor about a growing trend in personalized healthcare called *individual vitamin compounding.* In this process, your doctor takes blood or hair samples and sends them to a lab for analysis. The generated report tells you exactly what your body needs, detailing your vitamin and mineral deficiencies as well as any you have in abundance. Your doctor takes this information, and in conjunction with a compounding pharmacy or supplement manufacturer, provides you with an individually prepared supplement with the vitamins and mineral quantities tailored to your body's specific needs.

This type is more expensive than your off-the-shelf-brands, but it can be *less* expensive than taking several different vitamins. If you want something tailored specifically to your needs, neither too much nor too little of certain nutrients, it's well worth it. Insurance companies still haven't cooperated in helping out with vitamin supplements, but don't let them dictate your health. Hopefully insurance companies will eventually agree that choosing a supplement based on deficiencies should be classified as a medical need.

such as vaginal itching, a fishy odor, discharge, and discomfort), which is one of the most common vaginal infections. Replenishing the vagina with probiotics helps restore the balance.

The two main probiotics (and where to get them)

The two primary types of bacteria — *lactobacilli* and *bifidobacteria* — help maintain a healthy balance of intestinal flora:

- **Lactobacillus:** This bacteria breaks down protein, carbohydrates, and fats in your food. In the process, it produces lactic acid. Many forms of bacteria and yeast (like Candida albicans) don't get along well with lactic acid. Lactobacillus maintains the ratio of good to bad bacteria by creating its own antibiotics (acidophilin, lactocidin, and acidolin) to keep toxic bacteria — such as E. coli, Helicobacter pylori, and clostridia — at bay.

  Lactobacillus also produces B vitamins and butyric acid, which help you absorb nutrients from food, and is especially helpful in absorbing lactose products. Most of all, lactobacillus reduces your chances of developing diarrhea, constipation, gas, and bloating.

- **Bifidobacteria:** This probiotic is the most common probiotic in the large intestine. Often called bifidus, bifidobacteria aids in digestion, fights infection, reduces severe diarrhea commonly associated with rotavirus, and is associated with a lower incidence of allergies. These bacteria are also important in the production of B vitamins.

These two primary bacteria have several forms, and you can find the most common ones in the following foods:

- **Sweet acidophilus milk:** Sweet acidophilus milk has lactobacillus acidophilus added but isn't fermented, so it doesn't have the acidity and flavor people associated with fermented products.

- **Fermented yogurt:** Yogurt is a semi-solid fermented milk product that must be marked as made with live cultures to be considered probiotic. Fermented yogurt is also made into drinks.

- ✔ **Miso soup:** Use warm water only, because boiling water can destroy the good bacteria.

- ✔ **Pickles:** Must be naturally fermented without vinegar.

- ✔ **Sauerkraut:** Must be raw, non-pasteurized, not canned; no vinegar used in processing.

In addition to finding probiotics in food, you can purchase supplements over the counter in most health food stores, pharmacies, and grocery stores. They come in a variety of forms, including capsules, liquids, and tablets. Preparations made specifically for infants and children contain targeted bacteria at lower counts. If manufactured carefully and stored properly, probiotic bacteria can remain viable in dried format and reach your intestines alive when you consume them.

One criticism of probiotics sold over the counter is that they may not contain enough bacteria to actually do any good, so always look for the supplement with the highest number of bacteria. According to one study, a minimum of one billion live cells of lactic acid bacteria is required to do any good, and the product shouldn't require refrigeration, because refrigerated products may not be stable at room temperature.

People who take immunosuppressive medication should *not* take probiotics, because they may cause serious infection in the immunosuppressed.

306

Using Herbs and Plants for Health and Healing

Hundreds of years before you picked up your medications at the local drive-through pharmacy, people were trying herbs and other plants as cures for various illnesses. Many medicines had their basis in plants, and here are a few:

- ✔ **Foxglove plant:** This plant is the origin of digitalis, which is used to treat heart conditions.

- ✔ **Aloe vera:** This plant is an ingredient found in many ointments today and has anesthetic, antibacterial, and anti-inflammatory properties.

- ✔ **Rosemary:** This herb can increase circulation, relieve headaches, and help fight infections.

Herbal products available today still may use the leaves, flowers, stems, berries, and roots of plants to prevent and treat illness. However, while some herbs may have restorative properties, many can be downright dangerous if you mix them with prescription medications. One known interaction between herbs and prescription medicine occurs with birth control pills. Some of the herbs to avoid while using birth control include chasteberry, red clover, black cohosh, St. John's wort, licorice, hops, dong quai, and wild yam. Most of these herbs contain natural estrogens that can interfere with the body's hormonal regulation and therefore with birth control pills. Discuss with your doctor all the herbs that you're taking or planning to take so that any potential interactions can be addressed.

The FDA regulations for dietary supplements (including herbal remedies) are much different from the regulations of prescription meds. Although many of today's prescriptions contain botanicals (plant life), they're synthesized in large laboratories, and they adhere to standards and guidelines specifically designed for pharmaceutical manufacturing. This lack of regulation explains why the same herbal remedy from one manufacturer may not have the same effect as one produced by another.

Table 8-3 provides a list of common useful herbs, benefits, dosage, and cautions or interactions you must heed if you're taking any medications.

Table 8-3	Common Herbs that Ease Aging Woes		
Herb	*Benefits*	*Dosage*	*Cautions/ Interactions*
Arnica	Anti-inflammatory; can be used to reduce bruising and aches, and helps heal wounds	Used only topically as a gel or cream to be applied as needed	External use only; poisonous if taken internally.
Black cohash	Root used to treat arthritis-type pain, and also used to treat menopausal symptoms (hot flashes, vaginal drying and anxiety)	Usually 40 mg daily	Rarely causes headaches and gastritis at higher dosages. There are no interactions with any medications.
Cascara sagrada	Bark acts as natural laxative	Daily use for chronic constipation; typical dose is 300 mg	Could interfere with some heart medicines. May cause abdominal bloating.

Herb	Benefits	Dosage	Cautions/ Interactions
Chamomile	As a tea, relieves nausea, heartburn, colic, and indigestion; is a mild sedative, relaxant, anti-spasmodic; has anti-septic, anti-inflammatory, pain-relieving, and tension-reducing properties	Depends on what form you're using — cream, pills, or capsules	Generally considered safe; mild local reactions from topical use can occur, including, itching, rash, and swelling.
Comfrey	Topically, it relieves severe skin sores (diabetic ulcers, bedsores), brown spider bites, and staph infections	May mix in peroxide for infections	External use only; very toxic if taken internally.
Cranberry	Tannins in the juice cure/prevent mild to moderate bladder infections	300 to 500 mg tablets twice daily	Deemed safe, but large quantities may cause diarrhea. Can interfere with antacid medications.
Donq quai	Relieves menopausal symptoms and pre-menstrual (PMS) symptoms; increases women's energy	500 mg tabs up to 4 times daily, but will be different if using the other forms	Not for use with fibroids, breast cancer, or when pregnant; don't mix with warfarin (anti-coagulants), St. John's wort, and some antibiotics

Herb	Benefits	Dosage	Cautions/ Interactions
			(such as sulfon-amides, quinolones). Can cause a hyper-sensitivity reaction in children.
Echinacea	Boosts immune system; prevents cold and flu; acts as mild anti-bacterial agent	2 to 4 capsules per day	Don't mix with some heart, anti-fungal, HIV, and anti-anxiety medications.
Garlic	May help lower cholesterol and prevent blood clots that lead to heart attacks; in raw form, acts as antibiotic	4 grams of fresh garlic or 8 mg of oil	Capsules may increase blood-thinning effect of anti-coagulants; may decrease blood sugar; don't take with diabetes medication.
Gingko	Improves short-term memory; acts as anti-oxidant; increases blood flow and vascular (blood vessel) tone; improves immune system	120 to 240 mg daily	May increase effect of anti-coagulants (aspirin, Coumadin, heparin and warfarin), provoking serious bleeding disorder.

Herb	Benefits	Dosage	Cautions/ Interactions
Ginseng	As a tea, reduces stress, boosts energy, improves stamina; may help lower cholesterol	200 mg per day	Can cause nervousness and excitation; overuse can lead to headaches, insomnia, and heart palpitations; can increase blood pressure; don't use with prescriptions for high blood pressure or Coumadin.
Hawthorn	May help reduce angina attacks by lowering blood pressure and cholesterol levels	160 to 900 mg per day	Don't mix with digoxin, a heart medication; may lower heart rate too much.
Propolis	Boosts immune system; acts as powerful antibiotic; considered a *total healer,* adding to longevity	Take daily to help maintain health	Reactions to the topical use include rash and itching.
Saw palmetto	Part of an herbal treatment for benign prostatic hypertrophy (BPH) in men	320 mg of extract or 1–2 grams of crushed saw palmetto berry	Some hormonal medications can interfere with saw palmetto.

Herb	Benefits	Dosage	Cautions/ Interactions
St. John's wort	Acts as anti-depressant for mild to moderate depression and anxiety	120–360 mg once a day; it may take 2 to 3 months to receive the full potential	Don't mix with kava, other anti-depressants, HIV medications, oral contraceptives, some heart or blood-thinning medications, or tamoxifen.

*mg = milligram

 The quality of an herbal supplement is only as good as the raw herb and its manufacturing process, so make sure that the label reads *certified organic* before you buy. The name of the certifying agency should also be specified on the label. This guarantees that the product is free of any genetically modified ingredients.

Part IV
Getting Physical

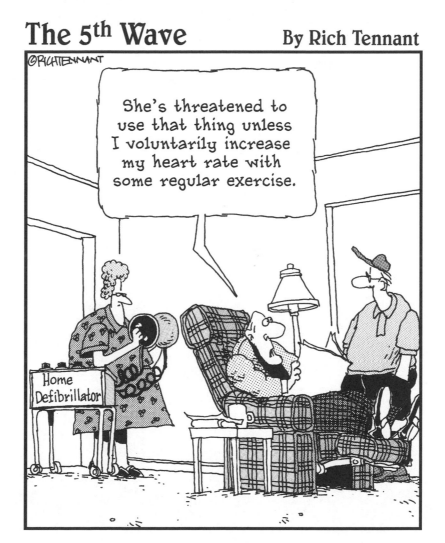

In this part . . .

You discover the importance of fitness, which helps you stay active, maintain a healthy weight, and exercise regularly. In this part, we tell you how to get in shape and stay in shape to stay young (or at least feel young). Having a healthy body, heart, and muscles is a guarantee to feel better!

Chapter 9

Maintaining a Healthy Weight and Fitness Level

....

In This Chapter

▶ Surveying body mass and the consequences of extra pounds
▶ Knowing your present health before setting future goals
▶ Getting on track with your personal plan
▶ Resorting to weight-loss surgery
▶ Keeping off the pounds

....

It's a sad story, but the vast majority of folks nowadays are on the fast track to fat like a runaway freight train in a summer blockbuster movie. The saddest part isn't so much the daily discomfort and inconvenience as it's the cumulative effects of lugging around those extra lipids. That added weight can actually take years off your life and possibly plague your days with illness and disease. We guarantee that membership to this club has more drawbacks than bonuses.

So what's a person to do? The good news is that obesity-related diseases and illnesses are preventable for the vast majority of people if they just lose the excess pounds and

315

maintain a healthy body weight — this is also an excellent way to add healthy years to your life. And contrary to popular assumption, very few people actually have a genetic predisposition to weight gain because of variations in hormones and metabolism. This means that you have hope, although the sooner you act, the better. The solution is simple, but we agree with you: It sure ain't easy sometimes.

Please don't sigh and flip to the next chapter. In this chapter we arm you with a lot of information so you understand how your weight affects your overall health and life expectancy, and we take you through the process of reaching your fitness goals even when they seem overwhelming (minus all the fad diets and overhyped weight-loss strategies, of course!). So join us for the ride — we promise that you'll find it well worth your effort in the long run.

Understanding Healthy Body Weight

Determining your "perfect" weight from a table can be difficult for the simple reason that everybody is different. Some people have bigger bone structures, more muscle mass, and/or carry weight in different areas of the body. These variations in people's frames make using any tool that categorizes someone as overweight or obese difficult.

Your ideal body weight is the eventual weight that your body adjusts to when you have a consistently healthy approach to eating and exercise. Your body wants to naturally maintain this weight based on your physiologic makeup. It may take some time to determine this number if you have weight to lose or if you're underweight now.

 The most common method for determining your ideal weight is the *body mass index* (BMI), a mathematical calculation of a person's ideal mass (weight) based on his or her height and weight. Don't confuse BMI with *BMR (basal metabolic rate),* which is the amount of energy used while at

316

rest and is discussed in more detail in Chapter 7.

The BMI doesn't discriminate between muscle, fat, or bone. People who know that they're at their ideal weight based on their nutrition and other fat measurements can and should ignore the BMI; if you have a greater amount of muscle than most people, this generalized calculation isn't going to apply to you.

In general, however, a person's BMI score is a relatively good tool for people between the ages of 18 and 65. It isn't accurate for pregnant women, weightlifters, competitive athletes (their extra muscle adds extra weight even though they aren't overweight), or people with various chronic illnesses (they can suffer from muscle wasting and malnutrition).

Calculating body mass

Figuring out your body mass index sounds like an exercise in quantum physics, but don't despair; plenty of online tables do the work of calculating your BMI for you, given your height and weight. However, if you're the mathematical type who wants to check your figures against the tables, you can figure out your BMI in either pounds and inches or kilograms and meters:

✔ **Pounds and inches:** Calculate BMI by dividing weight in pounds (lbs) by height in inches (in) squared, and multiplying by a conversion factor of 703.

Weight (lb) ÷ [height (in)]^2 × 703

Example: Weight = 170 lbs, Height = 6' (72")

Calculation: $[170 \div (72)^2] \times 703 = 23.05$

✔ **Kilograms and meters:** You can calculate the BMI using the metric system by using weight in kilograms (kg) divided by height in meters (m) squared. Most often the height is measured in centimeters, so you have to convert the centimeters (cm) to meters by dividing the height by 100.

Weight (kg) ÷ [height (m)]^2

Example: Weight = 70 kg, Height = 183 cm (1.83 m)

Calculation: $70 ÷ (1.83)^2 = 20.10$

Recognizing unhealthy body mass

By BMI standards, people with a body mass index of less than 18.5 are underweight, and those with a BMI of 20 to 25 are within range of their ideal body weight. For the most part, the higher the BMI, the higher the associated health risks. If your BMI goes over 25, you're creeping into the dreaded "overweight" category. Following is a breakdown of the categories of BMIs that are outside the ideal range:

✔ **Underweight:** A person with a body mass index (BMI) of 18.5 or less is considered underweight. Just as with being overweight, the BMI is a tool and having a low BMI may not mean that you're unhealthy. Often underweight individuals are perfectly healthy. If you experience any symptoms such as fatigue, thinning hair or nails, irregularity in periods (women), continuous weight loss, abdominal pains, or any other symptoms, see your doctor for further evaluation.

✔ **Overweight:** A person with a body mass index (BMI) of 25 to 29.9. Approximately 127 million adults (or 60.5 percent) in the U.S. are overweight. About 1 billion people in the world are overweight.

Childhood obesity is already an epidemic in several countries and becoming one in many others. About 22 million children under the age of five are overweight, while obesity among children ages 6 to 11 has doubled since 1960.

✓ **Obese:** A person with a BMI of 30 to 39.9. About 60 million adults (or 25 percent) in the U.S. are obese and 300 million obese adults exist worldwide. This number doesn't include children — one of the fastest growing obesity groups.

✓ **Morbidly obese:** A person 100 pounds over his normal weight or with a BMI of 40 or more. In the U.S., 9 million adults (or 5 percent) are morbidly obese. This group has a definite increase in obesity-related illness and mortality. The good news is that people in this BMI category *can* lose the weight, just like the people in the other weight categories. Get motivated and consult your physician to get a weight loss plan.

The Tolls of Extra Weight

Being just "a little bit overweight" doesn't mean that you can sit back and feel safe from the serious health concerns associated with being overweight. The most important fact we want you to take away from this chapter is that if you're even a little overweight, you are just that — over your healthy weight — and you should try to get down to a healthy weight.

The majority of researchers feel that being overweight shares the same health risks as being obese. It's easy, especially in today's overweight world, to ignore a little extra weight, especially if you're the thinnest one in your family or in your circle of friends. But this tendency can give you a false sense of comfort that can be dangerous to your health.

From a health-risk standpoint, there are only three categories: underweight, healthy weight, and overweight. You can have disease at any weight, and being underweight can be a serious health concern if associated with weight loss from bulimia or anorexia. The majority of weight-related disease, and the fastest-growing weight sector, is related to the overweight category.

Most people aren't aware of the range of medical conditions directly associated with being overweight or obese — from the mildly unpleasant heartburn to death from stroke or heart disease. Yes, it's *that* serious. According to the Journal of the American Medical Association, obesity is the second-leading cause of preventable death in the U.S., right after smoking. The heavier a person is, the less mobile he becomes, which then leads to a more detrimental, sedentary lifestyle. Weight gain and poor nutrition precipitate lack of exercise and becoming sedentary, which then increases risk for illness and disease — it's a vicious cycle.

Approximately 30 illnesses and diseases are linked to being overweight. The following represent only a handful of these medical conditions:

- ✔ **Arthritis:** Pain, stiffness, and loss of mobility of the hands, hips, back, and especially the knees are worse in people with a BMI of 25 or greater. The joints are put under a greater load of pressure that makes osteoarthritis (OA) more prevalent in obese people. Losing just 10 to 15 pounds is likely to relieve symptoms and delay disease progression.

- ✔ **Cardiovascular disease:** Obesity (BMI of 30 or

more) increases a person's risk for heart disease due to its effect on blood lipid levels. The American Heart Association recognizes obesity as a major risk factor for heart attack. Weight loss helps blood lipid levels by lowering triglycerides and LDL (lousy) cholesterol and increasing HDL (healthy) cholesterol.

✔ **Diabetes (type 2, adult onset, non-insulin-dependent diabetes):** The number of type 2 diabetics keeps increasing annually. As many as 90 percent of individuals with type 2 diabetes are reported to be overweight or obese. If you're overweight, losing as little as 5 percent of your body weight can reduce your high blood sugar.

✔ **High blood pressure:** More than 75 percent of high blood pressure cases are reported to be directly attributed to being overweight. For more on this subject, check out *High Blood Pressure For Dummies,* 2nd Edition (Wiley) by Alan L. Rubin, MD.

✔ **Sleep apnea:** Between 60 and 70 percent of people who have *sleep apnea* (they temporarily stop breathing while they sleep) are obese. Obesity is the largest risk factor for developing this condition.

✔ **Strokes:** People with a BMI over 25 increase their risk of *ischemic* stroke (from fatty deposits that obstruct blood vessels to the brain). Being overweight or obesity is associated with high cholesterol leading to atherosclerosis (narrowing of the arteries). Atherosclerosis is a direct risk factor for strokes.

In addition to those direct links, consider the following facts:

- ✔ National Cancer Institute experts concluded that obesity is associated with cancers of the colon, breast (postmenopausal), endometrium (the lining of the uterus), kidney, and esophagus.

- ✔ Forty-two percent of those diagnosed with breast and colon cancers are obese.

- ✔ Of all gallbladder surgery, 30 percent is related to obesity.

The good news is that being over your ideal weight isn't a disease with no cure, but rather a condition with multiple cures. Keep reading and see that achieving a healthy weight is something that's very attainable.

The government started recording life expectancy in 1900. The current obesity epidemic may well lead to the first downward turn in those numbers in the future. The *New England Journal of Medicine* already projects that obesity will decrease life expectancy by close to a year; other researchers see life expectancy numbers dropping by as much as five years in the near future.

Assessing Your Current Level of Health

No one ever said losing weight was easy. Okay, maybe some people say that, but they're usually people who have never had any weight to lose! Listing what you have to do to lose weight is easy; finding the right combination of what works for you can end up being a lifelong pursuit. It's an all out tug of war, with your body fighting to hang on to every pound. The more you fight with your body, the more your body's going to win.

So, where do you begin? You may be mentally ready to take on the battle, but how do you know whether you're physically ready and able to begin a serious weight-loss and exercise program? This section tells you how to get ready for the battle of the bulge — check in with your physician before checking in at the gym. We also look at what you need to know about your own health before you can tailor those workouts to be beneficial and safe. Finally, we cover your current weight and your goal weight to give you a good idea of the road ahead.

Evaluating your fitness level

Before beginning an exercise routine, ask yourself, "What's my baseline fitness level?" Translation: How active are you? Are you overweight? Do you exercise now? How many minutes a week do you exercise? Do you lift weights or do aerobic exercise? These questions give you, your doctor, and/or your personal trainer an idea of what your basic fitness level is.

The best personal fitness assessment comes from a personal trainer. Some gyms include the cost of an assessment as part of your membership, although others don't. You may also want to contact a local personal trainer specifically for this service.

Here are some elements the test may include:

- **Exercise history:** What type of exercise have you done in the last year? Walked to the mailbox at the end of the street? Or ran a half-marathon? Someone who's starting a fitness program for the first time is very different from someone who's just taken a 6-month hiatus after a long history of routine exercise.

- **Height and weight:** You may feel that we're beating this to death, but the quick and easy way to assess your body weight is the BMI. See the section "Calculating body mass," earlier in this chapter, to figure out how to calculate your BMI.

- ✔ **Body composition:** This element is much more pertinent to the experienced exerciser than the beginner. Some people can use a more detailed breakdown of their body, but, for the majority, a basic BMI (see the previous bullet) works fine initially.

- ✔ **Resting heart rate:** This number is important to know when figuring out your target heart rate during exercise.

- ✔ **Resting blood pressure:** Everyone starting an exercise program needs to check his or her blood pressure. Exercise can help lower blood pressure if elevated, but you need to have a medical doctor evaluate and manage any elevations prior to beginning an exercise routine. If your blood pressure is normal, you can monitor it yourself; many personal trainers also monitor blood pressure.

- ✔ **Flexibility test:** You don't want to hurt yourself and end up in worse health than when you started! Look at your range of motion and evaluate muscle weakness and tightness to avoid injury.

- ✔ **Strength and endurance testing:** This one tests muscle strength and the amount of time it takes to reach muscle fatigue. Having areas of the body that are weaker may cause problems with balance and posture.

- ✔ **Post-test consultation and goal setting:** Understanding your overall fitness level and areas of concern or concentration helps you observe your progress (or lack thereof). Setting goals keeps you on track and allows you to monitor incremental improvements.

At the post-test consultation, the following issues are determined:

- ✔ The level of weights you should begin using
- ✔ How many days a week you should train
- ✔ How long you should train each workout day
- ✔ Which muscle groups require the most work

Getting the green light from your primary physician

Checking with a doctor before starting an exercise routine or weight-loss program is much more than just a legal disclaimer, so don't let this advice go in one ear and out the other. Some conditions and symptoms may require medical attention prior to jumping into exercise, just to make sure that your new exercise plan is right for you. This is a safety precaution; always err on the side of caution and see your doctor if you have any concerns. In this section, we take a look at some important questions that help you decide whether your first step should be on a treadmill or into a doctor's office.

If you're starting an exercise routine that consists of walking or light weights and you have no medical conditions or complaints, you probably don't need medical clearance. If you're not sure whether you need to see a doctor before starting a new or restarting an old exercise program, go through this health questionnaire. A "yes" answer to any of these questions means that you should consult a medical doctor first:

- Are you over the age of 40?

- Are you overweight?

- Do you smoke?

- Have you been sedentary for a long time?

- Are you starting an exercise program that involves more than walking or light weights?

- Has a doctor told you that you have a heart murmur?

- Has anyone in your family died of heart disease prior to the age of 55?

- Do you have a high risk of coronary heart disease or stroke?

- Do you have any medical conditions, such as high cholesterol, diabetes, high blood pressure, or kidney disease?

- Do your ankles swell?

- Have you experienced severe pain in your leg muscles while walking?

- Do you get short of breath more than usual when you're performing routine tasks?

- Have you fainted or do you have dizziness?

- Have you experienced any abnormal heartbeats or chest pain either at rest or when exerting yourself?

You may have noticed that the first question in the list asks about your age. If you're over 40, you may be thinking, "Hey, I'm in the best shape of my life! Why are they singling me out?" Being over 40 doesn't mean that you're old.

You're on this list because some experts believe that people over 40, whether they're at risk for heart disease or other medical conditions, should have a complete physical examination before starting or intensifying an exercise program.

Relax; there aren't many situations where your doctor tells you that you can't exercise in some fashion. People with heart disease used to be discouraged from exercising, but studies show that, in many cases, exercise under medical supervision is helpful for patients with stable heart disease. In one study, patients with heart disease who were as old as 91 increased oxygen consumption significantly after 6 months of supervised treadmill and stationary bicycle exercises. Remember, though, that it's often difficult for a doctor to predict health problems that may arise as the result of an exercise program, so if you are at risk for any health problems, be aware of any related symptoms while you exercise.

After getting the green light to exercise, it's time to put your plan into action (before you change your mind).

Crunching your body composition numbers

The BMI determines body mass — not fat percentage. For the percentages, you need a *body composition analysis,* which splits your body weight into individual components: most commonly, lean mass and fat mass.

When people ask you what your lean body mass (lean muscle mass) is, you likely think that it is an indication of strength and muscle. *Lean body mass* is actually the weight of your tissues other than fat; muscles, bones, organs and fluids of your body, of which 50 to 60 percent is water. *Body fat mass* is the percent of the body that is fat and is an important number that sets the mark for the rest of the body analysis. To figure your body composition, you measure the percent of fat mass, and then subtract that number from 100 to get the percentage of lean mass.

The ideal fat percentages for men and women differ. Men have a normal range of 8 to 25 percent body fat while women should be in the range of 18 to 32 percent body fat. All the testing measures in the following sections are inexpensive options to discover more about your body makeup.

Measuring waist circumference; Or, accounting for the most dangerous form of fat

Just to make it more confusing, all fat isn't created equal — one type of fat has more potential health concerns than the other. People with central obesity (think beer bellies), or fat that is predominantly found in the abdomen (*visceral fat,* which is fat packed around the organs in the abdomen) tend to have more health-related illnesses than those with mostly *subcutaneous fat,* which is the type of fat just under the skin and is largely located in the thighs and buttocks. (See Figure 9-1 for an illustration.)

The difference in danger between the two locales of fat lies in two causes:

- ✔ Visceral fat, also known as "organ fat," is nearer to the body's most vital organs than subcutaneous fat, so this fat is the kind that leads to the bulging belly better known as a beer belly.

- ✔ Visceral fat contains properties that increase the risk of insulin resistance, which can contribute to diabetes.

The ideal waist measurement for women is less than 35 inches. For men, an ideal waist is less than 40 inches. Go over 35 inches for women or 40 for men, and you increase your risks for health problems — regardless of height. If your BMI is in the normal range but your waist measurement isn't, go with your gut, literally — your waistline over-rules your BMI on this one.

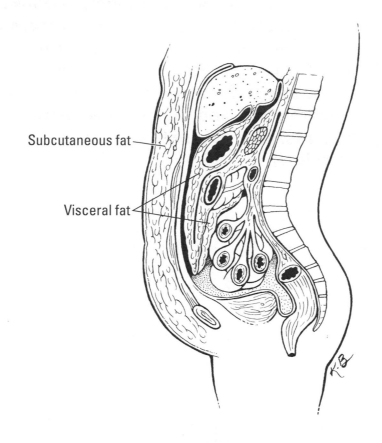

Subcutaneous fat

Visceral fat

Liposuction is often sought after a cosmetic procedure, but the fat it removes is just that — cosmetic. A study done by the *New England Journal of Medicine* found that because liposuction removes only subcutaneous fat, it doesn't have much effect on weight-related health risks.

Assessing overall fat and muscle percentages

A body composition analysis uses specific tools that calculate the percentage of body fat and muscle mass to determine a person's ideal weight. By far the most common tool is the simple skinfold caliper, a quick, cheap, and noninvasive device that most trained health or fitness professionals can use. It usually requires taking three measurements at different sites of the body (triceps, abdomen, and upper thigh) by pinching and measuring subcutaneous body fat at several points and then plugging these numbers into a formula that calculates body fat. Because the tool is manual, it may have a 3 to 5 percent error in measurement — the measurement can be affected by the skill level of the professional using the tool, and the measurement isn't accurate for obese patients. (See Figure 9-2 for an illustration of how the skinfold caliper is used.)

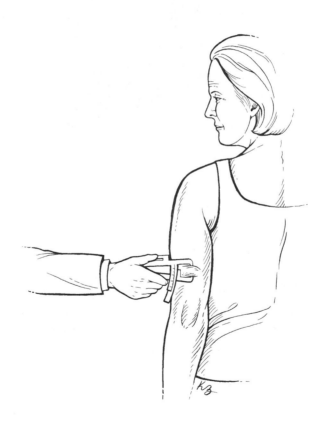

Figure 9-2:
A skinfold caliper is the simplest method for calculating your percentage of body fat.

Other less-common methods for measuring body composition include the following:

✔ **Bioelectrical impedance:** This is a fairly

inexpensive scale or handheld device that sends an electrical impulse through your body (don't worry; you can't feel it). It measures body fat by recording how easily the impulse is transmitted, because an electrical impulse travels through tissues with more water content (muscle) more easily than those with lower (fat). It gives a good sense of your body fat changes over time but it may not be highly accurate. Readings can be easily affected by hydration status (the amount of fluids consumed, especially water), and muscle mass. Muscular athletes typically get higher-than-actual results.

- **Underwater (hydrostatic) weighing:** This technique requires specialized equipment that includes a water tank with a mounted scale and chair and highly trained technicians to perform the test. While you're completely submerged in a tank of water, you breathe out all air from your lungs to decrease tendency to float. The test measures body density, which is compared to your weight on land. When performed correctly, this assessment has less than a 3-percent error rate.

- **Dual X-ray Absorptiometry (DEXA):** This device is quick, easy, and very accurate, but it requires expensive equipment typically found only in hospitals and research centers. The DEXA is an X-ray of the body that shows fat, muscle, and bone mass based on differing densities.

- **Bod Pod:** This fairly new device seems to have great promise. You sit in an enclosed egg-shaped pod for about 5 minutes while computers generate data from the sensors that determine the amount of air displaced by your body. These devices are available in most cities and are often used at local health fairs. Studies show that it's comparable to underwater weighing and DEXA, but it's likely more accurate. The major advantages are that the equipment is fairly inexpensive, it requires little training to operate, it's comfortable for people of all shapes and sizes, and it's quick and easy.

Custom-Designing Your Plan with Balance in Mind

With so many opportunities to supersize, and so many unhealthy food choices prominently displayed in grocery stores, making healthy food choices and sticking to them in the long run are harder than ever. It can be easy to yo-yo between starving yourself and stuffing yourself, instead of settling comfortably in the middle (which is where you really need to be). After all, whether you spend your life worrying about your weight or neglecting it entirely, you're not living healthfully.

The simple math is this: The cause of weight gain is eating more calories than you burn. Your body gains one pound for every 3,500 calories it doesn't use. People who exercise daily throughout their lives maintain their ideal body weight more easily than those who don't. We can't stress this fact enough.

Counting calories for weight loss

Eating right is the best thing you can do for weight loss. Exercise is always important, but what you eat and how much is much more important for maintaining a healthy weight. If you exercise heavily for one hour every day of the week, but don't change your diet, you may not lose any weight.

We all know the coworker, neighbor, or fellow gym attendee who exercises religiously for months, but just doesn't seem to lose any weight. Most of the time, the reason is lack of dietary modifications.

You can find a lot of dieting options out there, and most of them center on getting a good balance of protein and carbohydrates. Drop your calories down to between 1,200 and 1,800 calories based on exercise intensity and body size. The goal is to decrease your calorie intake by 500 calories below the minimum calories that you utilize in a day and then you lose 1 pound per week. This reduction in calories results in weight loss in most cases and 1 to 2 pounds per week is a healthy weight loss rate. (See Chapter 7 to calculate your individual caloric needs and see how much protein, carbs, and fat you should be taking in — and how much you shouldn't.)

Creating a safe and effective exercise program

The popular saying "What your mind can conceive, your body can achieve" is a great motto to live by. Use this book to set a solid plan and follow it. Everyone can live healthier and can improve in some areas.

After a doctor clears you to exercise, and you have some physical assessments done, you should be able to compile a personalized exercise program to follow. If you don't have the help of a personal trainer, set up a program based on your level of experience. This section guides the way, and Chapters 10 and 11 dig in a bit deeper.

Covering the bases: The components of a complete routine

A common misconception for people who are just starting a routine is to focus only on cardio. But in that case, your body burns the energy stored in your muscles first and burns fat only as a last resort. (We know — it's a frustrating arrangement!) So, a body transformation occurs most efficiently by *simultaneously* gaining muscle through strength training and losing fat through aerobics and diet. (See Chapter 12 for the lowdown on strength training and Chapter 13 for info on aerobics.) It's like a tricycle — all three wheels have to turn at the same time.

Keep these facts in mind as you build your personalized program:

- ✔ **Aerobic training:** Activities like walking, swimming, and biking are all good for the lungs and heart. See Chapter 11 for more information.

- ✔ **Strength training:** This is the only activity that slows muscle and bone loss while it promotes weight loss. See Chapter 10 for more information.

  Your body needs energy to sustain muscle mass because muscle cells are *metabolically demanding* (high-maintenance); for every pound of muscle you add, your body burns 30 to 50 more calories a day even at rest. How's that for a great bargain! (And those burned calories are more likely to come from fat reserves, which is really the whole point if your goal is to lose body fat.)

  If you're just beginning your strength training routine or are a novice, we recommend strength training 20 to 30 minutes two to three days a week. If you're an old pro, you're most likely strength training 30 to 60 minutes four to five days a week, so keep it up! Don't forget to incorporate five to ten minutes of flexibility training to stretch your muscle groups before and after your strength training.

People over 60 who want to reduce their risk of falls and injury should start by strengthening legs, arms, and core muscles with two to three days of weight training a week for three to four weeks before walking long distances or engaging in aerobic exercise.

✔ **Flexibility training:** To maintain good muscle health and reduce injury, we urge you to incorporate flexibility training through stretching, yoga, and Pilates. These activities not only feel good but also increase the range of motion of your joints — see Chapter 10.

Aerobic exercise with weight training using lighter weights and more repetitions is better than weight training alone using heavy, bulking-type weights and exercises.

In order for your routine to work and be effective, it has to be something you want to do and take full responsibility for. So, while you decide what kind of workout you want (weight training and aerobics), where you're going to get it (at the gym or on the bike trail), and which days of the week to devote to which activity (Monday: gym, Wednesday: rollerblade in the park, Thursday: swimming), personalize and work with your routine until it's comfortable. One trick to help you stay on track is to put your weekly plan on paper (or in your PDA) on a Sunday night before you start your week. That way, you're more likely to stick to it!

Then, of course, you start working out. Many people are wonderful at putting plans together — and terrible at implementing them! The best exercise plan in the world won't do a thing for you unless you actually *do* it.

People who have been sedentary for long periods (at least 6 to 12 months) may be at a higher risk for injury because muscle tone is weak, flexibility is limited, and balance is shaky. **Note:** Although most people consider walking the first step in becoming active, starting with strength training may be safer and more beneficial for people with limitations in their mobility (joint disease) or aerobic capacities (advanced lung disease).

If you haven't had much experience in the gym, start with some basic training. Many fitness centers offer circuit training, which consists of multiple machines with instructions and displays of the muscle groups that they target. You cycle through the machines, targeting all the muscle groups. You can increase the intensity as you go and concentrate on specific weak areas as you see fit. Aerobic activity can be worked into the schedule or you can alternate days between aerobic and strength training.

Factoring in your personality and lifestyle

When starting an exercise routine, you need to first evaluate your personality and lifestyle. If you create a routine that you don't enjoy, can't afford, or can't squeeze in, chances are good that you won't stick with it. Ask yourself the following questions:

✔ **What motivates me?** Motivation (or the lack of it) has the power to start and stop a routine as fast as you can spit the word out. We've met a lot of people who just won't do aerobic activities like running or biking, but they can play basketball or soccer for hours. Sports are a great source of exercise, and joining a league locks you into a schedule. Paying for a membership gets some people to commit to the gym because they want to get their money's worth. Make a bet or a deal with a colleague, friend, or partner that involves exercise or weight-loss goals. You can get motivated, but sometimes you have to be creative.

✔ **Can I stick to my guns all on my own, or do I need the support of a group class, support group, planned weight-loss program, workout partner, or personal trainer?** Some people wake up one morning, make a decision to stop living life in an overweight or simply sedentary body, and change their habits instantly. Others have a bit more trouble following through. Maybe they need to socialize and engage with others who have the same goals to continue toward successfully achieving those goals.

✔ **What type of programs meet my health needs and interest me?** Carefully consider what keeps you coming back for more. For some people, various classes at the gym are helpful; for others, the commitment to an upcoming 5K or a mini-triathlon piques their interest. Some people train for the next Iron Man competition, and others with limiting health conditions may set a goal to maintain their current health.

✔ **What resources are available to me, and how much money am I willing to spend?** You can find an exercise program for any budget. Remember that allocating funds for your health is an investment that can reduce medical visits, medications, and time off work. It could be the best money you spend!

✔ **What time of day is best for me to work out?** There's really no perfect time of day that maximizes your workouts. Some researchers have tried to designate a particular workout time based on hormones and body rhythms, but no solid data is available. Some environmental restrictions, such as heat, cold, or rain, may make certain times of the day safer (and make you less likely to cancel). The best time of the day is the time that's consistently available to you with the least interruptions. Many people say that they don't have the time to exercise. Our response? Ridiculous! If you can find the time for lunch, your morning coffee, a glass of wine before bed, or television, you can certainly find time to work out. You may have to set that alarm clock back an hour or work out during lunch a few days out of the week, while fitting in a quick meal before or after. You can even involve your family or partner to make sure that you get your exercise in.

When searching for time to work out, you're really talking about priorities. Everybody, we mean *everybody,* can find two and a half to three hours per week to exercise.

 People who work away from the home statistically cancel workouts more often if they go home before heading to the gym. After you hit the couch, forget about it. You need to plan your exercising before you go home — if you don't, plan on every excuse in the book entering your mind after you walk through your front door.

Getting the goods

You don't need to purchase expensive gym equipment to get a good workout. Sporting goods stores as well as major discount department stores have all sorts of products for at-home users or people who want companion pieces for their exercise classes. Many manufacturers feature products that run the gamut — from inexpensive starter kits to complete home gym systems with all the bells and whistles. Of course, you do the workout, but what could be easier? Here's a list of some basic equipment to get you started:

- **Handheld weights:** Hand weights (also known as *dumbbells*) are a must-have for any do-it-yourselfer. The most popular variety is vinyl-coated for comfort and easy grip and color-coded by weight. They range in increments from 1 to 10 pounds, and then go up to 12 and 15 pounds.

  If you're adding hand weights to your daily walk, go light because there's a risk of joint inflammation and injury, especially if you use heavier weights and don't do adequate warm-up. If you're doing bicep curls, try a few reps in the store. When your muscles fatigue at 15 repetitions, you've found a good starting weight.

- **Resistance bands:** These bands are easy to use at any age or fitness level and offer your muscles a full-range-of-motion workout. Resistance bands are long tubes that look like rubber jump ropes with handles. (Shorter versions come without handles, but we recommend the longer ones — the most popular and versatile variety — because you can always shorten them up for working out your arms.) Resistance bands are color-coded to indicate their strength (thickness).

- **Exercise stability balls:** Who would've thought that sitting on a big, round ball would be a workout? Seems like mere child's play until you try to balance yourself and realize that your body is using micro muscles you forgot you had! These balls offer numerous exercises and activities that activate and strengthen those hard-to-reach core muscles often overlooked during normal training. The balls come in a variety of sizes according to your height. The most common are 55 cm (for people who are 5'1" to

Finding a weight-loss program that works your body, not just your wallet

If losing weight is a losing battle for you, finding the best weight-loss program for you may be a bit like finding the proverbial needle in a haystack. People try programs and they lose weight, only to gain it back again — and then some. Statistics consistently show that 90 percent of dieters fail, mostly after spending large sums of money for programs and supplements. *Maintaining* is the key in the weight loss world, but maintenance in most programs is whispered about or promised with little success. Do your research to reduce the chance of becoming one of the failed-dieter statistics.

Before signing up for any weight-loss program, identify the factors that are most important to ensuring your success by considering the following questions:

✔ What does the menu plan look like? Are substitutions allowed? How many calories a day will you be eating? (Don't starve yourself; it isn't healthy. You should always be eating at least 1000 calories a day.)

✔ Does the program promote drinking 80 to 100 ounces of water a day? (If not, move on to another program.)

✔ Does the program encourage exercising a minimum of one hour a day, three days each week at some point?

✔ Does the program recommend checking with your doctor before starting any weight-loss or exercise program or is it medically supervised?

✔ Does the program provide education on food and nutrition?

✔ Will you take prescription appetite suppressants? Are they addicting? How long do you have to take them? Is there strict doctor supervision? Often use of appetite suppressants will lead to regaining the weight you lost after the medicine is stopped.

✔ How much does the program cost? What does the cost include? Can you find client testimonials? Can you speak with any of those clients?

If you have a hard time staying motivated and dedicated to a plan, ask about the support throughout the program. Choose one that addresses your needs based on these questions:

✔ Will you have a personal weight-loss counselor or coach to help you reach your goals and answer your questions? If so, what is that person's availability (weekly appointments, phone, e-mail, and so on)?

✔ Does the program include group support?

✔ Does the program offer a maintenance plan? If so, what's the format and length? What are the statistics on success rates?

Look into some of these healthy weight-loss programs:

✔ Jenny Craig (www.jennycraig.com)

✔ Nutrisystem (www.nutrisystem.com)

✔ The Trim Diet (www.trimlifestyle. com)

✔ Weight Watchers (www.weightwatchers.com)

5'7") and 65 cm (for people who are 5'8" to 6'1"), although we've seen them as small as 30 cm and as large as 85 cm.

- ✔ **Floor mat:** A *closed-cell* (nonabsorbent to wick away moisture) foam mat that's at least 5/8 of an inch thick is great to avoid slipping, and to provide comfort and support.

- ✔ **Workout DVD:** You can find an endless variety of workouts for every age, lifestyle, and fitness level. Try one from your local movie rental store or your public library before you buy it.

- ✔ **Good quality shoes:** A comfortable and supportive pair of sneakers is essential. You don't have to spend a fortune on the latest in technology trainers either. Make sure that your shoes have rubber soles and good arch support. More than anything, they should be comfortable. You may want to break them in before you wear them for your workout to avoid blisters. Good shoes are also important if you want to avoid knee pain. Many shoe manufacturers make cross trainers and other shoes for particular types of exercise. They need to be comfortably snug and have proper arch support and cushion to absorb the shocks of training. The wrong shoes can mean blisters, knee and back pain, and inflammation in the feet.

From trial to style: Making a (good) habit of it

Whatever the reason for *starting* an exercise routine, you need to have even better ones for *keeping* the fire burning. Too often, the smallest hurdle (a broken fingernail, a mild headache, or a friend saying, "Aw, do you have to work out today?") can put out that fire.

Unfortunately, the people newest to the exercise scene seem to get sidetracked the most easily and have the hardest time getting back. Why? Most likely because exercise hasn't become an established way of life, like brushing their teeth and tying their shoes. The longer a newbie delays returning to the schedule, the more he drags his feet going back to it.

So, having the right expectation from the get-go is critical. In general, you need to follow a routine for 21 days in order for it to become habit. And to achieve a healthy body weight and maintain it, you must truly believe that there are no short-cuts!

To help avoid this pitfall, keep these suggestions in mind:

- **Make exercise a priority.** Just like sleeping, eating, working, and spending time with your family — set a time in your schedule for exercise and stick to it.

- **Practice saying "no."** You can do this in a kind but firm way. When friends and family try to interfere with your workout plans, say no.

  Keep in mind, though, that your routine also affects the people closest to you; it takes them time to adjust as well. If you're consistent, you can ease resentment on both ends.

- **Implement a system of checks and balances.** Every decision you make requires some sacrifice to keep things in balance. (No one can have it all, do it all, or eat it all and reach their goals!) Balance is the key to life, and weight loss is no different. Trying to lose weight requires sacrifices every day — but those sacrifices are balanced by the rewards. You have to get yourself ready by recognizing the difficult situations that make it hard to make those sacrifices. For instance, don't have candy in the house if you love candy. Out of sight, (hopefully!) out of mind.

Sacrifice is important, but torture is unnecessary. Make sure that you have checks in place to increase your chances of success. If you like coffee in the morning, have the coffee, but also drink more water. If you like to have a beer in the evening, switch to a light beer. If you want to have dessert on occasion, work out 3 days a week to balance out those calories. To succeed in the fitness world, finding balance is essential. When you establish balance, it becomes habit and a new lifestyle.

Evaluating the success of your efforts (and rewarding yourself along the way)

Sometimes, despite their best efforts, people encounter the slump of discouragement and frustration, especially when they've tried to lose weight more than once, only to gain it back. To bounce back from those self-defeating thoughts and feelings, refocus with the following methods:

- ✓ Focus on the process instead of the end result.

- ✓ Focus on what went well today (or this week) and the successes.

- ✓ Use visualization and imagery techniques to focus on yourself at your goal weight, participating in an enjoyable activity.

- ✓ Focus on physical activity as an opportunity to do something enjoyable.

- ✓ Put away the scale for awhile and focus on making lasting lifestyle changes. As a result, the weight will come off.

Finding the rewards at the end of your rainbow of sacrifices is easy. Every time you reach one of your goals, reward yourself. Every positive action deserves a pat on the back. Get some new clothes or take a mini-trip. And make sure that you set reasonable goals, because the rewards are that much more valuable.

When Weight Just Won't Come Off: Considering Weight-Loss Surgery

If you can't lose weight despite your consistent dietary changes and physical activity, don't panic. Some people — although few — really do have medical reasons for weight gain and an inability to lose weight. Hormone imbalances, medications, and some genetic mutations can make weight loss difficult for some, and figuring out how to treat weight gain in these situations has become a major focus for many medical centers. If you've worked hard at weight loss and haven't seen significant results (meaning that you haven't moved out of the obese category after consistently following our advice in this book for six months and working with a physician to monitor your diet and exercise), you may want to consult a doctor who specializes in weight control.

If you're having a difficult time with your weight and have some other underlying medical conditions that raise the importance of weight loss, your doctor may decide that surgical treatment is the best option in your situation. But surgery should be the last resort for at least two reasons:

✔ Although it guarantees success (at least in the short-term), no surgery is without risk.

- Surgery isn't a miracle cure or quick fix for being overweight or, in most cases, even obese. Sure, it helps — but if a person resumes his bad habits after adjusting to life post-surgery, he can actually undo the benefits of the surgery by stretching out a stomach that's been made smaller.

- The financial costs are high. Sometimes insurance companies cover weight-loss surgeries, but with surgeries averaging $10,000 to $30,000, each person's provider must evaluate whether the benefits outweigh the medical risk and financial burden.

  The National Institutes of Health recommends that people with a BMI of 40 or greater (about 100 pounds overweight) and people with a BMI of 35 *plus* two or more significant obesity-related problems (like diabetes or high blood pressure) are appropriate candidates for weight-loss surgery.

We strongly advise that people considering weight-loss surgery (and we consider it *only* for the obese) exhaust *all* options first. A dedicated lifestyle of nutritious eating on a reduced-calorie diet with vigorous exercise should always be the first course of action.

If your doctor and you do decide to go the surgery route, your options include the following:

- **Stomach stapling:** This operation works on the premise that a smaller stomach pouch helps people lose weight because they feel fuller with less food. The size prevents people from overeating, and if they do eat too much, they feel ill.

- **Lap-band:** Like stomach stapling, lap-band surgeries are less drastic and, therefore, more popular than bypass operations. A small adjustable band is placed around the upper part of the stomach, creating a smaller pouch, which limits the amount of food that you can eat at one time. However, patients can cheat more easily than they can with gastric bypass and stomach stapling because the anatomy of the stomach isn't as strictly reduced. As a result, weight reduction tends to be more limited.

✔ **Gastric bypass:** This method involves taking the stomach and creating a small pouch that restricts the amount of food that can be ingested, and then attaching the small intestine directly to the pouch. About 10 to 20 percent of patients undergoing gastric bypass require follow-up operations to correct complications; the most common complaints are abdominal hernias. More than one-third of patients who have gastric bypass surgery develop gallstones.

Succeeding at the Hardest Part: Maintaining Your Healthy Weight!

Healthy eating is the biggest component of weight loss. Exercise definitely helps, and is most important for burning off extra calories from those situations when you stray from your normal dietary habits such as vacations, parties, or just dessert after a good meal out. Weight maintenance, on the other hand, is the result of successfully incorporating good nutrition and routine daily exercise into your lifestyle. Many people can lose weight, but they gain the weight back quickly. Becoming a yo-yo dieter, one who loses weight and gains it back, just to try to lose it again in what turns into a vicious cycle, isn't healthy and can become expensive if you have to buy new clothes or expensive diets and diet supplements.

Weight maintenance comes down to a few things:

- ✔ Making consistently smart food choices

- ✔ Staying committed to an exercise routine that's enjoyable and rewarding

- ✔ Maintaining plenty of balance and patience

- ✔ Weighing yourself weekly; what you don't know *can* hurt you

- ✔ Refusing to let "just a few little pounds" creep back up on you without taking immediate action

- ✔ Setting goals that work for you, not for someone else

Living life somewhere in the middle is apt to lead to more positive and long-lasting results than living in the extremes. And people who are able to successfully keep their weight down are the ones who have figured out how to make balanced choices. This isn't to say that you'll never eat another double fudge chocolate sundae — only that you've figure out how to make it part of your balanced choices.

Chapter 10

Strengthening Your Heart

● ●

In This Chapter

▶ Getting to the heart of it: The anatomy of your body's pump
▶ Understanding the anti-aging effects of aerobics
▶ Supporting your heart with a healthy diet
▶ Working your way to a healthier heart: Aerobics 101

● ●

It's hard to imagine that something the size of your palm is responsible for sustaining your life. The heart muscle is your body's engine, and of course, like any engine, it requires regular maintenance. The best maintenance plan for a healthy heart includes maximizing the good habits (like training and strengthening your heart muscle through aerobic exercise and eating heart-healthy foods) and minimizing the risk factors (like being overweight and sedentary).

Aerobic (which means "with oxygen") exercise is any activity that increases your oxygen intake, causing you to breathe faster or harder and your heart to beat faster. Aerobic activity includes many types of exercise that are of moderate to long duration and low intensity.

In contrast, *anaerobic* (which means "without air") exercise includes strength training and weight training; anaerobic activity doesn't increase oxygen output and is of short duration and high intensity. See Chapter 11 for more on anaerobic exercise.

In this chapter we show you how regular aerobic exercise can make and keep your heart healthy; why it's so important, especially as you get older; and just how much and what kind you need in order to reap the benefits.

Understanding the Anatomy of the Heart

For all its complexity, your heart is basically a pump made out of muscle, forcing blood to the lungs to be oxygenated and then pumping the oxygenated blood out to the rest of your body. Any problem that results in a weak pump affects blood flow throughout your body, and, as you age, different parts of your pump can start to break down or get clogged up.

Understanding the causes of a weak or damaged pump can help you keep your heart strong at any age. Understanding any problem areas your heart has is important if you want to try to prevent serious problems from occurring. Defects within its different chambers and blood vessels result in different types of disease, so it's helpful to understand exactly what's what when it comes to your heart's anatomy.

Your heart's main function is to continuously pump oxygen- and nutrient-rich blood throughout your body 24 hours a day, 7 days a week, sending blood to your lungs to be oxygenated and then out to the rest of the body. This fist-sized powerhouse expands and contracts to create that familiar beat 100,000 times per day, pumping 5 to 6 quarts each minute — about 2,000 gallons per day. That's a lot of love.

On the inside, your heart is a four-chambered, hollow organ that's divided into the left and right side by the *septum,* a muscular wall. (See Figure 10-1 for an illustration.) The upper two chambers (the left and right atria) receive blood from the veins; the lower two chambers (the left and right *ventricles*) pump blood into the lungs and the rest of the body. A weakness or blockage in any area can cause heart problems.

As the muscular walls *contract* (squeeze), they pump blood through your vessels:

- The right side of your heart pumps blood to your lungs to fill up on fresh oxygen and empty the body's waste product, carbon dioxide.

- The left side of your heart pumps oxygen-rich blood throughout a super highway of arteries in your body.

Here's a list of the major blood vessels that enter the heart:

- The **aorta,** the largest artery in the body, comes out of the left ventricle and delivers oxygenated blood to the body.

- The **superior vena cava,** a large vein, enters the right atrium, delivering oxygen-depleted blood from the head, chest, and upper extremities.

- The **inferior vena cava,** a large vein, enters the right atrium, delivering oxygen-depleted blood from the lower extremities.

- The **pulmonary artery** exits the right ventricle and takes oxygen-poor blood from the heart to the lungs where it's oxygenated.

351

- The **pulmonary vein** enters the left atrium to bring oxygen-rich blood from the lungs to the heart.

- The **coronary arteries** originate at the aorta and supply blood to the heart muscle.

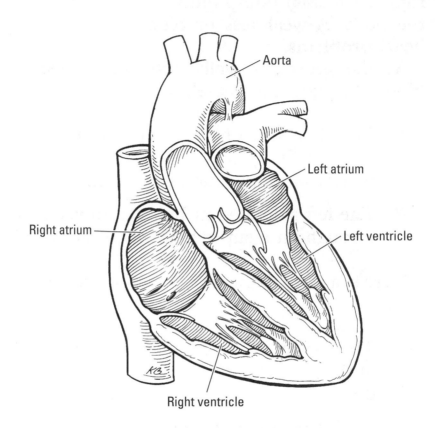

Figure 10-1:
The anatomy of the heart.

The Importance of Aerobic Activity and a Heart-Healthy Diet

Inactivity is one of the four major risk factors for *cardiovascular disease* (CVD); also known as *atherosclerotic* heart disease). In fact, people who are inactive have a 30 to 50 percent higher risk of developing CVD than those who are moderately active. The role inactivity plays in developing

CVD is complex, because the risk varies depending on what other risk factors a person has. However, because inactivity contributes to several risk factors of CVD, such as obesity, high blood pressure, and diabetes, it appears that increasing your physical activity can decrease your risk of CVD in several ways.

How inactivity damages your health

Being a "couch potato" may be one of the riskiest behaviors around, and one of the most commonly practiced. According to the Federal Drug Administration (FDA), one in four adults is sedentary, meaning that they sit around too much.

The heart, being a muscle, needs exercise to keep it strong and to keep the blood vessels that deliver blood to the heart working well. Some people have jobs that require constant walking or intense physical labor; others must find ways to be active when they get home, such as going to the gym, mowing the lawn, doing home improvement projects, or just taking a walk. The real problem begins when people who don't have active jobs also don't get any exercise at home. This fully sedentary approach to life is often combined with poor nutrition; the impact that both poor nutrition and inactivity can have on the heart can lead to serious heart disease.

How aerobic exercise improves your health

Want to increase your life span and your health without spending thousands of dollars? Want to try something that takes up just an hour of your time each day, a few days a week? A half an hour to an hour of aerobic exercise — which can be any type exercise that increases your heart rate for a sustained amount of time — three to four times a week can do the trick for you.

How can such a small amount of time a day yield such great results? The journal *Diabetes Care* reported that whether people lost weight, the ones who worked out 38 minutes a day lowered their blood pressure, heart disease risk, cholesterol, and AIC levels. The increase in activity equaled only about 2,200 extra steps a day.

Like all muscles, the heart becomes stronger and larger as a result of exercise; it can then pump more blood through the body with every beat and sustain its maximum level with less strain. The resting heart rate of people who exercise is also slower because less effort is needed to pump blood.

Regular aerobic exercise significantly benefits you in the following ways:

✔ **Aids in regulating blood pressure:** Regular exercise (at least 30 minutes of exercise on most, if not all, days) helps keep arteries elastic, even in older people, which ensures blood flow and normal blood pressure.

Sedentary people have a 35 percent greater risk of developing high blood pressure (*hypertension*) than athletes do, but you don't need high-intensity exercise to lower blood pressure. In fact, in one study, moderate exercise (jogging 2 miles a day) controlled hypertension so well that more than half the patients who had been on high blood pressure meds were able to discontinue them. So, even if you're not a competitive athlete, you can still get excellent benefits from less intense levels of exercise.

Studies also indicate that yoga and T'ai Chi, an ancient Chinese exercise involving slow, relaxing movements, may lower blood pressure almost as well as moderate-intensity aerobic exercises. (Check out

T'ai Chi For Dummies by Therese Iknoian and *Yoga For Dummies* by Georg Feuerstein, Larry Payne, and Lilias Folan [Wiley]).

High blood pressure is a major risk factor for stroke, so regulating your blood pressure is a good way to minimize your risk of stroke. The effects of exercise on stroke aren't well established, but most studies are positive. The following are some examples:

- According to one major analysis, men cut their risk for stroke in half when their exercise program roughly equated one hour of brisk walking five days a week. In the same study, exercise that involved recreation was more protective against stroke than exercise routines consisting simply of walking or climbing.
- A 2000 study of women also found substantial protection from stroke due to brisk walking or striding (not simply casual walking).

If you have high blood pressure, discuss an exercise program with your doctor before starting. In addition, you should:

- Work with your doctor to lower your pressure enough that you can control it with medications before you begin an exercise program.
- Avoid caffeinated beverages, which increase heart rate, the workload of the heart, and blood pressure during physical activity.
- Breathe as normally as possible through each exercise (holding the breath increases blood pressure).

✔ **Increases oxygen consumption:** Exercise increases the total number of red blood cells in the body to facilitate transport of oxygen. People who exercise the most often and vigorously have the lowest risk for heart disease, but any exercise is beneficial. Studies consistently find that light to moderate exercise is even beneficial in people with *existing* heart disease, as long as your doctor prescribes the activity, and in some cases, supervises the activity.

Progressive resistance training (like using hand weights) may be particularly useful. Even daily handgrip exercises can improve blood flow.

Only your doctor can prescribe an appropriate exercise program for your particular cardiovascular situation. Consult you doctor before starting an exercise program if you have any type of heart disease.

✔ **Strengthens muscles:** Aerobic exercises can help tone muscles throughout the body, which can provide several benefits:

- Improves overall circulation and reduces blood pressure
- Increases storage of energy molecules, such as fats and carbohydrates, within the muscles for increased endurance
- Increases the dilation of blood vessels in the muscle fibers, which improves blood flow through the muscles
- Strengthens muscles involved in respiration to facilitate the flow of air in and out of the lungs

✔ **Assists weight loss:** In 2002, a study on overweight adults confirmed beneficial changes in cholesterol and lipid levels, including lower LDL levels (bad cholesterol) even with very modest weight loss, suggesting that overweight people who have trouble losing pounds can still achieve considerable heart benefits by exercising.

Even people who performed low amounts of moderate- or high-intensity exercise, such as walking or jogging 12 miles a week, received benefits.

More intense exercise is required to significantly change cholesterol levels, notably increasing HDL (good cholesterol). An example of such a program is jogging about 20 miles a week.

✔ **Lowers the risk for type 2 diabetes:** Exercise lowers blood sugar, improves insulin sensitivity, and strengthens the heart — important issues for diabetics and people at risk for diabetes. One study found that adults who worked out 2 1/2 hours a week cut their risk of type 2 diabetes by 58 percent.

How heart-healthy foods help keep your clicker clean

Can you eat your way to good cardiac health? There's no question that a diet rich in fruits and vegetables is beneficial to heart health and can considerably reduce the risk of coronary heart disease. The exact reason is still unclear, but medical researchers theorize that antioxidants in fruit and vegetables lower LDL cholesterol levels in the blood. Foods with *anthocyanin, a flavonoid* (plants known for their antioxidant properties) in the skins of dark-colored fruits and vegetables, are best. See Chapter 7 for more on these foods.

The very large Harvard Nurse's Health Study, which followed more than 110,000 people over a 14-year period, found that people who averaged eight servings of fruit and vegetables a day were 30 percent less likely to suffer a heart attack or stroke than those who ate one and a half servings or less per day. According to a study by the United States Centers for Disease Control, only 27 percent of women and 19 percent of men report eating the recommended five servings of fruits and vegetables each day.

For other heart healthy food choices, consider that the fiber in unrefined (not processed) whole-grain foods can help lower your blood cholesterol. The American Heart Association recommends soluble fiber from whole-grain foods like bran, oatmeal, and whole wheat bread for a heart-healthy diet.

Another great dietary addition is omega-3 fatty acids, found in fish or fish oil supplements, some nuts (such as English walnuts), and vegetable oils. Studies support that omega-3 fatty acids lower triglycerides and reduce your risk of heart attack or stroke (blockage type), especially if you have known cardiovascular disease. You need to follow the recommended dosing, because people who ingest more than 3 grams a day can actually have an increased risk of hemorrhagic (bleeding type) stroke. Omega-3 fatty acids have also been associated with slightly lowering blood pressure.

 Substituting soy proteins for animal proteins may also help lower LDL cholesterol, according to the American Heart Association.

Aerobic Exercise — Ready, Set, Go!

Lucky for you, aerobic exercise comes in a wide variety of choices. For example, running a long distance at a moderate pace is an aerobic exercise, and playing singles tennis with near-continuous motion is generally considered aerobic activity. Other examples are swimming laps, biking, rollerblading, and cross country skiing. By getting your body moving through aerobic exercise, you breathe more deeply, making your heart work harder to pump blood.

The type of exercise — or exercises — you decide to concentrate on is up to you. Some forms of aerobic workouts are certainly more familiar, but finding an activity you enjoy is the key, as long as it keeps your heart rate elevated for a continuous time period. Check out your local health club for a schedule of activities; almost every one of them — from kickboxing to belly dancing to spin classes to yoga — can provide aerobic benefits.

Engaging in the joint-damaging, high-impact styles of workout isn't necessary. The same cardiovascular effects can be obtained through low-impact workouts like swimming and working out on an elliptical trainer, and you avoid the bone and muscle jarring that can result in strains, sprains, and muscle tears.

Although most healthy people of any age can safely engage in moderate levels of physical activity (such as walking, gardening, and yard work) without consulting a doctor first, some people — particularly those age 40 or over — should see a doctor for a medical evaluation before beginning a physical activity program, especially one that involves intense training. (See Chapter 9 for a checklist to help you decide whether you need to consult a physician before starting a new exercise routine.)

The time factor: How long and how often?

When people begin an exercise program, many begin exercising too hard and for too long. Doing too much too fast can result in muscle injury, and then you're sidelined for weeks while you heal. The American Heart Association recommends that you engage in moderate to intense aerobic exercise for 30 to 60 minutes three to four days a week. This recommendation supports similar exercise guidelines from the Centers for Disease Control and Prevention and the American College of Sports Medicine.

Some studies suggest that the greatest heart protection

isn't about the duration of a single exercise session; it's about the total daily amount of energy you use. In other words, the best way to work out may be with multiple short bouts of intense exercise. This advice can be particularly helpful for older people because they may not have the stamina for sustained exercise.

Starting off and ending right: Warming up and cooling down

Warming up and cooling down are important parts of every exercise routine. They help your body make the transition from rest to activity and back again, and can help prevent soreness or injury, especially in older people. Starting a workout too quickly can lead to muscle strain and injury, and stopping too suddenly can sharply reduce blood pressure, which is a particular danger for older people because they may become lightheaded and/or faint. Skipping a cool-down period may also cause muscle cramping.

Proper rest and recovery are also as important to health as exercise; otherwise your muscles can't improve or adapt adequately to the exercise.

When planning your exercise program, don't forget the following warm-up and cool-down tips:

✔ **Practice warm-up exercises for 5 to 10 minutes at the beginning of an exercise session.** Older people may need a longer period — typically at least 10 minutes — to warm up their muscles. A few warm-up options are to do some jumping jacks, jump rope, or go for a light jog or even just a short walk. The warm-up could be just a slower form of the activity that you're aiming to do. You just want to get the heart rate going and start warming the muscles.

If you want to stretch as part of your warm-up, be sure to do so carefully and do it after your initial warm-up — if you stretch cold muscles too quickly, you can injure them.

✔ **The cool-down is used to gradually decrease the heart rate until it's 10 to 15 beats above your resting heart rate.** This part of your routine should take about as long as the warm-up — 5 to 10 minutes. You may want to include lowering the intensity of the exercise you just performed. Stretching is a great option for the cool-down period. It helps to relax the muscles and increase flexibility. You should try to hold the stretches for about 20 to 30 seconds and cover all the major muscle groups. One theory is that cool-down stretching could reduce future injury, but it hasn't been proven.

The meat of the aerobic workout: Determining your target zone

Being confronted with fancy equipment for determining whether you're exercising in the "zone" or for figuring out what your "target heart rate" is may be enough to push you away from exercise forever — or have you sticking to something simple, like a walk around the block. Although any exercise is better than none at all, proper exercise gives you more bang for the buck in terms of cardiac benefits. Fear not — we're here to help you understand what your target rate, maximum rate, and VO_2 zone are and how to find them. It's easier than it sounds!

Identifying the terminology you need to know

If you're going to make exercise an important part of your healthy aging routine, you need to learn the lingo. Knowing how your heart rate and oxygen capacity can determine the quality of your exercise helps develop an appropriate routine. Determining what your heart rate should be based on your age and exercise intensity not only improves your aerobic workouts, but also keeps you from overdoing it and possibly harming your heart instead of helping it. Here's a look at some of the exercise terms that you may hear bandied about the gym:

- **Maximum heart rate.** This is the maximum rate that your heart should beat while exercising. Reaching rates beyond your maximum heart rate can be unsafe. The easy calculation is

  220 – your age = maximum heart rate

  Example: If you're 40 years old, 220 – 40 = 180 beats per minute

- **Target heart rate.** Target heart rate is measured as the number of beats per minute that you want to achieve for maximum exercise benefit. The target heart rate lets you measure your initial fitness level and monitor your progress in a fitness program. This approach requires measuring your pulse periodically while you exercise and staying within 60 to 85 percent of your maximum heart rate (your *target heart rate zone*). In your specific zone, you attempt to achieve a percentage of this maximum heart rate.

  Target heart rate = 60 to 85 percent × the maximum heart rate

  (Beginners start with 60 percent; moderate exercisers 75 percent; and advanced exercisers 85 percent.)

  Example: If you're 40 years old, your maximum

heart rate is 180 beats per minute. Take this number and multiply by 60 to 85 percent depending on your level of exercise.

180 (maximum heart rate) × 0.6 (60 percent for beginners) = 108 beats per minute

This number may seem low, but it's for beginners or a starting point for people who have an underlying medical condition. This number is increased gradually until you get to 85 percent.

Table 10-1 shows estimated target heart rates for different ages. Look for the age category closest to yours, and then read across to find your target heart rate.

A few high blood pressure medications, primarily beta blockers (propranolol, metoprolol, nadolol, and atenolol), lower the maximum heart rate and thus the target zone rate. If you're taking such medicine, call your physician to find out whether you need to use a lower target heart rate.

✔ **Aerobic capacity (VO_2 max).** This term describes the status of the cardiorespiratory system (the heart, lungs, and blood vessels) and is the maximum volume of oxygen that can be consumed by your muscles during exercise (which is why it's often called VO_2 max). The aerobic capacity represents your cardiorespiratory performance and your muscles' ability to extract the oxygen and fuel they receive. The higher your VO_2 max, the more oxygen is transported to exercising muscles and the longer you can exercise without exhaustion. So, the higher aerobic capacity, the higher your level of aerobic fitness.

To measure maximum aerobic capacity, you exercise on a treadmill, first by walking at an easy pace and then, at set time intervals during graded exercise tests, gradually increasing the workload.

Table 10-1	Target and Maximum Heart Rates According to Age	
Age	**Target Heart Rate (HR) (60–85%)**	**Predicted Maximum Heart Rate**
20	120–170	200
25	117–166	195
30	114–162	190
35	111–157	185
40	108–153	180
45	105–149	175
50	102–145	170
55	99–140	165
60	96–136	160
65	93–132	155
70	90–128	150

Creating an aerobic routine that meets your goals

Now that you know your target heart rate, you need a plan to reach your goal safely, without injuring muscles. Rome wasn't built in a day, and neither is a healthy heart!

When starting an exercise program, aim at the lowest part of your target zone (60 percent) during the first few weeks. Gradually build up to the higher part of your target zone (75 percent). After six months or more of regular exercise, you may be able to exercise comfortably at up to 85 percent of your maximum heart rate. **Note:** You don't have to exercise that hard to *stay in shape.* It's not necessary to be a marathoner (unless you really want to be) or to spend hours every day at the gym (unless you really love it there). Studies show that making exercise a habit and keeping your heart rate in the aerobic zone for 30 to 45 minutes most days gives you the cardiovascular benefits you need to reduce your risk of cardiovascular disease.

Based on your goals, follow these guidelines:

✓ If you're a beginner with a goal of improving overall fitness, losing weight, or reducing stress, exercise in the *healthy heart zone,* which is 50 to 60 percent of your maximum heart rate.

✓ If you already exercise regularly but are aiming to lose body fat, exercise in the *weight management zone,* which is 60 to 70 percent of your maximum heart rate. Build up to a workout of an hour of continuous exercise.

✓ If your goal is to improve aerobic capacity or athletic performance, exercise in the *aerobic zone,* which is 70 to 80 percent of your maximum heart rate.

✓ Competitive athletes may need to add interval training sessions during the week in the *anaerobic threshold heart rate zone,* which is 80 to 90 percent of maximum. This high-intensity exercise helps train muscles to handle lactic acid.

Exercising regularly at a heart rate intensity that's too high doesn't produce additional aerobic benefits; however, it does increase the possibility of an athletic injury.

To receive the benefits of physical activity, you don't want to tire too quickly. Pacing yourself is especially important if you've been inactive.

Chapter 11

Building and Fine-Tuning Healthy Muscles

When you think of exercise, you may think of walking, jogging, or cycling — but not strength training. Who, you, lift weights? Yes — although there's more to strength training than just lifting weights. The benefits of strength training for everyone at any age, not just body builders, have been studied in detail only over the past few decades. Strength training is more than just lifting weights to build muscle, although building muscle is excellent for staying in shape, maintaining your weight, and releasing endorphins, which make you feel good.

Strength training also makes your bones more dense, improves your balance (reducing the risk of falls), and can reduce the pain and disability of arthritis. In this chapter, we dissect your muscles, show you what happens on the inside when you do strength training, help you design a workable and effective strength-training program, and even give you tips on what to do when you've overdone it.

The Importance of Muscle Maintenance and Strengthening

Staying in shape as you get older is much more than a vanity thing. Keeping your muscles strong can help keep your whole body healthy, from your heart to your bones, and can help you live independently as you age. One of the greatest risks of aging is the increased incidence of falls; people who do strength training regularly are much less likely to fall and break a hip. Why? Because the more muscle mass you have, the better you protect your body against bone loss and joint deterioration — not to mention the fact that strength training for strong muscles also fosters growth in bone density.

Building muscle also decreases the amount of body fat you have, and body fat brings risks to your heart and cardiovascular system. So you definitely want to shed those extra pounds.

What happens to aging muscles

As people age, their skeletal muscle mass starts to deteriorate. Your *skeletal muscles* (also known as lean muscle) are the muscles that attach to your bones and are under voluntary control. These muscles include the biceps (more on the other two types of muscle later in this chapter).

As a result of deterioration, people begin to look, well, flabby as they get older. You may see these changes start as early as your 30s, but most people see the biggest changes between their 40s and 50s. You may find yourself staring in the mirror, wondering when your body started slipping south.

A recent study concluded that total muscle mass decreases by nearly 50 percent for people between the ages of 20 and 90. On average, people lose about 30 percent of their strength between ages 50 and 70, and another 30 percent of what's left per decade after that. Generally, people lose about 1 percent of their lean muscle mass per year after age 40.

There are four types of muscle weakening (called *atrophy*) that become more common as people age, and each type responds differently to strength training. They include the following:

- **Sedentary:** Muscle deterioration is a natural process, but a sedentary lifestyle can accelerate it. You can rebuild muscle mass lost from a sedentary lifestyle — all you have to do is get off the couch and do something physical! Some sedentary people include those who are bedridden, astronauts, and people with minimal physical activity.

  Statistics show that people confined to bed can lose around 1 percent of muscle strength for each day in bed. Physical therapy is often prescribed as treatment for people who are bedridden so that they don't have muscle loss. A person's recovery time from being bedridden can be improved if the proper actions are taken to prevent muscle loss. Interestingly, muscle loss also affects astronauts, who spend much time in a weightless state!

- **Age-related:** Age-related muscle loss is also called *sarcopenia,* which means "vanishing flesh."

Sarcopenia isn't an inevitable part of aging; it's the result of the loss of around ten ounces of muscle a year that isn't replaced due to a sedentary lifestyle. You can win this muscle back with a strength-training program.

✔ **Medication-related:** Certain medications, such as systemic corticosteroids (often prescribed for people with asthma or inflammatory conditions such as rheumatoid arthritis or lupus), can result in muscle weakness.

✔ **Disease-related:** Muscle atrophy from disease can be more difficult to overcome, especially when it involves nerve damage or disease of the muscle itself. The muscle loss in these situations is more damaging because you have almost no use of the diseased muscles. With the other types of muscle loss, you have at least some use of the muscle groups. Cancer can also result in a muscle wasting syndrome called *cachexia.* Diseases that cause cachexia often progress rapidly; many have no cure and are progressively disabling. Work closely with your doctor to prevent muscle loss if you have any of these conditions:

- Nerve diseases affecting muscles, including polio (poliomyelitis)
- Lou Gehrig's disease (amyotrophic lateral sclerosis or ALS)
- Guillain-Barre syndrome (self-limiting demyelinating polyradiculoneuropathy), which can cause short-term muscle weakness or paralysis

Other diseases affecting muscles include muscular dystrophy, congestive heart disease, liver disease, and

AIDS. If you have any of these illnesses, talk to your doctor about setting up a physical therapy program to help you retain as much muscle mass as possible.

In addition to general skeletal muscle loss, the following changes occur as you age:

- **Muscles take longer to respond to brain signals in your 50s than they did in your 20s.** As a normal course of aging, you begin to lose the muscle fibers that are responsible for making you move quickly. The speed of transmission of impulses from the brain to the muscles also slows down, so it takes longer to get the signal, "Hey! Move it!" Your muscles also can't repair themselves as quickly as they used to, due to a decrease in enzyme activities and protein turnover.

- **The water content of _tendons_ (the cord-like tissues that attach muscles to bones) decreases as you age.** This change makes the tissues stiffer and less able to tolerate stress.

- **Your heart muscle becomes less able to propel large quantities of blood quickly through your body.** As a result, you tire more quickly and take longer to recover. Check out Chapter 13 for info on keeping your heart muscle healthy and strong.

How exercise can help

Whether you're physically inactive due to your job and daily responsibilities, or you're a classic couch potato, or you've been bedridden due to a broken leg, your muscles start to rebuild as soon as you put them to work with some strength training.

You can delay or minimize the onset of age-related muscle atrophy if you incorporate strength training as part of your daily or weekly routine. You may notice that you have to work out a little harder just to keep from losing your lean muscle mass, but a nutrient-rich diet, strength training, and hormone supplements can help you keep and possibly build more muscles. Even 80-year-old muscles benefit from strength training, so it's never too late to start. Muscles that haven't been exercised can be revitalized at any time, whether you're 18 or 80 years old.

The longer your muscles have been inactive, the more slowly you must begin exercising them. If you haven't exercised or have any condition that has limited your activity for more than six months, you should consult your physician prior to any exercise. **Note:** The muscle, of course, must be healthy and already have some mobility.

Calling All Muscles: Report for Duty!

Think you don't have any muscles? You do — you have 640 of them! Muscles attached to bone is what allows you to move, and muscles are found throughout your body, and some of them act without your knowledge — or permission! Check out the following sections for further info on the different types of muscles in your body.

The three types of muscle

Muscle movement can be either voluntary and involuntary — *voluntary muscles* are those that you have control over; *involuntary muscles* do their own thing whether you want them to or not (and whether you're aware of them or not!). Within these general categories, you have three types of muscle:

- ✔ **Skeletal muscle:** This voluntary muscle is commonly referred to as *lean muscle mass* and is attached to bone. Skeletal muscle helps you move the various parts of your body — biceps, hamstrings, quadriceps, and basically any muscle you can tone at the gym.

  In this chapter, we focus primarily on your skeletal muscles because you have some control over strengthening them.

- ✔ **Smooth muscle:** This involuntary muscle moves food along your digestive tract and blood through blood vessels. For example, *peristalsis* is rhythmic movements of the muscles that force food from the throat into the esophagus and then into the stomach. It also allows you to eat and drink while swinging upside-down on the monkey bars!

  As for your smooth muscles, they pretty much take care of themselves. There really aren't exercises for beefing up your colon.

- ✔ **Heart muscle:** This involuntary muscle keeps your heart pumping without your having to think about it — imagine how stressful life would be if you had to concentrate on keeping your heart beating all day long!

  Your heart is clearly your most important muscle, but strengthening it doesn't involve weights; we cover it all on its own in Chapter 10.

The major skeletal muscle groups

In this section, we cover the major skeletal muscle groups, what they do, and the best ways to strengthen them for maximum muscle health. Here's a list of muscle groups and their jobs (see Figures 11-1 and 11-2):

- **Chest:** Help you breathe, lift a sagging chest, improve posture, and lift breast tissue

- **Abdominals:** Help hold in your stomach and support your back

- **Back:** Keep the spine in position, support your stomach, strengthen your core, strengthen your posture, and help with low back pain

- **Shoulders:** Lift, turn, and rotate the arms; keep the chest, back, and neck in line

- **Biceps:** Move the arms toward the shoulders and turn the arms. Also the muscle you flex when someone asks you to "make a muscle."

- **Triceps:** Straighten the arm. The lack of triceps toning allows your arm flab to jiggle when you wave goodbye.

- **Quadriceps:** Help you walk by allowing you to bend your knee; help protect against kneecap cartilage loss

- **Hamstrings:** Allow you to straighten your leg

- **Calves:** Lift the heel for walking

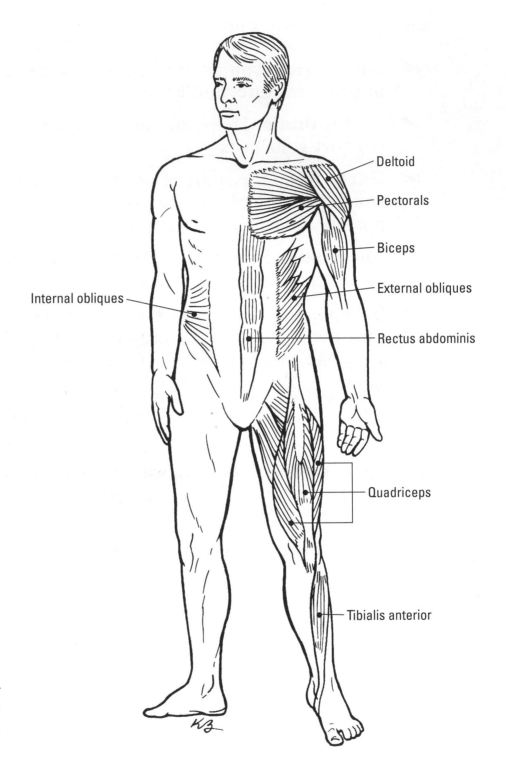

Deltoid

Pectorals

Biceps

External obliques

Internal obliques

Rectus abdominis

Quadriceps

Tibialis anterior

**Figure
11-1:**
*The body's
major
muscle
groups
(front).*

374

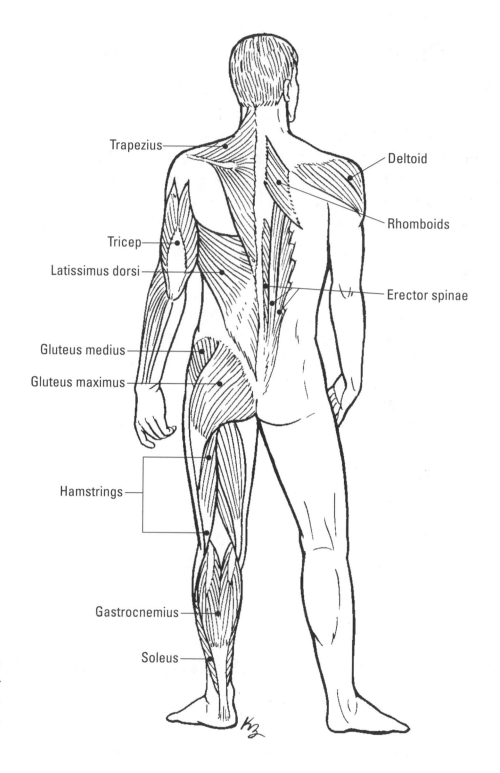

Trapezius

Deltoid

Rhomboids

Tricep

Latissimus dorsi

Erector spinae

Gluteus medius

Gluteus maximus

Hamstrings

Gastrocnemius

Soleus

Figure 11-2:
The body's major muscle groups (back).

The female monster-muscle myth and other hogwash

Women may worry that strength training makes their muscles bulky. Nothing can be farther from the truth. Most women don't have the genetic makeup or enough of the male hormone, testosterone, to bulk up like Popeye. That said, however, women are perfectly capable of developing strong, lean muscles. Pound-for-pound, female muscles are just as strong as a male's.

You may also have heard that strength training can be dangerous for women. More hogwash! Under a microscope, male and female muscle tissue are identical. Women are just as resilient as men and benefit from the same strength-training routines. Strength training also provides added protection against *osteoporosis,* a thinning of the bones that occurs after menopause (see Chapter 6).

Another reason some women stay away from strength training is because they're addicted to the scale. Have you ever heard a woman say that she's gained, not lost weight, after a couple of weeks of weight training? The reason behind the weight gain is that muscle is denser than fat. So, you may weigh more for a few weeks as your body adjusts its fat and muscle ratios. Soon enough, however, you notice that your pants aren't as tight around the waist. People start telling you that you look thinner. Our best advice? Throw out the scale! Evaluate yourself by the way your clothes fit and the way you feel.

The Two Types of Muscle-Related Training

Muscles live to work for you. The more you put into them, the more they'll work for you. Unlike any human-built machine (like a car or a computer), the more you rev up your muscles, the bigger they get and the harder they work for you. That's where strength training (sometimes called *strength and resistance training;* see the nearby sidebar "What's in a name? Strength versus resistance training") along with flexibility for stretching, stamina, and agility come into play.

To minimize confusion, we use the term *strength training* throughout this book to refer to both because, in all actuality, if you're strength training, you're inherently resistance training.

Strength training

Unlike aerobic exercise, which increases your heart rate, strength training concentrates on using your muscles to exert or resist force. This process can be done by using free weights, using weight machines — or other equipment that offers resistance when you push or pull against it, such as elasticized bands called resistance bands — or by doing exercises such as pushups. You can choose the option that works best for you.

Within each of the options for strength training are several other options, and it can get confusing trying to decide where to start. The following descriptions may help you:

- **Free weights:** With nothing more than a pair of dumbbells, free weights provide you with a variety of options to spice up any workout for many of your muscle groups. All you need is a little desire, creativity, and good form. A basic starter set of free weights is also fairly inexpensive and so small that you can store the weights very easily.

  Be sure that your form is correct so you get the maximum benefit *and* don't injure yourself. With some guidance, practice, and a little common sense, you'll be building your biceps in no time.

✔ **Weight machines:** These are a great choice for strength training, particularly if you belong to a fitness center. Machines are safe, smooth, and easy, and they specifically target one muscle or group of muscles. They're often set up in a specific routine to quickly exercise all the muscle groups.

Some people go this route in an attempt to bypass the personal trainer. The machines can guide you through the movements to achieve better form than dumbbells or bar bells.

Machines are great for beginners, because they don't have much of an intimidation factor. You select the seat height and the appropriate weight, and you follow the machine's range of motion to guarantee that you hit your target muscle. Because beginners aren't familiar with proper form, these machines also help prevent injuries by controlling the movements. Most gym staff members are more than happy to help you get started. Also, if you want some great

What's in a name? Strength versus resistance training

Chances are you've heard of both *strength* training and *resistance* training and are a bit fuzzy on the difference between the two — and for good reason! Strength and resistance training are largely interchangeable terms:

✔ Strength training is weight training.

✔ Resistance training is a specific form of strength training in which you perform each effort against an opposing force (elastic or hydraulic resistance).

guidance on starting a weight-training program, *Weight Training For Dummies,* 3rd Edition, by Liz Neporent, Suzanne Schlosberg, and Shirley J. Archer (Wiley), is your ticket.

✓ **Low-impact resistance training:** With resistance training, you only pull or push to get a rewarding workout. The beauty of resistance training is its low impact on your joints, because it allows you to create a full range of motion. Resistance training comes in the following forms:

- Swimming, with or without water weights and swimming gloves, and other water exercises
- Bicycle riding
- Elliptical machines (look like a cross between a stair-stepper, cross-country ski machine, and bicycle without a seat)
- All-in-one resistance machines (allow you to work a number of different muscle groups without switching machines)
- Stair steppers
- Resistance bands (used for strength training and available in graduated amounts of tension for isolating muscle groups)
- Calf raises and pushups (easy exercises, good for stretching and strength training)

✓ **Exercise balls:** This equipment works the core muscles, which helps you improve your balance and coordination by strengthening muscles in your upper legs, back, and abdominal region.

 Water exercises offer another type of low-impact training. Many fitness centers even offer classes. Water aerobics is for people who want to develop muscle and increase their strength but don't want to worry about their balance or the impact on their joints (or how to use those machines in the gym). You can buy weights for your arms or legs to help increase resistance as you exercise in the pool.

Flexibility training

Flexibility is the other half of the equation in strength training. Although you can have muscle strength and not be flexible, it doesn't necessarily make for easier living. What good does it do a 55-year-old woman to bench press 50 pounds if she can't bend over and tie her shoes? In addition to improving your balance and range of motion, flexibility training helps prevent and treat injury.

Exercise routines that include flexibility and range-of-motion movements not only strengthen muscles but also calm the mind. The goal of these exercises is to lengthen the *fascia,* a fibrous tissue that covers all muscle, allowing the underlying muscle to move and grow. The following programs provide this essential training:

- **Stretching:** Think twice before skipping this step, which people often skip. Stretching is a great way to give your body a gentle wake-up call (as opposed to a blaring revelry at 0500) or an effective warm-up. More than just being nice to your body, the benefits of stretching include

  - Preparing your joints for motion to help you avoid injury in the muscles you work
  - Helping reduce muscle soreness and cramping because it increases your flexibility after a workout

- **Yoga:** Yoga can make you more fit and improve your flexibility, strength, and endurance. The most familiar form of yoga works primarily through various levels of postures (from the Cat to the Corpse) combined with breathing exercises.

If you want to kick it up a notch, add the most physically challenging style of hatha yoga in *Power Yoga For Dummies* by Doug Swenson (Wiley). You still benefit from flexibility, strength, and endurance, but you turn up the heat with aerobic intensity for an empowering mind and body workout.

Don't be fooled into thinking that yoga is just for women and old people. Yoga stretches can be challenging even for the fittest individuals. (For more information on yoga, read Chapter 15.)

- **T'ai Chi:** For nearly 5,000 years, people have practiced T'ai Chi as a way to prolong life, build strength and stamina, improve concentration, and achieve psychological balance. This form of training can also help you increase balance and flexibility while you tone your muscles. People of any age can enjoy T'ai Chi.

  If you're 60 years or older, find out whether your community offers T'ai Chi programs for seniors. Because recent statistics show that T'ai Chi helps reduce falls, many states are funding these programs, making them free to the public.

- **Pilates:** Once thought of as just for professional dancers, this great activity combines elements of yoga, dance, gymnastics, and boxing with a little modern creativity thrown in. With Pilates, you can tone your muscles, improve balance, lengthen your spine, strengthen your core muscles, and improve flexibility and coordination.

TIP If you're not as hip as you want to be on the exercise trends of today, check out these other insightful books published by Wiley:

- *Stretching For Dummies* by LaReine Chabut
- *Yoga For Dummies* by Georg Feuerstein, Larry Payne, and Lilias Folan
- *Yoga with Weights For Dummies* by Sherri Baptiste and Megan Scott
- *T'ai Chi For Dummies* by Therese Iknoian
- *Pilates For Dummies* by Ellie Herman

Putting Your Strength- and Flexibility-Increasing Plan into Action — Safely

If you're not careful, your workout can leave you in worse shape than before you started. Your first thought when starting a strength-training program should be "safety first." Unfortunately, many folks put safety last, at least until they drop a dumbbell on their foot and are sidelined from strength training for weeks.

Sprains, strains, pulls, and other injuries can all wreak havoc on an exercise routine, so start slow, watch your form, and follow the suggestions in the next sections. If you do injure yourself, we also tell you how to take care of yourself to get back on your feet as quickly as possible.

Moving through your training and individual workouts

Planning your training workout can be complicated if you look at all the conflicting information on the Internet.

Don't worry about the differing opinions too much; the most important thing is to just get started, and you can refine your routine down the road. Here are some other important tips to keep you moving forward safely and effectively:

✔ **Alternate between upper and lower body on the days you strength train.** For example, work out your upper body (your arms, chest, and back) one day, and then your lower body the next time you train. When you strength train, you actually create tiny tears in your muscles that need to heal before you lift again. (For this reason, don't work the same muscles two days in a row.) This important process

---

Preventing accidental falls among older adults

It's a frightening reality. More than one-third of adults 65 and older fall each year. Of those who fall, 20 to 30 percent suffer moderate to severe injuries that make getting around or living alone more difficult and increase the chance of early death. Older adults are hospitalized five times more often for fall-related injuries than injuries from other causes.

The most common fractures are of the spine, hip, forearm, leg, ankle, pelvis, upper arm, and hand. Many people who fall, even those who aren't injured, develop a fear of falling. This fear creates a limit of activities, which leads to reduced mobility and physical fitness, which in turn increases the risk of falling.

How can older adults prevent falls? Improve lean muscle mass and exercise! Muscle helps support the body's frame, and regular exercise supports the strong muscles with balance, circulation, strength, and confidence.

is key to your program because it allows your muscles to come back just a little bit stronger each time.

✔ **After six or more weeks of consistent strength training, add more weight and change the order of your workout to make it more challenging.** For example, if your workout consists of a routine to work different muscle groups, change the order of your workout. You may want to change the time of day as well.

After you have some of the basics incorporated into your training routine, you may be interested in improving your training by refining how you rotate muscle groups. To help you achieve your best results from every workout, follow these suggestions:

✔ **Always warm up.** Do 10 to 15 minutes of light cardio (like walking or jogging), and don't forget the all-important stretching to avoid injury — see "Flexibility training" for more info on the importance of stretching. After you're actively exercising, your body is warm, so it's not necessary to stretch between reps or exercises.

✔ **Work large muscle groups before small ones.** If you wait to work the largest muscles last, you'll be too tired, so work your muscles in this general order: quadriceps, hamstrings, calves.

✔ **Work one muscle group before moving on to the next muscle group.** For example, perform all your quadriceps exercises first before moving on to the hamstring for maximum muscle buildup and minimum muscle fatigue.

When you're starting out, choose one exercise for each muscle group and do one set of 12 to 15 repetitions of each exercise. After a few weeks, you may want to slightly increase the weight as well as perform another set. At this point, individuals looking to increase strength may reduce the number of repetitions to about 10 to 12 as they increase the weight lifted.

✔ **Make sure the weight is right for you.** It's not about how heavy the weights are. The goal is being able to lift a weight heavy enough that your muscle is tired or fatigued after 12 to 15 reps.

Muscle responds to resistance. Use a weight that's too light and your muscles don't work hard enough; use a weight that's too heavy and you can damage your skeletal muscles and joints. For example, if you're doing a bicep curl with a 12-pound dumbbell, your goal is to do 12 to 15 repetitions per set. If the last few are a bit of a struggle, you know that the weight is making your muscle work. If you can't make it to 10 reps, then go lighter. If 20 reps is a breeze, add more weight accordingly.

✔ **Get used to using weight machines (if you exercise at a gym) before you use free weights.** Free weights require a bit more coordination and the use of more muscles to stabilize your body. Condition your muscles using weight machines before moving on to free weights.

✔ **Focus on your form.** Good form is more effective than using heavier weights, which leave you prone to injury. So for the first few weeks, focus on doing each exercise correctly. If you're using the right form, you can maximize your workouts with lighter weights and in the long run actually accelerate muscle strength. Also, talk to one of the staff at the gym or hire a personal trainer to be sure your form is correct. Proper form is critical. See the next section for tips on how to get proper form.

Preventing injury

If you're new to strength training, make sure that you talk to a professional first about your general fitness and health. In Chapter 9, we discuss key factors that determine whether you should consult your doctor before beginning an exercise program. If you don't fit those parameters but are new to strength training, and if you can afford it, we recommend that you have at least a couple of sessions with a personal trainer to show you proper form, give you helpful guidance, and answer any questions you may have.

In addition, buy or rent helpful videos to show you visual techniques on form. To maximize your workout and help prevent injury, follow these guidelines:

- ✔ **Align your body correctly.** If you're standing, your feet should be shoulder-width apart with your knees slightly bent.

- ✔ **Mind your movements.** Your movements should be slow and controlled. You aren't racing. Count to four, pause, and then return to your starting position.

- ✔ **Don't forget to breathe.** Your muscles need oxygen, so don't hold your breath. Breathe in at the beginning of the lift and exhale gently through your mouth during the release of each weight.

- ✔ **Especially in the beginning, be careful not to overtrain.** "No pain no gain" is *not* the motto for someone just starting an exercise program — you can damage your muscles and joints if you overdo it. A muscle injury in your first week of strength training can bum you out in no time, making it harder to get back in the gym and back on track. We want you to succeed, so stick to a plan.

Overtraining not only causes muscle injury, but can also make you lose your edge because if you've been progressively working out according to a routine and you get injured, it takes time to recover from your injury. During that time off, you'll slowly begin to lose what you've gained. In essence you'll have to start not where you left off, but farther behind.

✔ **When you stretch, reach until you feel a bit of tension and hold it for 10 to 15 seconds.** Slowly ease into the stretch to give your muscles time to adjust. Never bounce or hold the stretch until you feel pain.

Recognizing when you need to back off

You may be pushing too hard. Here are some signs to look for to indicate you're overdoing it:

✔ Your performance goes down while your effort goes up

✔ You start losing body weight

✔ You start getting infections

✔ You're constantly tired

✔ Your heart rate is elevated and you have an unpleasant burning sensation in your muscles

- ✔ You have difficulty sleeping
- ✔ You've lost your appetite
- ✔ You feel nauseous

If you think you're overworking your muscles because you're experiencing one or more of these symptoms, stop working out and see your doctor.

Body transformation occurs by simultaneously gaining muscle through weight training and losing fat through aerobics and diet. Particularly if you're overweight, begin weight training as part of your doctor-approved routine today. Many people falsely believe that adding weight training will either make you look heavier or impede your weight loss.

Here's the truth: Weight training helps promote weight loss because muscle mass increases your metabolic rate, which directly aids in fat loss. For every pound of muscle you add, your body can burn 30 to 50 more calories a day at rest. Those burned calories are more likely to come from fat reserves, which is really the whole point if your goal is to lose body fat.

Preventing and Treating Muscle-Related Injury

Even the best-trained athletes get hurt. While we're not encouraging you to injure yourself, you may sustain a sprain or strain from time to time. When it happens, you need to treat the injury properly and not make it worse by continuing to push ahead. In this section, we list some of the most common strength-training-related injuries and recommendations for treating them.

If you injure yourself or experience persistent pain or swelling *and* your symptoms don't improve within a day or two, seek proper medical attention.

Joint aches and pains

You may feel a little sore all over if you're a workout newbie. Your body experiences many changes as it adjusts to the new demands you're placing on it, so be gentle if you're sore the first couple of weeks. It's better to ease up than to quit.

If you continue to feel pain in your joints during a particular exercise, stop and ask a fitness instructor for help. Chances are you may not be in proper form. If your form is fine and you still feel joint pain, skip that exercise for now. Ask the fitness instructor for an alternative exercise or for a suggestion for warming up the joints to reduce the stress. If an alternate exercise also causes pain to that particular joint, stop exercising the joint until you can speak with a medical professional.

Very often the cause of joint pain is inflammation of the tendons, called *tendonitis,* or other soft and connective tissue. (Tendons connect muscle to bone.) Ice therapy for 15 minutes three to four times a day can reduce inflammation.

Muscle strains and pulls

If you pull or strain your muscle, it's going to hurt pretty badly because you're stretching your muscle fibers — like a rubber band — beyond their limits and they tear. Yowza! Many actions can lead to muscle pulls, but the painful results are all the same.

Sometimes when you have a severe pulled muscle or injury, you may notice that your urine is brown. This happens due to the excretion of the protein myoglobin that's released when the muscle is damaged. Other symptoms are

389

Relieving muscle soreness that isn't injury-related

That all-over body ache you get after a strenuous weight-lifting session may be partly due to tiny tears in muscle fibers and a buildup of waste materials in the muscles. Rest assured — these tears are completely normal and heal on their own. In the meantime, try one of these suggestions for relief:

✔ **Soak in a hot tub:** Rest your muscles and take a warm soak in the bathtub to loosen your muscles and get blood flowing. Try applying heat in the first 48 hours by bath, water bottle, or heating pad. Be careful, though — never go to sleep with a heating pad on.

✔ **Drink plenty of water:** Always keep your body hydrated, particularly after a workout. Water can help keep your muscles from cramping. Also, try eating a banana to get some extra potassium because potassium is essential for muscle activity.

✔ **Get a massage:** There's nothing like the power of healing touch, and a great massage by a licensed therapist (or even a gentle rub from someone special) can make a tremendous difference to your muscles — and mind, body, and spirit — after a strenuous workout.

✔ **Take an anti-inflammatory:** If you're still feeling muscle pain and soreness after a few of these suggestions, you may want to try an over-the-counter anti-inflammatory such as ibuprofen, aspirin, or naproxen. If you're still having pain, your doctor may prescribe a higher dose anti-inflammatory.

Talk to your doctor if you continue experiencing muscle pain or soreness after five to seven days.

swelling of the muscles a day or two after the injury, stiffness, and of course pain.

To treat muscle pulls, use the *RICE* method:

- ✔ **Relative rest:** Whatever you were doing to cause the muscle pull — *stop!* You won't feel much like doing that again anytime soon anyway. All you need right now is some good, old-fashioned time for the muscle to heal. Several days to several weeks isn't an unusual timeframe, depending on how many muscle fibers you tore.

- ✔ **Ice:** Apply a bag of ice for 15-minute intervals several times a day. This step reduces the swelling and pooling of fluids from leaky muscle cells and blood vessels.

- ✔ **Compression:** Use an elastic bandage for compression to lessen the swelling and constrict the injured blood vessels.

- ✔ **Elevation:** Let gravity do some of the work for you by keeping your muscle elevated above your heart. This step helps keep fluids from pooling in the injured area, keeps swelling down, and helps plasma and fluids return to your heart.

Use the RICE method for the first 12 hours after you pull a muscle because this timeframe is when most of the swelling occurs. After the swelling is under control, apply heat to increase blood flow and promote healing.

Dealing with a sprain

Although people often use the terms interchangeably, sprains and strains are two different things. A *strain* is an injury to a muscle; a *sprain* is an injury to a ligament that attaches bone to bone.

Sprains can result in a lot of swelling. A severe sprain may tear the ligament completely, and the joint will be swollen and discolored, and unable to bear weight. You need to see your doctor to distinguish among a severe sprain, strain, or fracture.

Treatment for sprains is similar to treatment for strains or pulls: rest, ice, compression, and elevation (see the preceding section).

Part V

Sharpening the All-Important Mind and Spirit

The 5th Wave   By Rich Tennant

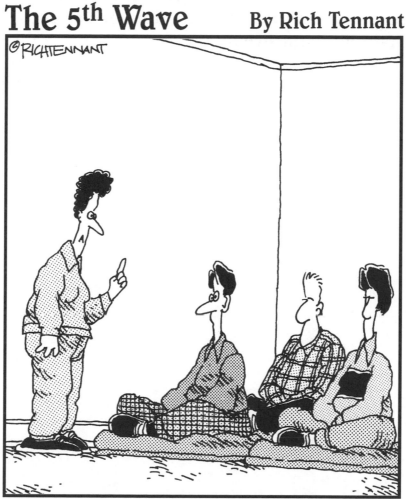

"Here's a tip – if you hear yourself snoring, you're meditating too deeply."

In this part . . .

A positive attitude, a spiritual connection, and a sense of general well-being significantly enhance the quality of life for adults. You can improve your mind and memory through mentally stimulating exercises.

In these chapters, you discover ways to keep your mind and spirit razor-sharp, decrease stress in your life, get a good night's sleep, and maintain your livelihood.

Chapter 12

Keeping Your Mind and Memory in Tip-Top Shape

Your brain — you can't live without it, but you may not appreciate it. It guides you through tasks as simple as deciding what to have for breakfast (No! Not the doughnut!) and as complex as putting together an unassembled child's toy. Brain power sends humans into outer space and to the bottom of the ocean, regulates all your bodily functions, and helps you cross the street safely, but you may take all these functions for granted until the brain stops working as well as it once did.

The brain is the most complex and vital of all organs of the human body. Your brain is command central for intelligence, and it defines and discerns your senses, regulates your body movement, and controls your behavior. It's also responsible for the storage and retrieval of all your precious (and not-so-precious) memories.

Your brain has tremendous — some scientists would say almost unlimited — potential to learn, remember, improvise and create, and its secrets are better understood today than ever before. But your brain does change as you age, as you know all too well if you've ever gone into a room and forgotten what you went there for. Understanding how and why those brain changes occur helps you minimize their effect on your daily activities.

Want to keep your brain young, healthy, active, and beautiful? We can't help with the beautiful part, but in this chapter, you go inside your brain for a look at how it works and how to keep your brain functioning at maximum potential as you age. We also touch on some brain changes outside the normal range that may concern you, such as Alzheimer's, dementia, stroke and Parkinson's disease.

Starting at the Top: Basic Brain Anatomy

You could read brain textbooks for years, and still not scratch the surface in discovering what the brain does. In all honesty, scientists still don't understand all the inner workings of the brain. In this section, we describe the basic anatomy (no, there won't be a test) and functioning of the different parts of the brain. We try to break down the brain anatomy simply, so you can get an idea of the complex computer that runs your body. Understanding which part of the brain controls which activity may help you understand why certain activities cause you difficulty as you become older.

 Researchers have discovered more in the last decade than the previous century because of the advancement in technology and funding for newer projects. The baby boomers have ignited the demand and accelerated the efforts to get more information on the brain. This group is interested in being active both mentally and physically past the traditional retirement age. Many are working into their 60s and 70s and are thriving on new options for healthy aging.

Dividing the brain into three governing areas

The brain divides into three areas: the forebrain, midbrain, and the hindbrain. The hindbrain controls your basic involuntary functions, such as heartbeat and breathing as well as balance and coordination; the midbrain helps control reflexes and your senses; and the biggest part of the brain, the forebrain, controls higher functions such as thinking, planning, and emotions. In the next sections, we explain the brain and its divisions in detail.

The forebrain, your body's command central

The forebrain is the largest part of the brain, covering most of the top of your head, and also the most developed, controlling most of the intellectual activities. Collectively, the forebrain functions to control cognitive, sensory and motor function, and regulate temperature, reproductive functions, eating, sleeping, and the display of emotions.

The forebrain consists primarily of the cerebrum, which is typically the part of the brain that you see in pictures. The cerebrum is divided into two hemispheres that have different responsibilities but are always in communication through a large network of nerve fibers (these hemispheres are physically separate entities). The unique functions that each hemisphere controls are as follows:

- **The right side** of the brain controls the left side of the body. It controls spatial orientation (the ability to

397

know where you are) and facial recognition, among many other things. The right side of the brain allows for music, art, and other creative activity.

✓ **The left side** of the brain controls the right side of the body. It generally controls language functions. Where the right side controls creativity, the left side of your brain is the more analytical side, used for math and logic.

The left and right hemispheres of the cerebrum are divided into four lobes, which drive most of your body's functions. The following details of the actions of the lobes as well as their location in your brain may be helpful (see Figure 12-1):

✓ **Frontal lobe:** The front-most portion of the brain is responsible for high-order functioning, reasoning, production of speech, and has influence on personality, emotions, and movement.

✓ **Temporal lobes:** Located laterally on the brain (your temples), the temporal lobes contain the primary audio cortex, where information from the auditory nerve from the ear is processed. This area is associated with perception, memory, and speech.

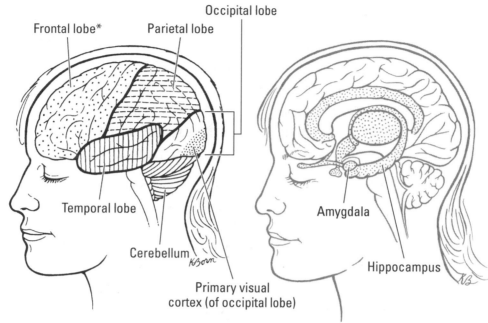

Figure 12-1: Basic brain anatomy.

*All lobes of the brain are paired structures.

- ✔ **Parietal lobe:** Located on the top-back surface of the brain, the parietal lobe is primarily concerned with integrating sensory information and spatial orientation.

- ✔ **Occipital lobe:** The occipital lobe, located at the back of the brain, is devoted almost entirely to visual processing.

The forebrain further breaks down into specific parts with crucial duties:

- ✔ **The amygdala:** This part contains a large number of opiate receptors that help control emotion and is responsible for emotional integration of sensory input and memories.

- ✔ **The diencephalon:** The diencephalon is the

399

posterior part of the forebrain. It contains the hypothalamus and thalamus.

- The *hypothalamus* regulates and drives emotions, and stabilizes your internal environment.
- The *thalamus* relays sensory signals, processes memory, and generates emotional status. It also coordinates information with the temporal lobes and serves a primary function in memory.

✔ **The hippocampus:** This part is responsible for the processing and coordination of memory function.

✔ **The limbic system:** The limbic system encompasses a number of brain structures involved with the endocrine and autonomic nervous systems. The amygdala, hippocampus, hypothalamus, and thalamus (see previous bullets) make up just a few of the many areas of the limbic system.

The midbrain, where senses are stimulated

The midbrain, also called the mesencephalon, is the uppermost part of the brainstem. It extends from the base of the brain to the spinal cord and contains the tectum and tegmentum. The midbrain serves as a motor relay center and contains auditory and visual reflex centers. It is involved in functions such as vision, hearing, and eye and body movement. One disease that is associated with the midbrain is Parkinson's disease, which affects the substantia nigra area of the midbrain. Some of the important parts of the mibrain are

✔ **Cerebral peduncles:** These two bundles of fibers carry signals between the cerebral cortex, brainstem, and spinal cord. They also relay information to and from the cerebellum.

- **Substantia nigra:** Found at the base of the midbrain, the substantia nigra receives input from numerous other brain parts and is involved in relaying signals concerned with motor function to parts of the brain, as well as serves as a source of dopamine production.

The hindbrain, your center for equilibrium and more

The hindbrain, located at the rear of the brain, includes three major divisions: the cerebellum, medulla, and pons, which together function to support many of the vital bodily functions explained in the following list:

- **Cerebellum:** The cerebellum coordinates musculoskeletal movements and stores memories of movement patterns. It indirectly regulates motor control by comparing intention with performance and making necessary changes to the nervous signals that go to the muscles.

- **Pons:** The pons, which means bridge, connects the brainstem and the cerebellum. The pons accepts information from the visual centers of the brain and relays this info to the cerebellum to aid in equilibrium and muscular movements. The pons also plays a role in arousal and sleep.

- **Medulla:** The medulla lies between the pons and the spinal cord. It's responsible for essential bodily functions such as breathing, swallowing, and maintaining muscle tone.

The hindbrain also contains the upper part of the spinal cord.

Understanding how the brain communicates with the body

Although neurotransmitters sound like they belong in your iPod instead of your brain, they're actually essential components in getting signals from one part of your brain to another. *Neurotransmitters* are chemicals that are used to transmit, intensify, and alter electrical signals between a neuron and another cell. There are a range of specific chemicals involved in various aspects of mental and physical functioning. You couldn't live without these neurotransmitters:

- **Acetylcholine:** This chemical affects voluntary movement of muscles, behavior, inhibition, and memory. Alzheimer's memory loss may be associated with decreased or blocked acetylcholine levels.

- **Dopamine:** Dopamine excites and controls voluntary movement and emotional arousal; Parkinson's disease symptoms may result from decreased or damaged dopamine levels.

- **GABA (gamma aminobutyric acid):** GABA is responsible for inhibition of motor neurons.

- **Glycine:** Glycine impacts spinal reflexes and motor behavior.

- **Neuromodulators:** These chemicals are responsible for sensory transmission, especially pain.

- **Norepinephrine:** This one is responsible for wakefulness or arousal. It is released from the adrenal gland and is most prevalent in the sympathetic nervous system.

- **Serotonin:** This neurotransmitter affects memory,

emotions, wakefulness, sleep, and temperature regulation. It's part of the brain's reward system, producing feelings of pleasure.

Sixty percent of all adults over age 40 have some degree of neurotransmitter deficiency for several reasons. Aging neurons make smaller amounts of certain chemicals. Also, as you get older, your body doesn't respond as well to the signals as well as it used to, for some of the following reasons:

- ✔ **Prolonged emotional or physical stress:** Your body is designed to handle short bursts of stress. Chronic stress takes a toll on the "fight or flight" stress hormones and neurotransmitters of the sympathetic nervous system, eventually depleting them. The neurotransmitter epinephrine and the hormone cortisol, which are released in stress situations, lead to decreases in memory and learning when chronically stimulated under stress. Researchers are continuing to look into their roles in chronic stress and how this effects aging.

- ✔ **Chronic dieting:** This habit is a common self-induced form of neurotransmitter depletion because of its affect on serotonin levels. Serotonin deficiency increases cravings, moodiness, and poor motivation. Many of the fad diets are at higher risk of serotonin involvement.

- ✔ **Disrupted sleep:** There are several neurotransmitters responsible for sleep, especially serotonin. Serotonin converts to melatonin, which is the main sleep hormone. When serotonin levels are low, melatonin levels will also be low. This results in disrupted sleep, causing fewer neurotransmitters to

403

be produced, perpetuating a vicious cycle.

✔ **Hormone imbalances:** Hormones are highly influential on neurotransmitter release. Aging in both sexes is associated with progressive declines in hormones and associated effects on energy, sleep, mood, libido, and weight.

Premenstrual syndrome (PMS) is a classic example of how low serotonin levels can temporarily shift each month. Mood, appetite, and sleep can be severely disrupted one to two weeks before the menstrual cycle.

A Microscopic Look at the Aging Brain

Keeping your brain function intact is probably high on your list of things to do as you age. Age can affect the complicated system of hormones, neurotransmitters, and nerves. In fact, the changes that can occur in the brain can be much more debilitating than some of the physical aspects of aging such as muscle and bone loss. In the next section, we look at exactly what happens to your brain as you age.

Normal physical changes

The ability to study the brain used to be limited to autopsies, but new brain imaging techniques have led to increased observation of age-related effects on the brain's structure and appearance.

The brain shrinks, the white matter thins, and the vital messengers in the brain diminish. Sounds scary, doesn't it? But relax! In most instances, you can compensate for age-related brain changes. You can expect the following as your brain ages:

✔ The brain's weight and volume decrease.

On average, the brain loses 10 percent of its weight, starting after the age of 20 with the abundance of loss coming after the age of 60.

✔ The *sulci* (grooves) on the surface of the brain widen.

✔ The brain starts to generate fewer messengers (the neurotransmitters).

✔ The brain can get accumulations of abnormal brain fibers made of protein, which are called *neurofibrillary tangles.* These plaques can cause Alzheimer's symptoms and are thought to contribute to age-related memory deficits.

✔ The accumulation of deposits of amyloid, an insoluble fibrous protein, in the brain cells is called *senile plaques.* Research is still not conclusive as to whether these plaques are part of normal aging.

How physical changes manifest through your mentality

There's a saying related to aging that goes "Of all the things I've lost, I miss my mind the most." This saying is a humorous way of stating that memory loss is a common part of aging. One of the biggest fears people have of aging is losing their ability to think and remember. In regards to aging and the mind/body connection, a few categories of people exist:

✔ People who have a strong healthy body but are losing their minds

✔ Folks who are sharp as a tack with a deteriorating body

✔ The strong-bodied and strong-minded

The good news is that most people will be able to keep their cognitive faculties as they age unless they develop Alzheimer's or some other disease.

Can you live into your 80s or 90s with your mind still sharp? As long as your brain itself remains healthy, the older version of you can stay as mentally sharp as ever, although certain activities may take you longer than they used to. The next sections help you determine whether changes you experience are cause for concern or part of the normal aging process.

Changes in mental function that are part of normal aging

Despite common belief, your memory doesn't worsen as you age. Memory does, however, change with age and these changes don't necessarily mean deterioration. In fact, memory becomes more accurate with age; you're just a bit slower at the processing part.

The most common normal change associated with aging is the ability to retrieve newly acquired information. In other words, your long-term memories remain intact, where as your short-term memory slows down.

So, when do all of these brain aging and short-term memory glitches start to occur? About 60 percent of people age 50 and older notice greater difficulty remembering names, dates, and other specific details. Memories associated with a specific time and place are most commonly effected. Thankfully, these small memory lapses — which are called *brain farts* as young adults or *senior moments* as you get older — aren't usually signs of a neurological disorder, such as Alzheimer's disease, but instead the result of normal changes in the structure and function of your brain.

Understand that memory difficulties caused by the normal aging process are minor, even if you find them frustrating. (Most people don't have difficulties with their activities of daily living, but for the less fortunate there are also many things you can do to protect and improve your memory; we cover them in the section "Keeping Your Brain Young" later in this chapter.)

Changes in mental function that may signify a health concern

Aging alone isn't the only cause of mental changes. Depression, dementia, side effects of drugs and alcohol, strokes, and head injury also cause mental changes, but these diseases aren't a universal occurrence. This leads us to the question, if some mental change is normal as you age, when should you be concerned and seek medical advice?

Don't panic. Ask yourself (or someone else, if you're not able to assess for yourself) if you're having any of the following changes in behavior or thinking processes. Often the mental changes that aren't part of normal aging progress much more rapidly leading to more elective doctor visits. If you notice one or more of these signs in yourself or a loved one, or if someone tells you they've noticed these behaviors in you, see your healthcare professional for a full evaluation:

✔ **Forgetting things more frequently than you used to (especially if a friend or family member tells you):** This may not seem like a big deal, but forgetting things can be annoying, and, in some cases, like taking medications, it can be dangerous. You may stop taking medications or take the wrong ones or forget directions and get lost while driving or walking.

✔ **Forgetting how to do familiar tasks:** Your nutrition may suffer if you can't prepare food properly or if you eat the same thing every day. There's also the danger of forgetting to turn off the stove or leaving water running.

✓ **Difficulty learning new tasks:** You need to be able to master new tasks to compensate for some of the normal changes that occur with age. In brain disease, the ability to learn and compensate are compromised, which can make daily activities difficult.

✓ **Being told that you told the same story within the same visit:** This isn't particularly dangerous, although it may annoy your friends and relatives!

✓ **Difficulty managing money, medications, and bills:** Aging adults are already major targets for money schemes and fraud. Those with brain disease or deterioration are even more susceptible to making bad purchases or losing track of their money. Families should make sure that there are safeguards in place to protect from these situations.

✓ **Changes in personality such as anger or avoidance:** Often the frustration of losing the ability to care for yourself is frightening and can cause people to lash out or become reclusive. This can lead to depression and stressors that can make mental deficits accelerate.

✓ **Decreased hygiene:** Being unable to bathe and take care of other hygiene issues can lead to infections in areas, such as the urinary tract or skin. Infections in aging adults with brain disease can cause worsening symptoms and can be difficult to diagnose because the changes may be assumed to be from the disease itself. Untreated infections can spread into the bloodstream and cause more serious infections with a high mortality rate.

There are other causes of abnormal mental function besides brain disease. Infections, medications, and other diseases can cause similar symptoms, so make sure that you or a loved one is evaluated by a doctor to get an accurate diagnosis if symptoms appear suddenly or seem to become worse.

Identifying and Coping with Brain Disease

Recognizing abnormal mental changes in yourself or someone you care about can be frightening, but it's important to identify them early and get treatment to prevent as much loss of brain function as possible.

Many diseases that cause altered mental behaviors result from direct damage to areas of the brain. Some of the diseases that can occur as you age are dementia (a loss of mental ability severe enough to interfere with normal activities of daily living), Alzheimer's (a specific type of dementia), stroke, Parkinson's, and Huntington's Chorea (a genetic disease where symptoms don't appear until middle age).

Damage to the brain from stroke, Alzheimer's, or diseases such as Parkinson's have different effects depending on the area of the brain that's damaged. These damages are covered in the following section.

Recognizing the most common forms of brain disease

Brain disease encompasses a large group of symptoms that collectively result in loss of both mental and physical function. These symptoms can occur gradually or quickly and in some incidences can be slowed once the cause of the brain disease is identified. Brain disease can cause a decline in memory and cognition, balance, speech, gait, or even some autonomic brain functions, such as blinking, smiling, and swallowing.

Dementia

As many as one percent of people age 60 suffer from dementia, and the frequency of dementia has been estimated to double every five years thereafter. *Dementia* isn't a specific disease; it's a group of symptoms. To be diagnosed with dementia requires more than just memory loss. People with dementia have attention, orientation, memory, judgment, language, motor and spatial skills, and function defects severe enough to seriously affect their daily lives. Some of the most common causes of dementia are Alzheimer's disease, vascular dementia (damage to the blood vessels leading to the brain), brain injury, and brain tumors.

There are several marked differences between memory loss associated with aging and dementia. With normal aging, you're consciously aware when you can't remember something. You can also compensate for the loss of a word by substituting the idea with a similar concept. The person who has dementia may not be aware of these problems even when it is severe enough to change a person's mood and personality.

Vascular dementia occurs when blood flow to the brain is interrupted for any reason and is sometimes called multi-infarct dementia. Brain cells can die from lack of oxygen, causing symptoms such as muscle weakness, speech difficulties, and other mental disturbances. Vascular dementia is the second-leading cause of dementia after Alzheimer's. Whether it's small blockages (strokes or mini-strokes) or just severe blood vessel disease, when blood and nutrients can't get to the brain, cognitive impairment occurs.

A person with dementia should be under a doctor's care. For some people in the early and middle stages of Alzheimer's disease, certain medications can be prescribed to possibly delay the worsening of some of the disease's symptoms. See a healthcare professional for a full evaluation if you notice one or more of these signs of dementia in yourself or a loved one:

- **Recent memory loss:** Many of the problems associated with dementia are caused by memory loss. Everyone forgets things for a while and then remembers them later. People with dementia often forget things, but they never remember them. They not only forget an object but also the context surrounding that object.

- **Difficulty performing familiar tasks:** People with dementia may forget how to cook a meal that they've prepared multiple times. They may have problems with dressing, color coordinating, and personal hygiene (all routines in the past).

- **Problems with language:** Folks suffering from dementia may forget simple words or use the wrong words or even add unusual words. This often makes conversations hard to follow.

- **Time and place disorientation:** People who have dementia get lost often. They can drive away, forget where they're going, and then get lost trying to return home. Some get confused whether it's night or day.

- **Problems with abstract thinking:** Dementia sufferers may forget what numbers are and what has to be done with them.

- ✔ **Misplacing things:** Some people may put things in the wrong places. Often they're trying to hide objects and then forget where they hid them. Hiding objects is a response to feeling the loss of control and insecurity based on memory loss. As the disease progresses, they have difficulty remembering who they know and who they can trust. They don't realize that this hiding things to "keep them safe" may backfire when they can't remember where they hid them — or even that they hid them.

- ✔ **Changes in mood:** People with dementia may have fast mood swings and can cover many in a short period. Some folks can become very angry, sad, and then seem happier than ever.

- ✔ **Personality changes:** These folks may become irritable, suspicious, or fearful.

- ✔ **Loss of initiative:** People who have dementia may become passive and don't like to go places.

Alzheimer's disease

Alzheimer's disease is a specific form of dementia that currently affects more than 5 million Americans, most over age 65. Twenty percent of dementia cases are diagnosed as Alzheimer's, which first appears between the ages of 40 and 60 in some people and affects only 10 percent of people in their 60s, but affects nearly 50 percent of those in their 80s.

Alzheimer's gradually destroys a person's memory and ability to learn, reason, make judgments, communicate, and carry out daily activities. As Alzheimer's progresses, individuals may also experience changes in personality and behavior, such as anxiety, suspiciousness or agitation, as well as delusions or hallucinations. Currently, there's no cure for Alzheimer's, although a few drug treatments slow progression in some people.

Alzheimer's causes a buildup of extracellular plaque in the brain, neuron loss in the cerebral cortex and deep cerebral regions, and brain atrophy (see Figure 12-2). An abnormal collection of a protein called amyloid is found in the areas of the brain crucial to learning, memory, and maintaining a sense of time.

A Canadian study done in 2002 showed that Alzheimer's was frequently preceded by a decline in verbal memory one to two years before the disease became obvious, so it's important for a person to be tested for Alzheimer's disease early in the disease process. That testing can help in early identification and treatment of potential Alzheimer patients.

Alzheimer's can be difficult to diagnose, especially in its early stages; it is not just a more severe form of dementia. The diagnosis of Alzheimer's disease not only requires memory deficits but also another cognitive deficit, such as language disturbance.

Sometimes it can be hard to tell the difference between normal age-related changes and signs of one of the brain diseases. The table below lists a few of the differences between normal aging and Alzheimer's.

Someone with Alzheimer's disease symptoms	Someone with normal age-related memory changes
Forgets entire experiences	Forgets part of an experience
Rarely remembers later	Often remembers later
Is gradually unable to follow written/spoken directions	Is usually able to follow written/spoken directions
Is gradually unable to use notes as reminders	Is usually able to use notes as reminders
Is gradually unable to care for self	Is usually able to care for self

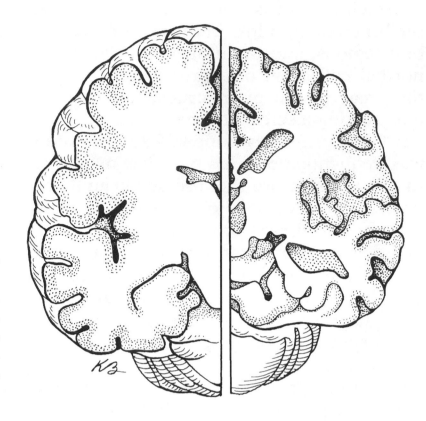

Parkinson's disease

Parkinson's is a progressive, degenerative brain disease caused by the loss of dopamine-producing brain cells. The part of the brain where these nerve cells are located, the *substantia nigra,* is responsible for controlling muscle movement. Normally these nerve cells release dopamine, a neurotransmitter that signals other parts of the brain to coordinate muscle to make controlled movements. Loss of these nerve cells leads to difficulty with muscle movements. Everyone will experience some loss of these dopamine-releasing nerve cells, but people with Parkinson's lose more than 50 percent of their cells.

Parkinson's causes tremor, muscle rigidity that results in a "mask–like" facial expression, postural instability, and bradykinesia (slow movements). Depression, emotional changes, and difficulty swallowing and speaking are also common symptoms. This is a progressive, disabling disease, but many people have many quality years of life after diagnosis.

Much research has been done on the cause of Parkinson's; it's believed to be a combination of genetic and environmental factors. Some medications and other diseases can cause Parkinson's–like symptoms in people who don't have the disease. There's a familial link for the disease, although it's a weak link.

Huntington's disease

Huntington's disease (HD), first described by Dr. Huntington in 1872, is still a disease with many unknowns. This genetic disease is a progressive, neurologic disease that unfortunately doesn't show symptoms until you're in your late 30s or older. In HD, a reduction in the amount of the neurotransmitters acetylcholine and GABA affects the amount of dopamine in the brain. The increased amounts of dopamine and the muscle movements are the opposite of Parkinson's, where there's a deficiency of dopamine. The initial symptoms start with clumsiness and then develop into strange posturing and uncontrollable movements.

Most HD patients also develop progressive dementia and memory loss. HD is usually fatal within 15 to 20 years after symptoms begin. Death is a result of disabilities, such as swallowing, which can lead to choking, or by secondary infection from a impaired immune system.

HD is a genetic disease caused by a dominant gene (a genetic trait is considered dominant when the disease is present in a person who has only one copy of that gene, received from one parent) which means that anyone that receives the gene from either parent will develop the disease.

Sizing up your risk for brain disease

Some of your risks of developing brain disease are within your control, and then some are simply a result or your genetic make-up. Of course, common lifestyle choices consistently found to be a risk of disease can also cause brain disease. We discuss the specific risks for the common brain diseases in the following sections.

Risk factors for dementia

Dementia has the same risk factors common to people who suffer strokes. In fact, a study of over 8,000 people by the University of California–San Francisco indicated that cardiovascular risks such as smoking, high cholesterol, hypertension, and diabetes at midlife were also risks for development of dementia in later life. Folks with all four risk factors were almost two and a half times more likely to develop dementia, and each single risk factor resulted in a 20 to 40 percent increase. People with severe or repeated head injuries also have an increased risk for dementia.

Risk factors for Alzheimer's

A family history of Alzheimer's and increasing age are considered risk factors for development of Alzheimer's disease, but they don't always lead to memory loss or dementia. Lifestyle and environment actually seem to be more influential than genes for some individuals.

Even though a known cause of Alzheimer's isn't yet found, a number of factors have been found to occur frequently in Alzheimer's patients. Experts suspect that some combination of the following can predispose a person to develop Alzheimer's:

- Family history of the disease (especially a parent or a sibling)

- Heart-disease risk factors — high blood pressure, smoking, obesity, diabetes, high cholesterol

- Previous head injury

- Environmental toxins

- Advancing age

- Stress

- Genes

    A gene variant called APOE E4 may be a risk factor, but only about 30 percent of people with Alzheimer's have this gene; other people with Alzheimer's don't.

The presence of any of these risk factors doesn't mean that you'll get Alzheimer's disease. In fact, researchers can say only that these factors have been associated with many Alzheimer's patients. Take "advancing age" as an example. It's listed as a risk factor only because Alzheimer's disease usually strikes individuals after age 65. Aging alone doesn't cause the disease and what does is still not quite known.

To find out more about Alzheimer's, go to www.alz.org on the Web, or check out *Alzheimer's For Dummies* (Wiley) by Patricia B. Smith, Mary M. Kenan, PsyD., Mark Edwin Kunik, MD, MPH, and Leeza Gibbons.

Risk factors for Parkinson's disease

Age is the biggest risk factor for Parkinson's and is more common in people over age 60, affecting 1 in 200 persons. Gender statistics show that more men than women are diagnosed with Parkinson's disease. There's a very slight (less than 5 percent) hereditary risk if you have a first-degree family relative. There has been concern that low levels of estrogen in post-menopausal women that choose not to take hormone replacement could result in an increased risk of Parkinson's.

Risk factors for Huntington's disease

HD, a chromosome defect, is found in approximately 5 in 100,000 people and affects men and women equally. HD is an *autosomal dominant disease,* which means you need to have only a copy of the gene from one parent to inherit the disease. Nearly all cases of HD are found in people with a family history of the disease; it's possible to test for HD genetically, but is controversial because there's no cure and can cause significant distress if you have no symptoms and are found to be a carrier. You should see your medical doctor and a genetic counselor for more information.

Understanding the treatment options

Brain disease is a feared development of aging. It can follow a slow progression or become disabling very rapidly, leaving you feeling hopeless and scared. The good news is that treatments can sometimes improve quality of life for years. Make sure that you get a thorough evaluation to determine treatment options that are available and to make sure to rule out other causes of your symptoms. Some of the treatments for the common brain diseases are as follows:

- **Dementia:** Treatment options include the following:
  - Surgical treatment of a brain tumor
  - Medical treatment for an infection or stroke
  - Prescription of vitamins for a deficiency

- **Alzheimer's:** Treatments for Alzheimer's include
  - Drug treatments to increase the level of acetylcholine in the brain:

Menantine (Namenda)
Rivastigmine tartrate (Exelon)
Tacrine (Cognex)
Donepezil (Aricept)
Galantamine (Reminyl)

- Promising research currently under investigation to create new drugs to prevent neuron damage before it occurs, preventing Alzheimer's instead of treating symptoms after they appear

✔ **Parkinson's disease:** Many treatment options include

- Medications that provide symptomatic relief in a majority of Parkinson's patients. Patients are often given levodopa-carbidopa (Sinemet), a combination drug; levodopa is converted to dopamine in the brain and carbidopa slows the breakdown of levodopa so that more of it reaches the brain. This drug is most effective against rigidity and bradykinesia, less so against tremors.
- Drugs called anticholinergics may help reduce tremors, and drugs that mimic the action of dopamine in the brain, such as bromocriptine, may also be used.
- The FDA recently approved a treatment called deep brain stimulation (DBS), which involves planting electrodes into the brain. The electrodes are then connected to a small electrical device called a pulse generator that can be externally programmed to help reduce symptoms.

✔ **Huntington's disease:** Treatment options include the following:

- There's no one treatment for HD.

419

- Drug treatment is usually directed at decreasing symptoms.

Keeping Your Brain Young

So, you want to be as young as you *think?* There are certain steps you can take to keep the cobwebs in your mind at bay as you get older. At least the signs of an aging brain aren't as visible as gray hair and wrinkles! In this section, we provide you with ways to keep your brain power strong.

Preventing age-related memory loss

The brain changes that come with age are inevitable — but they don't have to slow you down or trip you up. What can you do to minimize the impact of neurotransmitter deficiencies, as you age? There are some medical, natural, and nutritional ways to increase and balance neurotransmitters when they do get out of balance.

 Be sure to consult with your healthcare provider before taking any medications, supplements, or beginning any other therapies for treating any perceived neurotransmitter deficiencies.

Check out these ways of staying alert and preventing memory loss:

- **Exercising your mind:** Similar to the way your body needs physical activity, your mind needs to be exercised, too. Mental stimulation and exercises can actually protect against cognitive losses. Most severe mental decline is from the disease processes instead of normal age-related function loss because as you age, the brain is able to make new connections if it's challenged and taken care of. Here are a few ways that you can challenge yourself:

- Play a musical instrument.
- Do crossword puzzles or other challenging board games.
- Socialize with family and friends.
- Start a new hobby.
- Stay interested and up to date on current events.

✔ **Staying physically active:** Regular exercise can improve blood flow to the brain. Exercise increases your metabolism and energy levels, which can help improve your attention span. If you exercise for as little as 30 to 45 minutes three times a week, studies show that you can improve age-related declines in your cognitive abilities.

✔ **Eating brain foods:** Neurotransmitter health requires the same balanced diet as the rest of your body — protein, carbohydrates, and fats. Three neurotransmitters are especially important to keep your brain functioning well:

- **Acetylcholine:** Foods rich in this chemical include egg yolks, peanuts, wheat germ, liver, meat, fish, milk, cheese, broccoli, cabbage, and cauliflower.
- **Dopamine:** These foods include all proteins, such as meat, milk products, fish, beans, nuts, and soy products.
- **Serotonin:** Serotonin-rich foods are carbohydrate-based, such as pasta, starchy vegetables, potatoes, cereals, and breads.

What else can you ingest to make that brain of yours healthy? Here are some tips:

- Eat a diet rich in fruits and vegetables. Many of these foods contain *antioxidants* — substances

421

that protect and nourish brain cells. Antioxidants may help prevent cholesterol from damaging the lining of your arteries and slowing blood flow to your brain.

- Eat foods rich in omega-3 fatty acids like salmon and other cold-water fish. Eating fish at least once each week seems to protect against the cognitive decline associated with aging.

- Drink plenty of water. The brain is comprised of more water than any other organ in the body, at about 90 percent. Staying hydrated is essential for concentration and mental alertness, but how much water is enough? A good rule of thumb is to drink half of your body weight in ounces of water. If you drink coffee or alcohol, you have to add those ounces onto the total.

- Eat smaller, more frequent meals to increase your mental alertness. By eating smaller meals, there's less variations in the blood flow to the digestive tract and also more balance in blood sugars.

✔ **Drinking alcohol only in moderation:** People who drink heavily for years are at a higher risk of developing memory problems and dementia. We don't recommend drinking more than one to two drinks per day for men and one or less per day for women.

✔ **Stopping smoking:** Smoking is associated with dementia and one Dutch study found that smokers had twice the risk of developing Alzheimer's compared to those who never smoked. Smoking also has an increased risk of strokes, the other common type of dementia (multi-infarct).

✔ **Managing your stress:** Stress can cause the release

422

of enzymes and hormones that can affect judgment and memory. Protein kinase C, cortisol, and corticosterone are a few that are thought to have a memory-impairing effect. These hormones are released in the body under normal stress situations, but it's not until they hang around too long as a result of chronic stressors that they affect memory. A certain amount of stress is normal, but finding ways to manage and reduce stress helps keep these hormones in a normal cycle.

- ✔ **Protecting your head when exercising:** Head trauma can increase your risk of developing Alzheimer's disease. People who participate in sports such as running and swimming, which have a reduced risk of head trauma, have lower rates of memory loss. Take precautions to protect your head; for example, wear a helmet when riding your bike or performing other extreme sports.

- ✔ **Getting enough rest:** New evidence suggests that a regular pattern of eight hours of sleep per night helps protect you against age-related memory loss. Getting enough sleep can be a problem as you get older because of the age-related changes in sleep stages and sleep hygiene (see Chapter 14 for more info on age-related sleep changes). Sleep experts say that having a regular sleep routine can improve cognition. Several studies discuss the similarities of sleep deprivation and age-related memory loss, but they're still researching the long-term effects of poor sleep and memory loss.

Improving Your Memory

What you consider a poor memory may just be less-than-effective habits when it comes to taking in and processing information. Barring disease, disorder, or injury, you can improve your ability to discover and retain information.

What type of memory are you losing?

Memory loss with normal aging results from the subtly changing environment within the brain. It's not clear exactly how much is actual memory loss and how much is the inability to quickly process the request for the information. After a certain period of trying to remember something, you may give up or recall that piece of info when it's no longer needed . . . but it was there.

Memory studies have shown that about 30 percent of healthy people over age 60 have difficulty with declarative memory. To help explain the differences between age-related memory loss and memory loss associated with brain disease, we discuss the different types of memory below:

✔ **Declarative:** This refers to memory that's consciously available. It's the type of memory that stores facts such as names, places, and times. Declarative memory is also referred to as conscious or cognitive memory and what most people refer to when they're experiencing lapses in their memory function.

✔ **Nondeclarative or procedural:** This type of memory relates to skills and routines. It consists of memory associated with motor learning, habits, perception, intuition, and conditioning. This area isn't affected much by aging.

✔ **Sensory:** This type of memory involves retaining something you have just seen or heard. It gives you the ability to see something for just a second and memorize it. Sensory memory isn't affected by aging as much as the other types of memory.

- **Short-term:** Short-term memory allows you to recall something from several seconds to as long as a minute without repetition. This area can be significantly affected by aging. This type is also one that can be improved with memory games and brain exercises.

- **Long-term:** Long-term memory can store much larger quantities of information for potentially unlimited duration — sometimes a whole lifetime. This area is little affected by normal aging.

Try putting some new information in your brain "next to" something you know you won't forget so you can retrieve it more easily. For example, if you meet someone new and want to remember his name is Robert, think of someone from your past or a childhood friend named Robert and create an association, then lock it down in your memory.

Figuring out how to remember

A good percentage of aging adults develop age-related memory loss, while some end up with the more aggressive memory deficits seen in diseases like Alzheimer's. Learning tools to help increase your ability to remember and recall, however, can help you retain as much of your thinking ability as possible. The following hints may help you remember important information:

- **Create memorable mental pictures and notes:** You remember things more easily if you can visualize them. If you're reading something and you read it out loud, you may retain it easier. Try to relate substance to items, such as colors, emotions, and textures, which can make more of an imprint in the brain.

- ✔ **Group things:** Group any new information to already stored info because it's easier to remember the group.

- ✔ **Organize:** Place objects such as keys in the same place. Use calendars for events and recurring occasions. Take notes, especially on complex material, and add pictures and colors to the notes to increase recall.

- ✔ **Repeat learned items:** The more times you repeat things or say them, the better the memory. After you meet someone, repeating the name out loud increases your ability to retain.

 Exercising your mind is similar to exercising your muscles. Your memory is adaptable, pliable and you can get it in shape with a little knowledge, effort, energy, and a lot of fun! There are many Web sites dedicated to a variety of brain health programs for sharpening your noodle and maximizing your memory, as well as video games and some surprising other sources. Chapter 18 shows you a few that we found at the time of this printing.

Chapter 13

Decreasing Stress to Live a Longer, Better Life

· ·

In This Chapter

▶ Figuring out the different types of stress and how your body reacts

▶ Recognizing the signs of chronic stress and dealing with its concerns

▶ Understanding how to measure stress

▶ Seeking professional help for your stress

▶ Adopting proven stress busters

· ·

Are you stressed? Of course you are — all human beings are stressed, but that's not necessarily a bad thing. Stress is a necessary part of life. Hans Selye, MD, who did considerable research on the effects of stress on daily life, defined stress as "the nonspecific response of the body to any demand." This means that any event, from winning the lottery to slamming the car door on your hand, causes stress of some type.

Stress generally falls into one of two categories:

- Eustress, which is "good" stress, or stress occurring from positive events, such as moving into a new house or having a new grandchild

- Distress, which is stress resulting from negative events, such as losing a job or having health problems

Stress can be life saving; it activates the reactions that result in your jumping out of the way of a speeding car or grabbing onto a tree branch if you're falling.

However, if your stress reactions are activated too often, stress can become chronic. Instead of leveling off after the crisis passes, your stress hormones, heart rate, and blood pressure remain elevated. Extended or repeated activation of the stress response takes a heavy toll on your body and accelerates the aging process. In this chapter, we show you how to recognize and decrease chronic stress — as well as how to live well with the stress that's a necessary part of life.

Your Body's Built-In Response System: How It's Supposed to Work

Human bodies were designed for stress. The autonomic nervous system, consisting of the sympathetic and parasympathetic systems, continually attempts to balance your physical and emotional reactions to stress. Both distress and eustress cause physical and mental adaptations, such as an increase in your heart rate, dilation of your pupils, and a rise in your blood sugar. These responses are orchestrated by your sympathetic nervous system, and allow you to respond quickly to any changes in your world by helping you move faster, see better, and think quickly.

Each time your body experiences stress, the same biological and physiological responses are set off in a chain reaction known as the stress syndrome. Walter Cannon was the first to describe the body's basic sympathetic response to a stressor in the 1920s and then it was expanded on by Hans Selye in 1936. This sympathetic reaction became the first stage of the stress reaction syndrome.

Stress isn't meant to be a chronic condition. After the perceived "danger" has passed, the parasympathetic nervous system normally takes over, allowing your body to revert back to its normal "non-stressed" state.

Here are the stages of stress:

- **Stage 1: Alarm:** The initial response to stress is the "fight or flight" response. Your sympathetic nervous system pumps out adrenaline (epinephrine), a chemical produced by the adrenal glands, which increases your heart rate and blood flow to your muscles and brain. Blood vessels under your skin constrict to prevent blood loss in case of injury. The pupils in your eyes dilate to improve vision. Then, a spike in blood sugar gives you a quick burst of energy. After the cause of the stress is removed, your body should return to normal. If the cause for the stress isn't removed, you move on to the second stage.

- **Stage 2: Adaptation:** In this stage, your body responds by building a resistance against and adapting to the stress. Adrenaline release slows and the effects of the alarm phase lessen. The adrenal cortex produces hormones called *corticosteroids* (cortisol and aldosterone) for this resistance reaction.

    During this phase you adapt to the stressor, whether it's a loud startling noise or someone assaulting you. Most of the time the stressor resolves, the alarm phase slowly resolves, and the sympathetic and parasympathetic nervous systems equalize. When your body experiences an excess exposure to this stage without periods of rest, you become prone to fatigue, irritability, and lethargy, and your concentration lapses.

✔ **Stage 3: Exhaustion:** In the final stage, your body has run out of its reserve of energy. You reach the point of *adrenal exhaustion,* as your adrenal glands, which produce the hormone adrenaline, become depleted. Blood sugar levels drop and this combination leads to decreased stress tolerance, progressive mental and physical exhaustion, illness, and eventually collapse, which has an aging effect due to wear and tear on your body. You have now become the victim of chronic stress. (This stage isn't typically reached with minor stressors.) The reactions to stressors differ from person to person and you may reach exhaustion quicker than someone else.

The adrenals are walnut-sized glands located on top of each kidney, and are important control centers for many of the body's hormones. The outer layer of the gland, called the adrenal cortex, produces hormones, including cortisol, DHEA, estrogen, and testosterone. The centers of the glands produce adrenaline, the hormone named after them.

Observing the Tolls of Chronic Stress

In today's fast-paced world, many events can initiate a stress reaction. If your life lurches from perceived crisis to crisis, your ability to wind down after the immediate danger has passed becomes damaged. This reaction happens quite often with today's busy lifestyles. Chronic stress occurs when acute stress responses keep your body on alert continuously, not allowing it to return to a state of *homeostasis,* the scientific name for the balanced state of health. If you're faced with continuous stressors, over time, the sympathetic system becomes overwhelmed. When that happens, stress can cause serious mental and physical health issues. Chronic stress can be especially damaging as you age.

Recognizing chronic stress is the first step to combating its negative effects on your life. After you identify the symptoms, you can develop techniques to cope with it without being overwhelmed by it — in this section, we familiarize you with the gamut of common symptoms.

The physical effects

Chronic stress can take a heavy physical toll. The ongoing stress response causes the hypothalamus and pituitary gland to release a chemical known as ACTH (adrenocorticotropic hormone). ACTH, known as the "stress hormone," stimulates the adrenal gland to produce and release cortisol and stress can keep cortisol at an increased level.

Cortisol is responsible for helping with many of the body's functions, but the functions are different when cortisol is released in response to stress than when it's released in normal situations. Normally, cortisol helps with glucose metabolism, controlling inflammation, boosting the immune system, and regulating blood pressure. Cortisol released under stress can give you an extra burst of energy and can depress your response to pain. However, when cortisol release is prolonged due to chronic stress, it can have adverse effects on your body. (See "The mental and psychological effects" section in this chapter for more about cortisol's negative stress effects.) Cortisol levels are typically lowest during the night and highest in the morning, with a peak level at around 7:00 a.m.

Some studies show that 43 percent of all adults suffer adverse health effects from stress. Seventy-five to 90 percent of all doctor's office visits are for stress-related ailments and complaints.

Stress can contribute to many physical problems:

- Arthritis and vague aches and pains

- Asthma or breathlessness

- Being accident-prone

- Clenched muscles

- Diabetes

- Fatigue

- Headaches and migraines

- Heart problems, such as a racing heart

- Hypertension (high blood pressure)

- Increased use of alcohol, tobacco, and other drugs

- Insomnia

- Premature aging of immune system cells that causes accelerated aging in the following areas:

  - Impaired cognitive performance
  - Suppressed thyroid function
  - Blood sugar imbalances such as hyperglycemia
  - Decreased bone density
  - Decrease in muscle tissue
  - Higher blood pressure
  - Lowered immunity and inflammatory responses in the body, which leads to more frequent colds,

432

upper-respiratory infections, and other illnesses

- Increased abdominal fat, which is associated with heart attacks, strokes, the development of higher levels of "bad" cholesterol (LDL) and lower levels of "good" cholesterol (HDL)

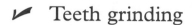 Rapid weight changes

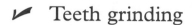 Skin conditions, such as acne breakouts, hives, rashes, and excessive sweating

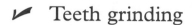 Stomach problems, such as constipation, diarrhea, indigestion, and nausea

 Stress is no longer believed to cause stomach ulcers, but stress is still thought to aggravate and exacerbate up to 45 percent of ulcers.

 Teeth grinding

Continual stress response and the hormonal influences can produce inflammation and are most commonly associated with worsening of autoimmune or inflammatory conditions such as rheumatoid arthritis, systemic lupus, and inflammatory bowel disease. Some hormones, including the glucocorticoids, are known to be *immunosuppressive,* meaning they suppress your immune system — not something you want when you're trying to heal.

The mental and psychological effects

Too much stress can upset your mental health. For example, the persistent stress-induced elevations of cortisol, which affects hormone neurotransmitters and the formation of free radicals, can contribute to age-related disorders including Alzheimer's disease and late-life depression.

The following are some general mental and psychological effects of chronic stress:

433

Putting your happiness hormones to work

Studies show that optimistic people are happier than pessimistic people, and being happy is good for your health. When you're happy, your endocrine glands secrete hormones that create pleasurable feelings into your bloodstream. While pleasurable feelings are nice, these hormones do far more than just make you feel good. They also can boost your immune system, reduce stress, modulate your appetite, and increase the release of sex hormones. Two of the most important hormones for happiness and good health are listed here:

✔ **Endorphins:** Released by the pituitary gland, endorphins are known as the "happy brain" chemical. Endorphins are natural opiates that promote feelings of intense pleasure; the euphoric state known as a "runner's high" is caused by endorphin release. Exercise, laughter, and certain foods — such as chocolate (but didn't you always know that?) and chili peppers — also cause endorphin release. Endorphins also act as a natural painkiller; they're three times more powerful at blocking pain than the narcotic morphine.

   Endorphins bind to the opioid receptors in neurons that cause pain sensations. (These are the same receptors that painkillers like morphine bind to.) Endorphins block the release of neurotransmitters, which means pain signals can't reach your brain.

✔ **Seratonin:** Serotonin is a neurotransmitter that's manufactured in your brain and gastrointestinal tract using the amino acid *tryptophan,* which is the chemical in your Thanksgiving Day turkey that makes you sleepy and gives you a feeling of well-being. Serotonin helps with sleep, calming anxiety, and relieving depression.

✔ **Mental symptoms**

- Persistent negative thoughts
- Indecisiveness
- Poor memory
- Boredom
- Loss of concentration
- Bad dreams
- Poor decision making

✔ **Emotional symptoms**

- Irritability
- Anxiety and worry
- Mood swings
- Crying spells
- Tension
- Lack of enthusiasm
- Cynicism
- Feelings of alienation
- Loss of confidence
- A general sense of dissatisfaction

✔ **Behavioral symptoms**

- Unsociability
- Restlessness
- Changes in eating habits
- Changes in exercise habits
- Changes in sleeping habits

Understanding the Big Picture: Why Chronic Stress Is a Concern as You Age

The relationship between the mind and body's reaction to stress and its effect on your mental health is complex, particularly as you age. Stress often accompanies change, and certainly many changes accompany aging — both internally and externally. Changes in socioeconomic status, physical health and abilities, and family support are among the stressful life events commonly experienced by people as they age. The body is already experiencing normal age-related changes and when you compound that with chronic stress reactions, the results can be dangerous for some.

The effects of chronic stress are especially serious as you age; here are a few reasons why:

✔ **As you get older, your brain slowly loses its ability to regulate hormone levels.** As we explain in the previous section, stress makes hormone levels go all out of whack anyway, but those unbalanced levels are prolonged with age, which directly leads to health problems — the longer your brain has been exposed to stress hormones, the more possibility for damage.

For example, high, prolonged levels of cortisol in the bloodstream accelerate the aging of healthy muscle and bone, and slow down healing and normal cell regeneration. The raised blood pressure and heart rate end up placing stress on the heart's vessels and accelerate the onset of heart disease. In addition, an excess of cortisol over your lifetime can damage the *hippocampus,* a part of your brain that's crucial for storing and retrieving memories (see Chapter 12). Studies show that high cortisol levels correlate to poor memory.

✔ **The normal biological responses to stress, such as rapid heartbeat and an increase in blood pressure, don't return to normal as quickly as you age.** Long-term stress creates added wear and tear on the body. In fact, data suggests that long-term stress can increase a person's risk of heart attack and sudden death (in persons already susceptible to these health issues).

✓ **When the levels of stress neurotransmitters rise in response to chronic stress, parts of the immune system are impaired.** Duration of illnesses or infections can be prolonged due to changes in the white blood cells (immune cells). These effects suppress the immune system as a whole and leave the body susceptible to viral infections.

Women in particular are more susceptible to an overload of stress hormones as they age. In fact, the impact of age on cortisol levels is nearly three times stronger for women than for men. So, as women continue to be employed in higher-stress occupations, they need to pay special attention to the potential effects of stress on the body.

Measuring Stress

Are you feeling like you're more stressed than usual, or more stressed than other people? Have you reached the point where everything seems to send you into a state of adrenaline-pumping emergency? A simple self test can help you identify the times when your stress levels are shooting out of control, as well as give you some tools for calming yourself down.

If your stress levels are out of control, a professional evaluation may help you get a better handle on the stressors in your life, as well as give you guidance on how best to manage them — we explain how to seek that guidance in this section as well.

Paying attention to your stress response

Much of the stress of daily life can be planned for ahead of time. Do you drive to work every day? It's a pretty safe guess that traffic is going to be a daily stressor for you. Baby-sit your grandchild once a week? Spilled milk and temper tantrums may be on your weekly stress list, too.

Staying in tune with your body and becoming more aware of stress symptoms when they first appear can help you begin to relax before your stress levels are out of control. Watch for the following signs of increased stress:

- ✔ **Are you a clencher?** Check your body for tension to see whether you're clenching your muscles. Start at the top of your head and work your way down. Feel the muscles in your face, jaw, and neck. Move down to your shoulders, chest, and back. Keep moving your way down to your arms, hands, and torso. Do you feel tension in your thighs, calves, feet, or toes?

- ✔ **Do your hands get cold?** Place your hand on the side of your neck just above your collar. If your hand is noticeably cooler than your neck, your hand temperature indicates that your body is probably stressed.

- ✔ **Do you sweat?** Excessive sweating is an involuntary stress response caused by the secretion of certain stress hormones. Many people perspire when they're tense.

- ✔ **Does your pulse race?** If your heart is beating above 100 beats per minute (bpm) without exertion, chances are good that your body is responding to stress. Most people at rest have a pulse rate between 60 to 80 bpm, although some have a resting pulse as high as 100 bpm.

✔ **Do you have rapid breathing?** Rapid, shallow breathing indicates tension. When you're tense, you tighten your stomach muscles and breathe through your chest, which isn't very expandable. When you're relaxed, your breathing is slow and deep with your stomach muscles relaxed.

✔ **Do you ruminate about things?** If you're constantly thinking about the same thing over and over in your mind day in and day out, it may also be a sign of a stressor. Ruminating can be a tipoff that you need to reduce the amount of time that you're focusing on something.

Defusing your stressors

Some stressors are inevitable and tough to completely eliminate — wild children at home, a difficult boss, and a long, hectic drive into the office are just a few examples. You may not be able to get a grip on how to handle these stressors without help; if you could do it alone, most likely you would've taken care of it already.

Sometimes brainstorming with a friend or family member can help you find a solution. For instance, if you have a nightmare commute to and from work, find a co-worker who's willing to carpool, or offer to pay for gas and catch a ride with someone. (Make sure that riding with the co-worker doesn't cause more stress than it relieves!) Consider taking the bus or train part of the way. If you're stressed at home, talk to your family to find ways to allow you to balance your need to be with the family against your need for some occasional downtime. You may find that taking the train home gives you time to both unwind and avoid the stress of driving through hair-raising traffic — two stressors eliminated in one easy change!

The important point is to recognize your stressors and then look for ways to modify them. Coauthor Dr. Agin sees a large portion of his patients for issues regarding stress and how to cope. It's a common problem; just acknowledging the stress is the first step toward making the decisions that can help you control it.

Working through Stress with a Professional

Sometimes chronic stress has such a stranglehold on your life that you need professional help in releasing its grip. Fortunately, medical professionals and therapists can help you recognize and deal with stress that's become too much for you to handle. You may find some of these tools used at stress management workshops as well.

A professional may use interviews and standardized stress questionnaires to help assess the frequency and amount of stress in your daily routine and then guide your therapy and treatment accordingly. The following are just a sample of the kinds of evaluations and therapies available:

- ✔ **Daily Stress Inventory:** The Daily Stress Inventory is a self-reporting tool for patients. They provide a daily assessment of the sources and personal impact of relatively minor stressful events. This test concentrates on recognizing the small but cumulative stress-inducing events of daily life — things you don't consider major sources of stress. Because these are everyday events or activities, you may not realize the stress that they can cause. Tools like this one point out these stressors and can open your eyes to the fact that you may have more on your plate than you thought.

- ✔ **The Hassles and Uplifts Scales (HSUP):** This test presents a new way of looking at stress by measuring attitudes about daily situations categorized as *hassles* and *uplifts*. In it, you see the many items that you consider to be hassles and find ways to balance these items with the uplifts. This tool steers away from measuring major life stressors and concentrates on finding ways to evaluate and more effectively cope with the highs and lows in your everyday life.

- ✔ **Biofeedback:** Biofeedback uses machines (electronic instruments) to monitor your body's specific, often unconscious physiological activities and habit patterns. The doctor uses your reactions to create awareness of your physical responses to stress, which helps teach you to modify your reactions. A biofeedback stress test performed by a physician measures the following vital signs:

  - Heart rate
  - Blood pressure
  - Breathing rate
  - Brain waves
  - Muscle tension
  - Skin resistance
  - Temperature

When you're aware of the physical changes that accompany stressors, you can recognize the beginnings of stress before it gets out of hand and utilize stress-release techniques until your body is no longer reacting adversely to the stressor.

Making Personal Strides to Reduce Stress

Learning to manage and reduce your stress load may improve the quality of your life, and give you a better chance to live a long and healthier one. Lots of tools, tips, and techniques can help you reduce stress and figure out how to relax. Recognizing stress is the first and hardest thing for many people to do. Finding and focusing on sources of stress is helpful, because you're concentrating on what you can do to change rather than letting stress continue to grow until it's out of control.

Most of the time, if you need professional help with stress, it's because you let the unrecognized stress build for too long. If you're ready to start reducing stress on your own, think about your life, find the stressors, and then develop a way to manage them. Although the key to successful stress reduction is maintaining a positive attitude, picking a technique that works for *you* is critical. We encourage you to explore the techniques in this section and try a few on for size — you'll know when one fits.

With a little practice and creativity, you can reduce your stress levels and soon look forward to the newfound pleasure of relaxing your mind and body with the help of one of these stress busters.

Accentuating the positive

Researchers say that the people with more positive attitudes may deal with stress better and have a stronger will to live. People who feel good about themselves as they get older live about seven and a half years longer than the bitter, negative types.

How can you keep a positive attitude? Two things that help are

442

✔ Accepting that you can't control some events in your life

✔ Being assertive and positive instead of aggressive in stressful situations

Part of staying positive is being able to see humor in situations, including those that may normally stress you out. Laughter really is the best medicine when it comes to reducing your stress. Laughing reduces the production of cortisol (which accelerates aging) and increases the level of health-enhancing hormones like endorphins and neurotransmitters. Laughter also increases the number of antibody-producing cells and enhances the effectiveness of T cells. What that boils down to is a stronger immune system and fewer physical effects from stress.

Employing self-relaxation techniques

It's easy to say "Just relax" when your stress levels are building, but it's easier to do if you've developed some relaxation techniques. Try the following methods of self relaxation:

✔ **Practicing breathing techniques:** Deep, slow breathing — the kind that reaches all the way into your gut, moving your abdomen out and in — is one of the easiest and most cleansing stress relievers with a variety of body-benefits. Deep breathing helps oxygenate your blood, which "wakes up" your brain, relaxes your muscles, and quiets your mind. You focus on relaxing your body and releasing air on each breath. Deep breathing is easy to practice because you can breathe anywhere, and it works quickly to relieve your stress.

- **Meditating your way to peace:** Meditation builds on the technique of deep breathing and goes one step farther. After you master the technique of slow, deep, cleansing breaths to calm your body and restore and calm your breathing to a normal, relaxed state, you can begin to meditate. In some forms of meditation, your brain enters a state that's similar to sleep, but it carries some added benefits that you can't achieve as well in any other state, including the release of certain hormones that promote health. In other meditation techniques, the focus is on recognizing and accepting your feelings in the moment without trying to change them and without dwelling on them.

During meditation, you clear your mind of any focus or distraction. This enables you to detach from stressors and restores your body to a state of calm, essentially giving your body time to repair itself. Breathing returns to normal, so you use oxygen more efficiently. Your heart rate slows down, your blood pressure comes down, and anxiety levels decrease, so you sweat less.

A tremendous benefit of meditation for anti-aging is that your adrenal glands produce less cortisol, adrenaline, and noradrenaline, which have been associated with negative effects on aging. By relaxing the body in this manner, you prevent damage from the physical effects of stress. You also make additional positive hormones and your immune function improves.

Check out *Meditation For Dummies,* 2nd Edition, by Stephan Bodian and Dean Ornish, MD (Wiley), for more info.

✔ **Practicing guided imagery and visualization:** Guided imagery and visualization techniques involve envisioning a relaxing scene or picturing yourself achieving goals or increasing your performance in some specific way. People who practice guided imagery go into a deeply relaxed state that provides significant stress-reduction benefits, including physically relaxing the body quickly and efficiently.

✔ **Hypnotizing yourself:** Self-hypnosis incorporates some of the features of guided imagery and visualization (see the preceding bullet), with the added benefit of enabling you to communicate directly with your subconscious mind. Hypnosis can be a valuable tool in helping you overcome fears, withstand pain, or reduce stress in your life. Self-hypnosis, however, may take some practice and training with a professional to make sure that you discover how to initiate and then come out of the session.

✔ **Practicing progressive muscle relaxation:** By tensing and relaxing all the muscle groups in your body you can relieve tension and feel much more relaxed in minutes, with no special training or equipment. Follow these steps:

1. **Start by tensing all the muscles in your face, holding a tight grimace for ten seconds.**

2. **Completely relax the muscles from Step 1 for ten seconds.**

3. **Repeat Steps 1 and 2 with your neck, followed by your shoulders, and so on, all the way down to your toes.**
   You can do this exercise anywhere, and as

you practice, you'll notice that you can relax more quickly and easily, reducing tension as quickly as it starts.

✔ **Calming yourself with music:** Music can be a powerful tool to aid relaxation and relieve stress. Music therapy has shown numerous health benefits for people with conditions ranging from stress to cancer. Music has been found to have an impact on hormones and neurotransmitters in the brain and has direct anxiety-lowering actions. Listening to, performing, or writing music can lower your blood pressure, relax your body, and calm your mind. It's often used as part of stress-management programs or in conjunction with exercise and is used in a variety of healthcare settings with good results for dealing with illness and stress. Music therapy is an emerging field, one whose benefits are just now starting to be realized.

Exploring your thoughts through journaling

Writing in a journal is a therapeutic self-expression of your thoughts, feelings, and life events, and it can be a powerful tool for self evaluation. Keeping negative feelings and thoughts inside isn't healthy, but many people don't feel comfortable expressing themselves or don't have anyone to confide in. As a stress-management tool, journaling helps you detail specific stressors, as well as how you think and feel about them. Journaling allows you to clarify your thoughts and feelings in order to gain valuable self-knowledge.

To use journaling as therapy, write down all aspects of a stressor rather than just bits and pieces. Be consistent — don't skip several days or occurrences. Journaling for therapy is different from keeping a daily event journal in which you chronicle everything that you did in a day. Therapeutic journaling allows you to focus on issues that need to be addressed; these issues become evident as you write down things that come to mind after you've given yourself time to clear your thoughts. You'll be surprised at what thoughts are lingering in your brain that, when released and examined, can give you a wonderful sense of well-being and freedom from stress.

Journaling is also a great way to keep track of where you are in your life. By reading what you wrote only a year or two ago, you can see how much progress you've made in different areas of your life. It's also helpful to see that concerns that loomed so large a year or two ago are now forgotten. Journaling helps keep things in perspective.

Journaling can be a good problem-solving tool. Putting pen to paper has a tremendous way of helping you resolve problems and come up with solutions. Writing about traumatic events helps you process them by fully exploring and releasing the emotions involved and by engaging both hemispheres of the brain in the process, allowing the experience to become fully integrated in your mind.

Exercising away your stress

Exercise is one of your body's best natural cures for stress. It leads to the release of endorphins, which has a healing effect on the body and mind and protects against some of the harmful effects of stress. Researchers have found that those who exercise have fewer stress-related health problems, which provides a positive impact on healthy aging.

Exercise can be as simple as a walk around your neighborhood every evening or as complicated as working out with a personal trainer. Find the type of exercise that works for you and your body. For example, swimming is a great exercise if you suffer from arthritis and can't tolerate the joint-pounding strain of aerobic exercise. You may also find riding a stationary bike easier than running a marathon.

Yoga, anyone?

Yoga is an ancient path to spiritual growth. Today, yoga is a broad term for a series of personal stretches and exercises that bring together your physical, mental, and spiritual aspects of life. Yoga teaches you a series of stationary and moving poses called *asanas* and a form of breathing known as *pranayama,* as well as concentration techniques to help you get in tune with your body, your mind, and your emotions in the present moment. You can find a lot of different schools of yoga, but they all have the goal of attaining a state of wholeness and completeness.

Yoga is designed to balance the different systems of your body. By taking your mind off the causes of stress, and having you gently stretch your body in ways that massage your internal organs, yoga helps you create an inner peace.

People of all ages can benefit from regular yoga practices, and with the various schools and the ability to change the poses, yoga can be adjusted to fit physical limitations and other complications.

 For more information on yoga, check out *Yoga For Dummies* (Wiley) by Georg Feuerstein, Larry Payne, and Lilias Folan.

Working out in the bedroom

People often joke that the most uptight and stressed-out people may lighten up a bit if they just had sex. But there's truth there — the benefits of sex in stress reduction are plentiful. These benefits include deep breathing, lowering blood pressure, decreasing anxiety, getting a physical workout, and feeling a pleasurable sense of touch.

Most people feel the least like having sex when they're stressed out, but it's worth giving it some extra effort. Sexual activity releases endorphins and other feel-good hormones that put a smile on your face in no time. Sex has other health benefits as well (lucky you, right?), and we discuss them in Chapter 15.

Tossing out poor habits

When you're feeling stressed, it's natural to look for ways to cope. However, some of the things you turn to when stressed may actually be more destructive or create more stress on your body than you're relieving, creating a vicious cycle. Three coping mechanisms that fall into this category are caffeine, nicotine, and alcohol.

Eliminating caffeine

Consider eliminating or at least decreasing your caffeine intake. Caffeine is a drug and a stimulant and may cause your body to react as it would to stress by increasing your heart rate and blood pressure. Consuming caffeine may also accentuate the symptoms that you experience during panic attacks. We're not telling you to eliminate your morning wake-up routine, but be aware of caffeine's potential symptoms. Many people have no problems with coffee intake in moderation (2 cups per day), but too much coffee can have systemic effects that may mimic or potentiate stress. The other option for diehard coffee drinkers is to drink unleaded (decaf) fuel. If you can't give up caffeine altogether, find a balance between regular and decaffeinated by switching to decaf after two regular coffees.

Dr. Agin always tells his patients to avoid consuming anything that requires you to taper off. The need to taper means that you've become dependent on something and may experience withdrawal symptoms when you stop abruptly. If you do decide to eliminate caffeine, do so gradually, because you may have headaches, sweats, and some irritability.

Avoiding nicotine

During times of stress, smokers often reach for a cigarette to calm down, but nicotine is actually a stimulant. Nicotine increases blood pressure, heart rate, and respiration, and stimulates the central nervous system. Nicotine has a stimulatory effect on the brain and can cause the release of neurotransmitters and endorphins that give a temporary feeling of energy and well-being. Most smokers have become dependent on nicotine and need it to maintain normal moods. They often suffer from unpleasant feelings of irritability and tension between cigarettes, when nicotine levels in the blood are falling.

People often feel that they can't stop smoking when they're under stress because the act of smoking is therapeutic and reduces stress levels. Some also use smoking as a timeout from problem situations; this learned behavior is the largest reason people give for continuing smoking. Smoking in social settings may reduce stress by giving smokers something to do with their hands and something to look at. The laughter and the socializing can also be therapeutic, but smokers will attribute their stress reduction to smoking. Lastly, smoking may produce a short-term reduction of stress because it removes the stress caused by nicotine withdrawal symptoms from the last cigarette you smoked.

Nicotine withdrawal causes an initial increase in anxiety and stress, so choosing the right time to quit is important. Right before your daughter's wedding, for example, may not be the best time!

Holding alcohol consumption to a moderate level

The messages on alcohol use and stress are mixed. Some studies have found that alcohol itself can actually trigger the stress response. But other studies suggest that low levels of alcohol can reduce stress, tension, and anxiety. Moderate drinking has even been shown to improve your mood. So which is it? Does drinking help ease stress or make it worse?

Although low doses of alcohol have been shown to reduce stress, research has shown that alcohol induces some of the same physiological effects as other stressors:

- ✔ It interferes with the stages of sleep and can lead to sleeping difficulties (see Chapter 14 for more information).

- ✔ It numbs your emotions, impairing your ability to cope with stressful situations.

- ✔ In excess, it can lead to social isolation, anger, depression, and paranoia.

Alcohol isn't a healthy way of coping with stress. Drinking to deal with stress can interfere with work, relationships, and finances, and it can lead to more problems, like alcoholism and health complications. So, instead of drinking, which is avoiding the problem, try to make constructive changes that will deal with the problems directly and make you feel better about yourself without subjecting you to the health risks of heavy drinking. The various techniques we discuss in this chapter can help you develop better coping skills.

Bringing out the kid in you

Life should be fun, and participating in activities you enjoy is a great way to relax and decrease stress. Having hobbies

451

and outside interests keeps you connected and engaged with the world outside yourself.

Board games, puzzles, online games, crossword puzzles, and other fun activities can bring added joy and happiness to life, and they can be a great way to relieve stress. When you get really engrossed in an activity you enjoy, such as putting a puzzle together, you can experience a state of being know as *flow,* in which your brain is in a near-meditative state. This state benefits your body, mind, and soul.

Your stress level and your happiness benefit from at least one activity that you do regularly just for fun. Hobbies and games provide a fun way to sharpen skills, express your creativity, or just blow off steam.

Chapter 14

ZZZ . . . The Infinite Importance of a Good Night's Sleep

The business of helping people catch some ZZZs has mushroomed — to say the least — over the past few decades. Pharmaceutical companies promise immediate sleep with a tiny pill, while books on meditation and relaxation promise restful sleep with a simple "Ohmmm" and a lavender-scented candle. Mattress companies have cashed in, luring the weary with promises of a good night's rest based on numbers designating mattress firmness and materials that mold to your body, and major hotel chains tempt guests with soft pillow tops and ever fancier bedding. As a result, people feel like a good night's sleep is impossible without pharmaceutical aides, a guru, self-adjustable air mattresses, Swedish contour foam pillows, combed Egyptian cotton sheets, and half a dozen strategically placed body pillows.

And yet, even with all this help, sleep remains elusive. People can't get enough of it. We're not talking about the occasional restless night; we're talking *insomnia* (the inability to sleep well for an extended period of time, such as weeks and months) and the restlessness and early awakenings that often accompany aging.

Lack of sleep significantly affects a person's mental and physical health, even more so as the years creep along. In

The deadly danger of sleep deprivation

The fatigue that accompanies lack of sleep also makes you dangerous on the road. People who are tired are more likely to be involved in car accidents. Quite literally your life can depend on good sleep. Many studies make it clear that sleep deprivation is dangerous. Sleep-deprived people who are tested by using a driving simulator or by performing a hand-eye coordination task perform as badly as or worse than those who are intoxicated. Sleep deprivation also magnifies alcohol's effects on the body, so a fatigued person who drinks will become much more impaired than someone who's well rested.

Driver fatigue is responsible for an estimated 100,000 motor vehicle accidents and 1,500 deaths each year, according to the National Highway Traffic Safety Administration. Because drowsiness is the brain's last step before falling asleep, driving while drowsy can — and often does — lead to disaster. Caffeine and other stimulants can't overcome the effects of severe sleep deprivation. The National Sleep Foundation says that if you have trouble keeping your eyes focused, if you can't stop yawning, or if you can't remember driving the last few miles, you're probably too drowsy to drive safely.

this chapter, we cover the basics on the importance of sleep, its changes due to the aging process, and your own body's sleep rhythms, including a discussion on bona fide sleep disorders, the real spoilers in the aging process. So whether you're an okay sleeper or a major sleep-deprived soul lugging from one day to the next, this chapter can help you toward a better night's sleep — every night.

Why Adequate Sleep Is Crucial to Your Health

Sleep is nature's restoration period. While you sleep, your body restores your immune system, your nervous system, and even your muscular and skeletal systems. Certain hormones and brain-related proteins also restore while you sleep. So, if you don't sleep well or enough (or both), your body doesn't get the time it needs to rejuvenate itself, and it slowly lags behind in its optimal ability to function — over the long haul, you function less than optimally with many systems affected. Studies have shown that lack of sleep can lead to immune dysfunction and disrupted hormone regulation. Sleep deprivation is a form of stress on your body; you're not regulating the hormones that can lead to long-term problems with chronic stress (see Chapter 13 for more information on the effects of stress).

The end result? If you sleep well, you wake up refreshed and energized; however, if you don't get enough sleep, sleep too long, or the quality of your sleep is compromised, you may be affected in one or more of the following ways:

- You wake up grumpy and sluggish.
- You're downright unproductive.
- Poor sleep can affect your health, your relationships,

455

and your work.

- Prolonged poor sleep has also been linked to diabetes, obesity, heart disease, and premature aging.

- Sleep deprivation has been linked to anxiety disorders.

- You may not be able to deal with the small irritations of daily life.

- Drowsiness affects your work productivity, your ability to relate to others, and your attendance record.

- At home, you may be irritable and grouchy with your spouse, children, or friends.

- You can be a danger to yourself and others.

Men and women face different issues when it comes to sleep, but the end result is the same. It doesn't matter what the cause of sleep deprivation is; what matters is the quantity and quality of your sleep. Many things disrupt sleep quality or quantity; all make for painful days at the office, home, or wherever you're struggling to keep those lids open. Some notorious sleep problems are gender specific; for example, women deal with the following:

- **Pregnancy:** Sleep can be a problem for pregnant women, especially toward the end of pregnancy, when finding a comfortable sleeping position becomes difficult.

- **Baby's feeding schedules:** After the baby arrives, waking up in the middle of the night to feed and change the baby becomes a common occurrence for most women (and, yes, many men experience this too).

- **Menopause:** Women get hit again by the insomnia monster before and during menopause when nightly hot flashes can keep them awake for hours.

Men handle these situations:

- **Middle age:** Men get less restful sleep in middle age and that can contribute to conditions like diabetes and heart disease.

- **Sleep apnea:** Men are more at risk of developing sleep apnea — a life threatening and, at the very least, severely-sleep-depriving condition in which a person stops breathing repeatedly during the night.

- **Prostate problems:** Many men need to get up at night to urinate due to an enlarged prostate, and that interferes with good sleep.

How Sleep Does Its Job

Although you don't remember it, your sleep time is really a time of tremendous activity. A lot of maintenance work goes on in the body and particularly in the brain during those "off" hours. The body has a built-in cycle that's supposed to operate efficiently to get you sleeping well and prepared to face the next day, but several factors can alter this cycle and keep people frustrated and sleepy eyed.

In short, there are two types of sleep: rapid eye movement (REM) and non-rapid eye movement (NREM). NREM comprises four stages and accounts for about 80 percent of sleep. As you sleep, you enter into sleep cycles that contain both REM and NREM sleep. For the first 75 to 80 minutes, you're in NREM, and then you reach REM for about 15 to 20 minutes before the cycle starts over. The average person goes through four to six cycles per night. These cycles usually last around 90 minutes but can last up to 100 minutes and are important in figuring out the amount of sleep that you need. If you sleep well and don't use an alarm clock, you're likely to find that you wake up at times that are multiples of the 90-minute sleep cycle. For example, you may wake up after 4 1/2, 6, or 7 1/2 hours.

 Many sleep experts direct you to figure your sleep needs in 90-minute increments. You want to complete each 90-minute cycle, because the slightest alteration of these sleep stages is enough to make you feel sleep deprived.

The next sections cover what happens in each of the sleep phases.

The structured phases: NREM sleep (stages 1-4)

NREM sleep is known as dreamless sleep — how boring! So what's the purpose of NREM, you might ask? Your body is actually accomplishing some important tasks during NREM, although they may not seem very exciting. NREM puts you in relaxation mode; your pulse and blood pressure drop, and you have minimal eye movement during this stage. The body does its repair work during NREM, which is subdivided into four stages:

- **Stage one:** This stage usually lasts less than 10 minutes. Stage one is your body's introduction to sleep — your breathing, brain waves, and muscles slow down — your blood pressure falls. In this stage, you may experience muscle contractions (hypnotic jerks) that suddenly jolt you out of sleep. These muscle contractions sometimes make you feel like you're about to fall or trip. They're weird but perfectly normal and usually occur as you transition from being awake to going to sleep.

Your eyes are closed during stage one sleep, but if someone wakes you up, you often feel as though you haven't slept at all. People who suffer from insomnia spend more time in this first stage of sleep.

✔ **Stage two:** In this stage, your brain waves slow down even more, but they're occasionally interrupted by a cluster of fast-moving waves. Your eye movements, which were slowing down in stage one, stop altogether. You spend about 40 minutes of your sleep cycle in stage two sleep.

If someone wakes you up while you're in stage two sleep, you may not be particularly happy about it, but you won't be the walking dead either. When you take the occasional short nap, you enter stage two sleep. You awake refreshed but you couldn't survive on naps alone.

✔ **Stages three and four:** These two stages are characterized by the appearance of very slow brain waves (*delta* waves). Delta wave sleep is the deepest sleep you achieve throughout the sleep cycle. The main difference between stages three and four is the amount of delta waves that occur. Stage three usually contains less than 50 percent of the sleep waves as delta waves while stage 4 has more than 50 percent of it's waves as slow delta waves. Delta waves are mixed with faster waves in an up-and-down pattern. In these stages, it can sometimes take a very loud noise to wake you up.

When you finally reach stages three and four, your body does a lot of its repair work — the longer you stay in these stages, the more refreshed you feel in the morning. During this time, hormone levels and brain chemicals are restored. If someone wakes you up while you're in this stage, you're groggy and disoriented for quite some time. This is also the deep sleep when children wet the bed and sleepwalk.

You stay in deep sleep for about 20 minutes of each of your sleep cycles and then you move on to the most interesting part of the night — the dream stage.

The random dreaming phase: REM

The last sleep stage is REM sleep, which accounts for about 20 percent of sleep time and about 20 minutes of each sleep cycle. Throughout this stretch of sleep, dreaming occurs, your breathing quickens, your heart rate increases, your blood pressure rises, your eyes move just as if you were watching a movie, men develop erections, and your temperature regulation is impaired. If you're awakened during REM sleep, you may find that you're hot or cold (mostly hot) and have to adjust the covers accordingly. During this stage your muscles become temporarily paralyzed, but your brain activity increases to levels that are similar to when awake. Babies spend about 50 percent of their sleep in REM sleep.

Dreams rarely occur in NREM sleep, and most often are a function of REM sleep. Dreams can be images, sounds, or thoughts and often provoke emotional responses. Dreams can run scripts related to events that happened during the day or they can be quite dynamic containing many details, leaving dreamers wondering what may have caused them to dream specific topics. Researchers have a couple of theories about the reasons for these dreams:

✔ **The brain uses dreams as a mechanism for categorizing information and realigning brain-related pathways.** In other words, the brain performs certain housecleaning tasks that it can't do while a person is up and moving. Lending credence to this theory is the fact that REM sleep is most active during the first two years of life when a baby's brain is growing and developing.

🗸 **Dreams are associated with a person's emotions.** If you're very worried about a problem, there's a strong possibility that you'll dream about it at night. That's not always bad — often, a discovery or a way to solve that problem also shows up in a dream.

On the flip side, bad dreams or nightmares can be reminders of issues or fears that need to be addressed. In other words, dreams may act as a pressure-cooker, allowing you to vent your feelings in the safety of your sleep.

How Sleep Changes as You Age

As you age, you may become more prone to wakeful nights both because of natural age-related sleep cycle changes and other problematic causes. Quality of sleep can decrease because deep sleep (the delta sleep of stages three and four) decreases, and light sleep (stage two) increases (see the preceding section). Until recently, research on sleep problems focused on the elderly. However, new research indicates that sleep disruptions start in middle age — the time of life when people are most productive. Hormonal changes combined with work- and family-related stressors are a recipe for sleepless nights. There's conflicting evidence about the *exact* causes of age-associated impaired sleep, but it's clear that impaired sleep is a common complaint of the elderly.

As you get older, the following issues may contribute to poor sleep patterns:

✔ **Sleep hygiene:** Sleep hygiene is the practice of following simple guidelines to ensure restful, effective sleep that promotes daytime alertness and helps avoid the onset of sleep disorders. Poor sleep hygiene is the number one cause of sleep-related issues in all populations, including the elderly. Sleep is easily disturbed by outside influences and bad habits of the poor sleepers. Irregular sleep/wake times, caffeine, alcohol, and daytime napping are all common occurrences. Sometimes people are already practicing these bad habits while others grasp onto them for a desperate solution. (See the later section "Resuming Your Rhythm When You Veer Off Track" for more on this issue.)

✔ **Changes in the circadian rhythm:** Circadian rhythms are the powerful rhythms of the body that influence many different systems — sleep being one of them. A few situations — such as illicit drug use, travel across time zones, and brain diseases — can cause this rhythm to be out of sync and become a major difficulty (see the next section for a rundown of the circadian rhythm).

People tend to sleep more lightly and for shorter time spans as they get older, although they generally need about the same amount of sleep as they needed in early adulthood. About half of all people over 65 have frequent sleeping problems, such as insomnia, and deep sleep stages in many elderly people often become very short or stop completely. This change may be a normal part of aging, or it may result from medical problems that are common in elderly people and from the medications and other treatments for those problems.

✔ **Hormone changes:** Changes in a woman's body before and during menopause can cause severe disruptions to sleep, such as hot flashes, heart palpitations, and anxiety. Decreases in both growth hormone and melatonin, two important hormones for sleep regulation, is one of the biggest causes of sleep problems in the elderly.

✔ **Pain:** Pain is a common reason for poor sleep in older people. From arthritis to heartburn, pain or discomfort is a common complaint as you age. Even minor aches and pains rob older people of sleep.

✔ **Bladder control problems:** Frequency or loss of control of urination may cause awakenings in both men and women and seem to increase with age. Men frequently awake to urinate because of enlargement of the prostate, while women may lose some strength and control over the muscles of the bladder that results in the need for more frequent bathroom trips at night. Some people get to the point where they wear adult pads just to try to keep the problem from interfering with sleep, but it can still interfere with the quality of sleep even if you don't have to get out of bed. See your doctor for some possibilities to improve these conditions and your sleep.

✔ **Sleep disorders:** Conditions such as sleep apnea, restless leg syndrome (RLS), and insomnia are all commonly experienced as you age.

✔ **Prescription medications:** Some medications can interfere with sleep. Some antidepressants, nicotine, and beta-blockers can effect the stages of sleep and therefore how rested you feel.

Understanding Your Biological Clock: The Circadian Rhythm

Your body has a 24-hour internal clock (called the circadian rhythm) that controls your biological functions. Your personal circadian rhythm governs the time you wake in the morning and when you feel sleepy at night, as well as the times you feel most productive — essentially, it's your biological clock. (People who are most productive and happily awake in the wee hours of the night have a circadian rhythm that's opposite from most people — but it's normal for them.)

The more you understand — and listen to — your personal clock, the more rested you feel. This section is all about helping you find that rhythm and keeping you on schedule even when the occasional sleep problems threaten to throw you off course.

Seeing how the rhythm works and how it runs amok

Circadian rhythms work by influencing hormones that play a role in sleep and wakefulness, metabolic rate, and body temperature. The circadian rhythm affects more than just sleep, and researchers feel that it has a connection to certain diseases and medical events. For instance, researchers have found that more people have heart attacks in the morning than in the evening and more asthma attacks happen at night than during the day. Although researchers haven't proven the connection between these events and the circadian rhythm, there's a lot of interest in the possibility of such a connection.

Most people have a circadian rhythm a lot like their ancestors; however, that rhythm is all too often affected by artificial light, night shifts at work, time zones, medications, and other factors. This rhythm is controlled by the *suprachiasmatic nucleus* that lies in the hypothalamus of the brain. Some of the influences on sleep center on the body clock missing some of its clues, such as bright morning light or evening darkness. These changes can cause the rhythm to shift, and as a result, your suprachiasmatic nucleus produces hormones at the wrong time or stops producing the right amounts altogether if it's interrupted for long periods.

Here are some common reasons why circadian rhythms are off-balance:

- ✔ **Jet lag:** This condition of fatigue and insomnia is caused by travel across time zones. This travel disrupts the circadian rhythm, causing sleepiness and decreased daytime alertness. It usually resets in three to four days, but it can take a week to feel back to baseline.

- ✔ **Rotating work shifts:** You may be affected by this issue if you frequently rotate shifts at work, especially night shifts.

- ✔ **Night owls:** Night owls suffer from delayed sleep phase syndrome (DSPS). These folks stay up almost all night, functioning well when most other people wouldn't be able to recite the alphabet. That said, however, night owls have a hard time waking up for work, school, or social engagements.

- ✔ **Advanced sleep phase syndrome:** This issue (ASPS) causes folks to get sleepy in the very early evening but then wake up before the rooster crows. This experience is typical of aging.

If you feel that your circadian rhythm is off due to one of the above reasons see the section below, "Resuming Your Rhythm When You Veer Off Track" to improve your sleep or correct one of the sleeping syndromes. You can also check out www.sleepdisordersguide.com or www. clevelandclinic. org (type "DSPS" or "ASPS" into the search section) for more information on ASPS and DSPS.

Determining your own circadian rhythm

Just like your thumbprint, your sleep needs are unique. Some people can live on five to six hours of sleep each night, and others are positively grumpy if they don't get their eight hours of shut-eye. Some folks are night owls and a few oddballs (we can't handle it) wake up refreshed and perky at the crack of dawn (although the oddballs become increasingly less "odd" among older populations).

At some point, each person finds his or her own comfortable sleep cycle, whether it's forced by work, children, or the desire to maintain a cycle based on the least amount of sleep required to still feel well. After your circadian rhythm is established, it's delicate and resistant to change. You can likely recall an evening when you went to bed later than you normally do, but slept in longer to keep the total number of sleep hours the same. The strange thing is that you don't feel the same even though your total amount of sleep is adequate.

This example shows how the rhythm establishes the release of hormones that solidify your sleep; even small variations in the pattern can result in less-optimal sleep. If you're having trouble setting your rhythm based on when you feel you should be sleeping, try moving your bedtime forward or backward by one to two hours. If you have to work at falling asleep, give this a try; your circadian rhythm may be an hour or so out of whack.

In general, adults need about eight hours of sleep daily. The amount of sleep each person needs depends on many factors, including age. Here's a typical rundown:

✔ Infants generally require about 14 to 16 hours a day.

✔ Teenagers need about eight to nine hours on average.

✔ For most adults, seven to nine hours a night appears to be the best amount of sleep, although some people may need as few as five hours or as many as ten hours of sleep each day.

✔ Women in the first three months of pregnancy often need several more hours of sleep than usual.

 People who feel that they need more than eight hours of sleep often have complaints of fatigue, are taking more than one medication, or have other medical complaints. Even when they do get nine or ten hours of sleep, they seldom feel completely rested.

The amount of sleep a person needs also increases if she's been deprived of sleep in previous days. When you don't get enough sleep, you create a "sleep debt," and your body doesn't have overdraft protection. You end up paying for it one way or another. Your body isn't able to adapt to getting less sleep than you need; while you may think that you're used to a sleep-depriving schedule, your judgment, reaction time, and other functions are still impaired. Paying back sleep debt is impossible. Sleeping for a week can't reverse the toll of continuous sleep deprivation. You simply have to get back into a routine and get your circadian rhythm back to normal.

If you're sleep-deprived, no one needs to tell you — you can feel it! Experts say that if you feel drowsy during the

Workin' 9 (p.m.) to 5 (a.m.)

Some people, by virtue of their jobs, don't have the luxury of sleeping at night, no matter what their personal circadian rhythm is. Nurses, police officers, casino workers, and pilots are just a few professionals who have to be on the job when everyone else is getting some ZZZs.

Many people who work odd shifts gravitate to these times because they have circadian rhythms that fit being up all night; others work night shift because their job requires shift rotation, or because all newbies start on the night shift. If your circadian rhythm is set for the night, you're good to go. But what if the night shift is anything but natural for you — or, even worse, if your job requires rotating shifts? Try the following suggestions:

- Sleep at a regular time. You may be too wired to go right to sleep, so establish regular sleep hygiene, like a glass of warm milk, a warm bath, or listening to relaxing music for 15 minutes. Don't watch television or start reading the latest bestseller.

- Darken your room — really darken it — and buy one of the gradually lightening lights that simulates dawn.

- Turn off the phone! When Sharon worked nights, the ringing of the phone was the pet peeve of most of her fellow nightshifters. Why not just turn the thing off? If you have school-aged kids who may call with an emergency, try to have a nearby friend who can be your contact person; she can come pound on your door if you're really needed.

- Run a noise machine. The *white noise* — such as rainfall or ocean waves — that's emitted from sound machines is a gentle tone that can be found in nature. White noise combines the frequencies of sound from low tones to high

> pitches, making it useful to mask other noises and sounds. This is invaluable, especially during the summer when kids are out playing. Try to sleep in a back bedroom, away from the street, to cut down on noise.

day at any time (boring activities excluded), you haven't had enough sleep.

 An unscientific way of testing how much sleep you need is to go to bed and wake up at the same time every day. If you get to the weekend and find yourself sleeping in, your body's telling you that it has a sleep debt. If, on the other hand, you wake up wide-eyed and bushy-tailed on Saturday morning at approximately the same time as you do during the week, you're doing just peachy on getting your required sleep.

 If you routinely fall asleep within five minutes of lying down, you may have severe sleep deprivation, possibly even a sleep disorder. The widespread practice of "burning the candle at both ends" in Western industrialized societies has created so much sleep deprivation that what's really abnormal sleepiness is now almost the norm.

Recognizing abnormal sleep issues

Many times people with sleeping problems complain of multiple medical symptoms and problems. For example, they may say that they can't keep their eyes open during important meetings at work, or they may complain that they can't return to sleep after they awake at night. Truthfully, people can blame just about anything on lack of sleep, but for some it's more than just an excuse.

Good sleep hygiene (see the section "Resuming Your Rhythm When You Veer Off Track") can greatly reduce or eliminate some symptoms, such as waking up tired; however, some symptoms — such as gasping for air (sleep apnea) — can be serious or deadly; they require immediate medical attention. Others, like sleepwalking, can be symptoms of a serious sleep disorder or another medical problem.

Here are some signs that you may have a sleep disorder:

- Being unable to sleep at night or waking up numerous times during the night

- Being too tired to perform simple tasks

- Being irritable and unable to concentrate

- Snoring so loudly that you disrupt your sleep or the sleep of your partner

- Sleepwalking or talking in your sleep

- Gasping for air while you sleep

- Twitching in your legs at night

- Sleeping more than nine hours a night for an extended period of time

 A sleep disorder is any condition that prevents you from getting a good night's sleep for an extended period of time. If you haven't slept well for about two weeks, you may have a sleep problem. So, if you experience any of these symptoms for at least two weeks and you maintain consistently good sleep hygiene, consult your primary care physician to discuss your situation and possible treatments (more on that topic at the end of this chapter in the section "Seeking Professional Treatment").

Resuming Your Rhythm When You Veer Off Track

Some of the most common causes of sleeping problems are completely preventable and fall under one category: sleep hygiene. Sleep hygiene isn't specifically associated with cleanliness — it focuses on the everyday habits that induce good sleep. Often these routines are the first things investigated when visiting your doctor with a complaint that you can't sleep, and often they require very simple changes.

Some of the most common remedies for poor sleep are listed here. Remember, though, that these are general guidelines — *you* may be lucky enough to be able to drink a double espresso two hours before bedtime and not have it interfere with your sleep, but even if you can, you may not be sleeping as well as you *could* be!

 Here are some bedtime tips:

- ✔ **Reserve the bed as a sacred place for sleeping (or sex).** Don't watch television or read when you're in bed. The bed is a place for sleep; don't go there until you're ready for that commitment. Do your socializing and television watching in another room because these types of activities can stimulate your mind enough to affect your sleep. Or you may find yourself so caught up in reading a book that you can't put it down and are still wide awake reading until early in the morning.

- ✔ **Go to bed and get up at the same time every day.** The easiest way to reset your rhythm when it's been thrown out of whack by travel, late nights, or illness is to get back to your targeted sleep/wake cycle and stick to it. The body functions well on a fixed schedule. Your body can't set a consistent schedule, or circadian rhythm, when you go to bed at 11 p.m. one day and then 2 a.m. the next. You'll feel tired and often have difficulty sleeping. After you determine the time you want to go to bed and the time you want to wake up, you need to go to bed consistently at that time and set an alarm to get up at your desired time each morning.

✔ **Steer clear of the caffeine at least six hours prior to bed.** Some people are actually affected by caffeine longer than this timeframe, but six hours is a good rule of thumb. Remember that chocolate also falls into this category. Sorry, chocoholics!

✔ **Exercise regularly but at a reasonable time.** Yes, this advice is a constant for what ails you. Exercising regularly (at least 30 minutes a day; preferably in the morning) helps you sleep better at night. Remember to stay away from heavy exercise two to three hours before bed — the release of endorphins, which are natural stimulants, energizes and wakes your body up, and it can take a few hours to wind back down.

✔ **Eat your last meal or snack at least three hours before going to bed.** You don't want to go to bed starving either. The important point to remember is to avoid eating a large meal or high-sugar content meal before bed. This intake can cause heartburn and other gastrointestinal upsets that interrupt sleep.

✔ **Try not to nap during the day.** If you don't sleep well during the night, logically, you shouldn't sleep during the day so that you can establish a pattern. You may have to work hard at skipping that afternoon snooze to get into a good sleep pattern, but you can do it.

- ✔ **Avoid drinking alcohol four hours before bed.** Many people drink alcohol because they feel that it makes them sleep better. Yes, it can make some people fall asleep, but the problem is that it often keeps you in the lighter stages of sleep.

- ✔ **Consult your doctor about sleeping medications.** Don't take any sleeping medication — even over-the-counter ones — without consulting your doctor. Sometimes medications that make one person sleepy may make you wide awake, and some pills make getting up in the morning harder and can make your body dependent on the medication. You also don't want to *treat* sleeping problems if you can *solve* them — getting in sync may take a few days, but you'll feel better in the long run.

If you have recurring, disturbing dreams that are adversely affecting you, talk to your doctor to see whether he or she can help. Getting a detailed medical history dating back to when the dreams or nightmares started may help you see whether any life-changing events, medication changes, or other major lifestyle changes could be the cause. Your doctor will make recommendations based on how it affects your activities.

Getting Back to Sleep When Your Eyes Are Wide Awake

It happens to everyone, and is one of the most frustrating events of sleeping: You wake up in the middle of the night and can't get back to sleep. If this is just an occasional occurrence, don't worry too much about it. But if it happens often, you may want to review your evening dietary indiscretions, your bedroom's soundproofing, or your partner's snoring patterns to see whether you can figure out what's waking you up.

Hopefully the information in this chapter will cut those frustrating wide-eyed nights to a minimum, but if you still find yourself staring at the ceiling at 3 a.m., the following suggestions may help:

- ✔ **Write down your anxious thoughts.** Many people find it helpful to keep a journal to unload in. You can also write a letter to a person who's upsetting you, but you don't have to send it.

- ✔ **Remember that you can't fix things in the middle of the night.** Remind yourself that there's nothing you can do about a problem in the wee hours of the night; then convince yourself to set it aside until you're refreshed and have the ability to change the situation. Often, this self-talk is enough to help you break the worry cycle. In the morning, you may wonder what on earth you were so worried about — the nighttime has a way of magnifying problems until they seem insurmountable.

- ✔ **Get up.** If you find that you really can't go back to sleep, get out of bed and do something really boring. That means absolutely no Web surfing or television. If you just have to read, make sure it's nothing motivating or incredibly engaging — try the section of your local newspaper that least interests you. You don't want to stimulate your brain.

  You can also listen to a relaxation CD or take a warm bath. Also, keep the lights down as much as possible. Light is a stimulant — the last thing you need when you're having a restless night.

- **Shut off the TV.** Reading or watching TV can produce different stimulatory emotions such as anxiety, anger, and sadness. Any of these can get the mind going and the body stimulated. Practice relaxation techniques that focus on the tension of the relaxation of the muscles after a brief contraction. This starts at the toes and goes up the whole body.

- **Drink some warm milk.** Milk contains some of the amino acids (particularly L-tryptophan, a precursor to the sleep hormone melatonin that your body creates) that help you sleep. A half-cup of warm milk is often all you need to relax.

- **Drink chamomile tea.** Chamomile is a great tea because of its mild sedating effect. Much like warm milk, this beverage can be a great solution for a restless night.

- **Take a warm bath.** A warm bath just before bedtime is a signal to the body that it's time to relax. Adding lavender oil to your bath water or rubbing some lavender oil on your body after you bathe will help you sleep, too. Research suggests that some scents like lavender and chamomile trigger a sleep response.

- **Turn off the lights.** Research suggests that even the smallest bit of light coming from your clock radio, for example, can disrupt the secretion of the sleep-time hormone melatonin. Keep lights off as much as possible during the night. If you have to use the bathroom, use a night light. Make sure that your bedroom shades are drawn tight, so that light from outside sources doesn't enter your room. If you really want to induce deep sleep, put on an eye mask to keep out all light.

- ✔ **Try tension relaxation or meditation.** Start at your feet and work up to the muscles of your head, tensing and relaxing the muscles while focusing on relaxation. This technique can move you into a better position for sleep. Meditating is another positive option.

- ✔ **Breathe.** Shallow breathing is a sign of stress. If you're tense, inhale deeply to the count of four. Then slowly exhale while counting to four. The more oxygen you get, the more relaxed you become. Do this breathing routine 10 to 12 times; many people fall asleep in the middle of it!

Seeking Professional Treatment

We aren't trying to take job security from doctors, but most sleeping issues don't require professional help. Sleep issues account for many medical visits each year, and most people are looking for a simple "pill fix." But most people need just the information in this chapter to put them to sleep. If you still struggle to sleep after trying our suggestions, professional help is an option. Just remember that good doctors are going to explore your sleeping habits rather than just pulling out the prescription pad. If you've tried *everything* and sleep is still elusive, the following professional approaches may help.

Handling occasional sleeping problems

Many treatments can help you get better sleep. Some studies suggest meditation and cognitive therapy are effective and long-lasting treatments, and they don't require medication. However, physician-prescribed medication is necessary and a welcome relief for those people who've been sleep-deprived for years. The following list covers the wide range of sleep-related treatments:

- **Cognitive therapy:** Cognitive therapy addresses your thought processes and can be used for many other conditions, such as anxiety. For example, if you think, "Oh, no, if I don't get to sleep tonight, I'll never sleep well," you're setting yourself up for a sleepless night; you're conditioning your mind to believe that sleep is an anxiety-ridden activity. Cognitive therapy is about changing your belief system and allowing you to make more reasonable decisions about how much sleep you really need.

- **Progressive muscle relaxation (PMR):** This therapy uses imagery and self-hypnosis to relax the muscles in your body. With PMR, you contract and relax different muscle groups from your head to your toes. As you do the exercises, you're able to address tension in your body that keeps you from sleeping.

- **Meditation:** Guided meditations on CD take you on a journey of relaxation and self-hypnosis that can help you sleep better.

- **Supplements:** Herbs like chamomile, lemon balm, and valerian root have been used for centuries to induce sleep. However, no serious studies have indicated how effective these herbs really are. **Note:** If you're on medication for conditions like diabetes, arthritis, or heart disease, talk to your doctor before trying natural supplements. Some supplements may interfere with effectiveness of pharmaceutical drugs.

- **Pharmaceutical sleep aids:** If you're having a lot of difficulty sleeping, your doctor may prescribe a drug like zolpidem (Ambien), ramelteon (Rozerem), or eszopiclone (Lunesta). These drugs may stabilize your sleep rhythms so that your body can rest. After you get into a sleep routine, you're weaned off the medication.

Identifying and correcting sleep disorders

You can find several ways to treat sleep problems, and hopefully you see the difference between treating and resolving. Medications for insomnia and equipment for sleep apnea can treat problems, but proper sleep hygiene and weight loss can resolve them. If you do have a sleep disorder, shoot to find a resolution, not just a temporary solution when working on the treatment plan.

Medical conditions can have people flocking into their doctor's office begging for sleep remedies. Medical conditions may respond to simple treatments and solutions, but they may also require more serious medical intervention. The following sections include some of the most common sleep disorders for adults.

Insomnia

Insomnia is a general word to describe the inability to fall asleep. When you have insomnia, you may feel tired but you just can't sleep. Some people waken several times during the night or wake up and can't fall asleep again until the early morning. Acute or transient insomnia lasts from one night to a couple of weeks, but insomnia must occur on most nights for more than a month to be considered chronic.

Having a couple of sleepless nights when you're under stress is normal, but if sleepless nights become habitual — and you've already been through the sleep hygiene guidelines — talk to a doctor. When sleeplessness becomes a consistent problem, you begin to experience daytime

478

drowsiness that affects your work and other daily activities. Over time, insomnia can

✔ Lead to poor performance on the job

✔ Affect your personal relationships

✔ Leave you vulnerable to illness and disease

✔ Make you more accident-prone

Some effective treatments for insomnia include relaxation, cognitive behavioral therapy, and stress reduction. You may also need to take prescription and over-the-counter sleep aids. **Note:** With some prescriptions you run the risk of dependence, so talk to your doctor about your options.

Sleep apnea

The word *apnea* means "without breath" and is exactly what occurs when people are afflicted with sleep apnea. People who suffer from sleep apnea actually have episodes where they stop breathing during their sleep. These episodes can last for a few seconds to several seconds and can occur more than 100 times a night. People who have sleep apnea wake up feeling tired and irritable and may experience a sore throat or dry mouth when they wake up.

Some people with sleep apnea wake up gasping for air while others are aroused enough to breathe and then return to sleep without a clue to their problems. Oftentimes, if they don't remember these episodes, their sleep partners do — it's frightening to see and hear!

Sleep apnea is dangerous and has been implicated in conditions such as cognitive impairment, behavior problems, heart disease, and even sudden death. It's unclear whether the apnea itself or ongoing apnea and its associated heart

479

disease is what leads to sudden death.

The two kinds of sleep apnea are obstructive and central.

- ✔ **Obstructive sleep apnea** is the most common type, accounting for about 90 percent of sleep apnea. Obstructive sleep apnea occurs when the muscles in the back of your throat relax and then collapse.

- ✔ **Central sleep apnea** occurs when your brain doesn't send the proper signals to the muscles that control breathing.

The risks of getting sleep apnea include excess weight, having a thick neck, being male, aging, smoking, and the use of sleep medications. To determine whether you suffer from sleep apnea, your doctor may request that you do some sleep testing.

Some treatments for sleep apnea include oral devices that open the blocked airways or the Continuous Positive Airway Pressure (CPAPP) — a device that blows air into your nose at night. Surgery may be recommended for serious cases; for less serious cases, losing weight is often enough to put an end to sleep apnea.

Restless leg syndrome

People with restless leg syndrome (RLS) feel like they constantly have to move their legs to find a more comfortable position. However, no position feels right for long. Their legs feel tight and tingly, as if bugs were crawling up their calves. RLS negatively affects your sleep and may keep your partner from sleeping, too.

RLS seems to be more prevalent in women. Conditions like pregnancy, *anemia* (low iron), and depression may be the underlying causes. Other more serious conditions like

480

Parkinson's, diabetes, and rheumatoid arthritis may also cause RLS.

Behavioral changes that may minimize the problem include taking warm baths before bedtime, doing yoga stretches, and walking slowly. If the problem is anemia, an iron supplement may eliminate the problem entirely. The bottom line is that RLS is a very treatable condition, so see your doctor.

Chapter 15

Don't Worry, Be Happy: The Keys to Maintaining Health and Vitality

The power of positive thinking is more than just a cliché; it's supported by medical facts. Positive people live longer, healthier, happier lives than negative people. People who go with the flow and handle change with grace resolve conflicts and overcome health challenges better than those who resist change. Your outlook and attitude are the octane boosters that power you through each day giving your body the extra edge it needs to survive. Pessimistic people harvest stress, focus on failures, and are reluctant to keep moving forward. This approach to life affects relationships, work, and your health in the same negative way. Staying positive and keeping faith helps maintain a balance between the body and the mind. People who are emotionally and spiritually connected to a higher power have a stronger will to live, thereby increasing their longevity.

In this chapter, we examine the importance of maintaining a positive attitude as you age and examine its role in keeping you healthy, happy, and serene no matter what your age or circumstances.

The Importance of a Positive Attitude

Aging brings major life changes, and staying positive and happy isn't always easy during the years when you may lose people near and dear to you, have unexpected health issues, need to move out of the family home for financial or health reasons, have children move away, or retire from a job that meant the world to you.

Yet, contrary to popular opinion, aging and a negative attitude don't go hand in hand. One large study reported in the *Journal of Personality and Social Psychology* that as people age, they become happier rather than sadder and are able to regulate emotions more effectively than younger or middle aged adults. Even if you're not Mary Sunshine by nature, you can learn to develop a positive overall outlook.

Why bother? Although being optimistic isn't a surefire ticket to living into your 100s, several studies have shown that pessimism can increase your risk of dying at a younger age. Consider the following studies:

✔ A study done in the Netherlands involving nearly 1,000 participants age 65 to 85 showed that people who described themselves as being highly optimistic had a risk of dying that was 55 percent lower than the risk of pessimists during the ten-year study period. The risks of dying from heart disease were 23 percent lower for optimists during the same period.

- The Ohio Longitudinal Study of Aging and Retirement began in the 1970s with over 1,100 people and concluded more than 20 years later with over 600 people over age 50. The study showed that people with a healthy attitude toward aging lived more than seven years longer than those with a negative attitude.

- The Mayo Clinic reported that when psychological tests given to over 800 people were reviewed, pessimistic people were 19 percent more likely to have died in any given year than optimists.

Like everything else, you can carry optimism too far, which can have grave consequences. When you carry it too far, it ends up being more harmful than beneficial. Optimism can lead to a carefree attitude that results in unfortunate, but often avoidable problems resulting from taking risks when taking precautions would be the proper action. Excessive optimism can also lead to an overly trusting attitude, and some overly trusting seniors have been conned out of large sums of money by individuals or organizations. Again, balance is the key, and you have to have the right amount of positive thinking and common sense when it comes to your health, money, and other important life issues.

The bottom line? Being optimistic can help you live longer — but don't leave common sense at the door. In some situations, skepticism or a touch of pessimism may be the right choice.

Embracing a Healthy, Balanced Approach to Life

If you feel at times that life is a balancing act, you're in good company. Most people spend time trying to keep their lives in balance, because keeping life in balance, or a state of equilibrium, can lead to a happier, less stressful life.

Everyone's life brings unfortunate obstacles and difficult challenges, but life also brings rewards, opportunity, and satisfaction. When your scale starts to become imbalanced due to negative life events, the challenge is figuring out how to regain your balance so that you don't fall into patterns of negativity and pessimism, which increase stress and make bad situations worse. Finding balance may be very difficult at times, but looking for ways to maintain balance can keep you from getting overwhelmed and will lead to a healthier life even when you're under stress.

Turning around negativity

You may be convinced that a positive attitude can benefit your life, but how do you become a positive person if it doesn't come naturally? It's not as hard you think — being aware of your negativity is half the battle; figuring out how to turn negativity around is the other half.

Although a little negativity is normal in life, constant negativity can make you stressed, anxious, depressed, or bitter. It can wear away your self esteem and perpetuate a pattern of self-destructive behaviors. Some negative thoughts that can have negative effects on a positive attitude include

- ✔ **Worrying about what other people think about you:** Studies show that most of the time, other people aren't thinking about you at all, except to wonder what you think of *them.*

- ✔ **Preoccupation or obsession with stressors:** Although thinking through problems can be beneficial, constantly brooding about stressors produces only one thing — more stress! (See Chapter 13 for a load of specific stress-reducing strategies.)

485

✔ **Dwelling on the past and things you can't change:** You can learn lessons from the past, but constantly thinking about "what might've been" is unhealthy and unproductive.

✔ **Self criticism:** Self improvement is fine; putting yourself down isn't. After all, the world has enough people who feel the need to criticize, so why would you do that to yourself? You're your own best cheerleader, and you deserve the same respect and compassion from yourself that you give to others.

 Turning yourself from a negative to a positive person takes conscious effort and a lot of practice. Take these tips to heart:

✔ **Figure out how to recognize negative thoughts.** Stop entertaining them as soon as you notice them.

✔ **Replace the negative thoughts with positive ones by turning concerns "on their head."** Instead of thinking that you'll never be as productive at work as your friend, try to determine what it is that makes your friend productive. Positive attitude, the ability to say no when necessary, the ability to delegate? Which of those things can you modify in yourself to make yourself into a more productive person?

✔ **Put the negative thought into perspective.** If you find yourself using terms like "always" and "never" to describe situations — as in, "I'll never be promoted" or "She always gets the best assignments" — you may need to adjust your perspective on life. Very few things are black and white, and honestly examining your feelings, or writing them down, may help you see where you've fallen into negative thought patterns. Feelings are just that — feelings. They're not facts, and very often your feelings don't match the facts in a given situation. If you can find the discrepancies, you can begin to adjust your thinking.

Bringing out a mental "stop" sign whenever you find yourself drifting into negative thoughts and replacing them with positive ideas may be awkward at first, but within a few weeks, you may find that negativity is no longer a habit. And like many bad habits, negativity comes with health risks for aging that you can modify for a longer, more enjoyable life.

Being less confrontational

As you get older, you may feel like you spend half your life fighting with people — your younger boss, your kids, your spouse, the girl at the supermarket, your best friend. On one hand, you don't want your middle name to be "doormat," but on the other hand, being in constant conflict with other people is exhausting, it upsets your stomach, and it demolishes your hard-earned optimistic view of life. Some people — hopefully you're not one of them — feel that everything in life is worth fighting about, and so they spend most of their life in emotional turmoil. Learn to choose your battles — some things really aren't worth fighting about. Ask yourself, "Will this matter in a month?" If the answer is "no," why get yourself tied up in knots over it?

Conflict is, however, a part of life, one that some people never figure out how to handle well. Handling conflict means taking the high road sometimes and searching for the win-win solution in every situation. This resolution isn't the same as giving in. If everybody wins, everybody's happy, including you. Facing conflict and traveling the paths to overcoming it builds character and confidence. Defuse conflict by using some of these techniques:

- ✓ **Know what you believe and stick to it.** Have a core set of values — a balanced mix of self-awareness and confidence — while still being open-minded and accepting of other viewpoints. These values allow you to take a stand when moral or ethical issues arise and feel confident every time. Having a firm foundation of beliefs also lets you come across to others as committed, not defensive and antagonistic.

- ✓ **Look for common ground.** Keep focused on a positive, solution-based outcome. You may only agree to disagree, but you can do it without killing each other.

- ✓ **Realize that other people are human too.** Other people may often not live up to your expectation of them, so don't be surprised, disappointed, or upset to the point of argument when this happens. Being human, however, is a two-way street; you may not always live up to others' expectations — or your own! Cut yourself the same break that you'd give someone else when you're not living up to your expectations. And, if you're not living up to someone else's expectations, look at yourself with a clear eye instead of assuming that you're in the right every time.

- ✓ **Think carefully before setting yourself up for confrontational situations.** Do certain topics push your hot buttons with certain people? Then don't talk about them with that person, unless you're in the mood for a good argument. Does driving 12 hours in the car with your spouse turn you into someone who would argue that the sky isn't blue? Make alternate plans. (Maybe one of you could fly and the other could drive, or you could stop halfway and stay overnight.)

✔ **Figure out why this is upsetting you.** Every argument has a root cause, and often the thing you're actually arguing about isn't really the source of aggravation at all. Ask yourself "What's really causing this conflict, and why am I reacting the way I am?"

✔ **Always think win-win.** There's almost always a way for both parties to feel they've won. Put away your swords and look for a way for each side to walk away with a benefit. Resolving a conflict can be a great lesson in seeing an issue from another person's perspective, whether you agree with it or not. After you arrive at a win-win solution, accept it and implement it. Make sure that each person takes responsibility for agreeing with the decision.

✔ **Check your emotions at the door.** Conflict resolution is about problem solving, which is a logical process. Emotions color your perceptions and your logic and cloud the rational thinking that's essential to arriving at a solution.

✔ **Put your heads together.** Two heads are better than one, and three may be better yet. The more people focused on the solution, the better the odds of a successful outcome.

Staying Active and In Touch with the World

Staying active as you age means far more than riding your bicycle around the block every evening. Staying active and in touch involves both physically being involved in activities in your community and mentally being involved with the world around you. Being connected to your world is good for your health and mental attitude, and it can also benefit those around you.

Not sure where to start? Here are some suggestions.

- ✔ **Know what's going on in the world.** Read the newspaper. Watch the evening news. Subscribe to a weekly news magazine or read one at your local library. Being in touch with what's going on decreases feelings of isolation and gives you something more interesting to talk about with others than the state of your bowels.

- ✔ **Get a job.** Many seniors work part time not only to earn a little extra spending money but also to stay active. Love antiques? How about a part-time job in an antique store? Love books? Would working at a bookstore or the library interest you? Love to do woodwork? How about hitting the weekend craft shows and hawking your wares? Job opportunities are limited only by your imagination and, contrary to what you may think, many businesses love to hire seniors because of their positive work ethic and their maturity.

- ✔ **Help others out.** Volunteer opportunities are unlimited and many organizations are desperate for help. Hospitals are always in need of volunteers, and so are groups that help new citizens learn English. Many libraries have volunteer programs, and Meals on Wheels is always in need of drivers.

Want something more exotic? How about a mission trip (not all are religiously based) to a foreign country? You're never too old to hold babies or talk to teens in an orphanage. Many organizations offer yearly mission trips to the same area so that volunteers can make lasting connections there. Check out www.mmex.org or www.missionfinder.org for any number of organizations looking for volunteers for a week, a month, or a year, all over the world.

✔ **Get out and travel.** Going to a new place not only gives you something to talk about, but also sharpens your mind, stretches your map-reading skills, and is fun. Go on your own or with an organized group; you have no excuse for staying home when an organized tour does all the legwork for you.

✔ **Find a new hobby or expand an old one.** Do you love to sing? How about joining the local theater group (roles exist for all ages) or a barbershop quartet, or just singing in the church choir? Build model airplanes and join a local flying group. Crochet blankets or quilt. Join a book club — or start one in your neighborhood. There may be a dozen people on your street just looking for something new to do — ask around and you may find two or three folks with interests similar to yours.

✔ **Be civic minded:** Volunteer to man voting booths. Stomp for your favorite candidate — or become a candidate yourself! Neighborhood associations are often crying for help. Don't stay away because you don't know anyone — most times you'll be greeted with open arms if you offer help.

✔ **Use your computer:** The age group that's 55 and older has had the highest increase in computer usage. Yes, a lot of trash is on the Internet, but you can also find interesting chat rooms and instruction of all kinds; you can even take college courses online. There's more to the computer than playing solitaire, so check out the home and garden forums, the classic car boards, or the health chat rooms and talk to interesting people without ever leaving home.

✔ **Exercise:** You need to stay in shape to accomplish any of the other suggestions in this list. You can do many activities with friends while getting some exercise. Grab your golf clubs and walk nine holes of golf. It's a great way to socialize and exercise at the same time. Get a foursome and play tennis. If you want some alone time, head to the gym and get some quality personal time. The people over age 55 who exercise regularly are on a fraction of the medications that sedentary patients require. With the cost of medications today, using exercise to reduce some of your medication load is a great incentive.

Connecting with Your Spiritual Side

Some type of spiritual belief system is found in virtually every society on earth. People want and need to believe in something greater than themselves. Some studies have shown that spiritual beliefs and religiosity (participation in an organized religion) increase with age, leading to considerable research into the effects of religion and spirituality on health issues and aging since the 1990s.

You may concede that being spiritual or religious makes people feel healthier, but are there measurable results to support their belief? Yes, there are. Here are just a few:

- ✔ A 1992 study reported in the *American Journal of Psychiatry* stated that religious faith increased the ability of older adults to cope with illness, loss, disability, and mortality issues.

- ✔ A study reported in the *Southern Medical Journal* in 1998 reported that subjects who attended church once a week were 43 percent less likely to have been admitted to the hospital for any reason, and those who were hospitalized had markedly shorter stays.

- ✔ An article in *The Journal of Pain* reported that daily spiritual experiences were associated with more positive attitudes and resulted in a decrease in reported pain.

- ✔ A Duke University Medical Center in Durham study of over 4,000 participants over the age of 65 found that those who pray and attend religious services on a weekly basis, especially those between the ages of 65 and 74, had lower blood pressure than their counterparts.

So if this is all true, why aren't doctors out there prescribing religion and spirituality to their patients? Prescribing "religion" as treatment may cross ethical lines and also trivialize faith ("Want to get healed? Take this pill, go to church this weekend, and call me in the morning.").

Connecting with Others: The Significance of Support

Barbra Streisand sang it best, "People who need people are the luckiest people in the world." According to a social survey, the importance of family relationships and good health are the two highest-rated variables when measuring happiness. Why? The ability to form deep, lasting bonds with other people in which you can share life experiences, learn, grow, trust, and support one another fulfills a fundamental human need. The absence of such relationships and bonds leads to isolation and depression.

How do the relationships with the people in your life affect your attitude about getting older and how you spend your days? In this section, we look at how staying in touch with your nearest and dearest can be a blessing, positively contributing to both your mental and physical well-being.

Family and friends: Life preservers of the human kind

As you age, your family and friends may be your most critical lifeline. Numerous studies have shown that having a strong social network results in a longer, healthier, and happier life.

How can you stay in touch with family or friends who live scattered around the country or make new friends at a time when getting around can be difficult? Although keeping in touch with friends and family far away or making new friends may be difficult, the long-term results are worth it.

Keeping in touch with those nearby

When you live around the corner from family and friends, you may need to walk a fine line between being in touch and being in touch *too much.* Gauging the proper balance between closeness and too much togetherness isn't always easy, but, by using common sense, you can maintain close relationships without overstepping boundaries.

If you have close family and/or friends nearby, it may be beneficial for both of you to have definite times to get together instead of just dropping in and being dropped in on. Making "dates" to get together once a week, once a month, or once a day — whatever suits your particular lifestyle — gives both of you the freedom to plan your day and to know that you'll be seeing each other regularly.

Keeping in touch when miles separate you

Staying connected to loved ones who are hundreds of miles away has never been easier. With the advent of cellphones that transmit pictures instantly to text messaging to e-mails to phone hookups that allow you to see the person you're talking to, you need never be far out of touch with the ones you love.

And if you need to see people in person to feel connected, airlines offer dozens of flights a day to wherever you want to go. Airfares vary considerably, so get familiar with Web sites like www.travelocity.com or www.expedia.com, just to name two of many that offer discounted flights, hotels, and car rentals.

Although all the modern methods of connection are wonderful, don't forget one of the old fashioned — and certainly more permanent — ways of staying in touch — letter writing. Although it's becoming a forgotten art, letter writing not only is a way to stay in touch but also leaves a permanent legacy of your thoughts and day-to-day life behind.

Being a grandparent

If your children have children, being a grandparent can be

really fun. Grandchildren bring all the joy of children with none (or at least less) of the hassles! Being a grandparent (and a good one at that) takes practice but brings rewards almost greater than any other relationship as you age. If you don't have any grandchildren, you can always volunteer at school functions or get involved with organizations such as Big Brothers Big Sisters to develop meaningful relationships. Some hospitals also have an "Adopted Grandparent" program for hospitalized children.

What makes a wonderful grandparent?

✔ **Love your grandchildren unconditionally.** This one comes naturally to most grandparents!

✔ **Respect their parents.** This is often a tough one; respecting their parents means following their rules for child rearing, supporting them in their decisions, and not sneaking forbidden goodies to your grandchild behind their parents' backs.

✔ **Know your boundaries.** Holding back on visiting or being involved with grandchildren's lives can be hard, but their parents' wishes must be paramount. Visit as often as you're invited — not as often as you want — and your relationship will be much happier.

Making new friends

It can be harder, and a little scary, to forge new relationships as you get older. When you're younger, work relationships and parenting relationships lead naturally to friendships, but when you're older, meeting new people can be more difficult.

Finding new friends, however, can be fun. Here are some tips:

✔ Take classes at the YMCA.

- ✔ Join a gym.

- ✔ Find an organized sports league, such as bowling or softball.

- ✔ Join church or town social groups.

Adjusting when friends and family become caregivers

There's a very good chance that you may need the help of family and/or friends for daily care as you age. Statistics show that one in four families provide care for older family or friends. In fact, 85 percent of all long-term care is provided by unpaid caregivers.

As hard it can be to be a caregiver, it can be just as hard to be the person taken care of. Being dependent on others can lead to depression, anger with the person providing your care, and frustration at losing your independence.

 Even if you need help with daily care, you can maintain some independence. For example, you can

- ✔ **Make some of your own decisions.** What do you want to eat? Wear? Where would you like to sit? What time would you like to go to bed? There's no reason to give up all your decision making, unless your choices are inconvenient for the person doing your care. Making decisions helps keep you sharp and gives you some feeling of control over your life.

- ✔ **Keep in touch with the world.** Needing care doesn't mean you can't stay in touch with your world. Read the newspaper or check out the nightly news. Knowing what's happening in the world not only helps you feel connected but also gives you something to talk about at the dinner table.

- ✔ **Do as much as possible for yourself.** The trouble with needing help is that it's easy to escalate. Yes, it's

497

much easier to have someone else do your hair or pick out your clothes, but allowing others to "take over" leads to becoming passive and disinterested in your world. Using your hands and fingers less results in stiffness and loss of agility, so don't give up physical tasks just because others can do them faster or neater.

Love relationships: With or without them, how you age

You may have had the same partner for the last 40 years, or you may have a new love interest. You may be newly single, or still single after all these years and very happy. You can't argue with happiness, but some research suggests that having a partner may have its benefits.

According to a study done by the Center for Disease Control, which surveyed over 127,000 adults, married adults are healthier, smoke and drink alcohol less, are physically more active, and are less likely to be limited in activities of daily living. Many studies have come to similar conclusions, including the following:

- ✔ Married people are less likely to suffer from long-term illnesses and much less likely to die in hospitals as surgical patients.

- ✔ Married women at age 48 have an 8 percent risk of dying before age 65, versus a divorced woman's risk of 18 percent. A married man at age 48 has a 12 percent risk of dying before age 65, versus a divorced man's risk of 35 percent.

- ✔ Married people may be healthier because they have increased social support from their spouse, improving psychological well-being and immune function.

On the other hand, staying single doesn't mean that a person has to be alone or unhappy, nor does it mean that a person's health has to suffer as a result. Singlehood may be a choice, and a very happy one at that.

Is being single less beneficial from a health and happiness perspective? Consider these points:

- ✔ Marriage seems to benefit men from a health and emotional perspective more than women, possibly because single men engage in more risky behaviors, such as smoking and drinking too much.

- ✔ People who've always been single fare just as well as people who've been married, and both do better than those who've been divorced or widowed.

- ✔ Differences between married and single people are decreasing over time. This in part is due to the fact that some choose not to get married, but rather to be committed to someone. With the divorce rate increasing, many of the stats on health are changing due to the health effects of divorce.

- ✔ The degree to which marriage matters differs across cultures.

S-E-X: Why Getting It On May Help You Live Long

Getting older isn't all bad news. In fact, when it comes to having sex, you can be ageless, because sexual satisfaction is still possible at any age. Although age-related changes may necessitate some adjustments, where there's a will there's a way. For both men and women, physiological changes to the body make having sex a different experience as you age, but different doesn't mean worse; it just means adapting. After you understand what to expect sexually as you age, you'll see that sexual pleasure and intimacy don't have to fade along with the color of your hair.

Sexual activity is good for . . . everything

Sex certainly does have benefits. Regular and enthusiastic sex offers a host of measurable physiological advantages, probably more than anyone even knows. Sexual activity has positive effects on hormones, immune function, endorphins, and muscle strengthening; even if the effect is just a big smile on your face, sex does the body good.

Take a look at these examples of what sex can do for the body:

- ✔ **You live longer.** Men who reported the highest frequency of orgasm live longer than men who had less-frequent orgasms.

- ✔ **You have a reduced risk of heart disease.** Research shows that men who had sex three or more times a week reduced their risk of heart attack or stroke by half.

- ✔ **You can get some exercise.** A regular bout of sex burns around 50 calories — about the same as walking 15 minutes on a treadmill. The pulse rate in a person who's aroused rises from about 70 beats per minute to 150. However, don't substitute sex for other forms of exercise. You would have to engage in sexual activity for many hours to achieve the same aerobic benefits as other options.

- ✔ **You experience a sense of well-being.** Levels of

the hormone oxytocin increase during intercourse and in turn releases endorphins, which can give a sense of well-being and can even reduce pain because of the action of the endorphins and the pain receptors.

✔ **You get sick less.** People who have sex weekly have higher levels of an antibody called immunoglobulin A, which can be important for the immune system when fighting infections.

Recognizing the effects of aging on sex

Aging itself isn't responsible for diminished sexual desire. People still feel the need for sex, and as long as a partner is available, regular sexual activity is as normal as it is during any other time during your life. Just because people get older doesn't mean that they don't believe that sex still contributes to their physical and psychological health and well-being.

In most instances when people refrain from sex, it's not because of lack of desire, but is rather a functional problem that's wrongly assumed to be uncorrectable. Many men feel that it's just an inevitable matter of time before they'll have to jump in line to get their erectile medication while women assume that once menopause hits they'll need a firecracker under their derriere to get them interested in sex.

Studies show that the physical capacity for male erection and male and female orgasm continue almost indefinitely, even if achieving orgasm is desired but not always achieved. Research reveals that people over the age of 55 still engage in the same varied sexual practices they did when they were younger, such as masturbation and oral sex, in addition to intercourse. However, age does bring physical changes that need to be taken into account and adapted to if you want your sex life to remain lively as you get older.

Age-associated changes in men

Biological and physiological changes in men can impact their sexual function. These changes include the following:

- ✔ **A decline in levels of the hormone testosterone:** Testosterone is the male sex hormone responsible for creating and releasing sperm, initiating sex drive, and providing muscular strength. Between the ages of 15 and 18, testosterone levels peak. By the time men reach their mid- to late-20s, hormone levels start a slow decline. By the age of 40, some men notice a significant drop. At age 50, half of all men experience a significant reduction in testosterone levels, resulting in sexual side effects. For the majority of men with low testosterone levels, the major complaint is a diminished sex drive. Eighty percent of men who complain of a low libido also report the inability to maintain a strong erection.

- ✔ **The duration of the refractory period:** The *refractory period* is the length of time between ejaculations. As men age, this period of time increases. The refractory period varies widely between individuals over a lifetime, ranging from minutes to hours to days. When a man is in his youth, he may be able to ejaculate multiple times within the period of a few hours. As a man ages, he may not be able to sustain an erection, let alone ejaculate, for as many as 24 hours after his previous orgasm.

  There are several reasons for this. An increased infusion of the hormone oxytocin during ejaculation is believed to be chiefly responsible for the refractory period and the amount that oxytocin is increased may affect the length of each refractory period. Another reason may be a decrease in the amount of blood flow to the penis, because circulation can decrease as you age. Another chemical that could be responsible for the increase in the refractory period is prolactin. Prolactin suppresses dopamine, which is responsible for sexual arousal.

✔ **Erectile dysfunction:** One of the greatest fears for men as they age is erectile dysfunction. Fortunately for many, changes in lifestyle choices can eradicate the problem. Nearly half of men between the ages of 45 and 65 may have erectile dysfunction. The most common factor for these men is hormone deficiencies, poor dietary habits, lack of exercise, weight problems, uncontrolled or untreated high blood pressure, and diabetes.

   If you experience erectile dysfunction, talk with your doctor. Erectile dysfunction may provide a warning sign of coronary heart disease or diabetes. Erectile dysfunction doesn't cause heart disease, but it may indicate that the process of arterial blockage could be a problem in other areas.

Being aware of the sexual changes your body can go through as you age can help you be better prepared. Here are some additional age-associated changes men may experience and should address with their doctor:

✔ Decrease in the number and frequency of morning erections

✔ Reduced sexual arousal, both mentally (visual, psychological) and physically with respect to erectile and orgasm potential

503

Andropause

There's new interest in treating age-related hormone deficiencies in men, often referred to as *andropause.* In the past doctors often diagnosed male hormone-related issues as depression, early diabetes, or just old age. New testing of hormone levels and the subsequent treatments have shown promising results for people with low testosterone and human growth hormone (a hormone released from the pituitary that can decline with age). If you're deficient, treatment can improve libido, erections, energy, and weight and muscle management. If you think you could have hormone deficiencies, talk to your doctor about the available testing.

↙ Reduced duration and strength of orgasm

If you experience a loss of sexual desire and other related sexual side effects, speak with your healthcare provider. Treatment options may be available.

Age-associated changes in women

Menopause (the termination of menstrual periods) is the most dramatic change that affects women sexually as they age. Menopause usually occurs between 42 and 56 years of age with the average age being 50. During menopause hormonal production diminishes, the lining of the vaginal wall begins to thin and becomes more rigid, and the production of vaginal lubrication drops. The lack of vaginal lubrication can make intercourse uncomfortable and is a big reason that women lose interest in sex. However, many over-the-counter products aid in lubrication and some prescription options help, too.

A woman's capacity to achieve orgasm can remain at near peak levels well into her senior years, even though it may take quite a bit longer to achieve. Menopause doesn't negatively impact a woman's desire or interest for sex.

Solving sexual problems together

Both partners in a sexual relationship can experience sexual issues. The key to maintaining a positive relationship is to work together on issues that arise. The following may help keep things hot as you get older:

- **Lubrication:** To help with vaginal dryness, decreased erection, or atrophied vaginal tissues, use a little lube, such as KY jelly. A little goes a long way to solve these problems.

- **Patience:** It's probably going to take a little longer to get things going — for both of you. Take the time to enjoy what you're doing — enjoy longer foreplay. Sex isn't a race, anyway!

- **New underwear:** Liven things up a bit. Ditch the granny panties and the tighty whiteys for something more visually stimulating and fun. You can always pretend that you're buying those thongs for your granddaughter! Or shop online — no one will ever know.

- **Sex toys:** Don't be embarrassed; they sell these toys online now, and they may help by stimulating areas you didn't even know you had.

 Above all sex is supposed to be fun — let it be.

505

Part VI
The Part of Tens

The 5th Wave   By Rich Tennant

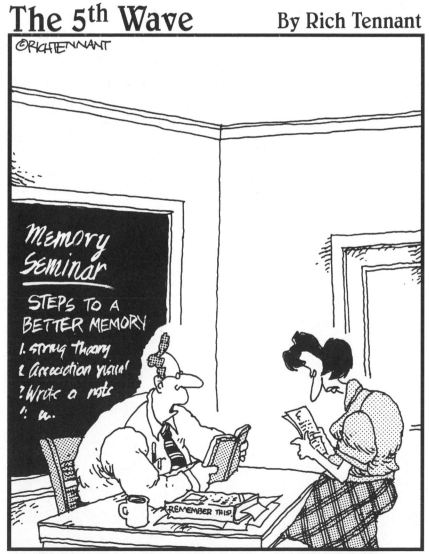

"Of course you're angry at me for springing a surprise memory quiz on you, but you've got to learn to forgive and forget."

In this part . . .

The Part of Tens includes short chapters packed with interesting and pertinent info. People like their info in short segments, right? If that's you, this part is for you.

In this part, you get the truth about ten myths of aging and a list of ten great food sources to help you age healthfully. We also show you how ten different memory games can exercise your brain, and we provide ten ways to make your home safer as you get older.

Chapter 16

Ten Medical Myths that Can Affect Your Health

....

In This Chapter

▶ Considering proactive choices: Sunscreen, good sleep, and exercise

▶ Knowing your risks for heart disease

▶ Avoiding the excesses: Herbs, extra calories, and second-hand smoke

....

There have always been old wives' tales related to health issues, passed down as family sayings or basic truisms. And then came the Internet, with its explosion of information, misinformation, myths, and just plain nonsense. Sorting out truth from fiction isn't easy when it comes to health issues. In this chapter, we look at some common misconceptions of healthy aging and give you the facts about some of the things you may have taken as gospel most of your life.

High Cholesterol Is Linked to Weight

If you're thin, it may not even occur to you to check your

cholesterol. The myth that people with high cholesterol are overweight can be a dangerous one. You can have high cholesterol and be as thin as a whispering willow. How can that be?

Any body type can have high cholesterol. Cholesterol comes from two sources: the foods you eat and what your body naturally makes based on heredity. You have control over the amount of cholesterol you eat, but cholesterol levels are influenced even more by your genetics. You should start getting your cholesterol levels checked at age 20 or earlier if you have a family history of heart disease. Take responsibility for your health by learning how to interpret the numbers, including HDL (good) cholesterol, LDL (bad) cholesterol, and triglyceride levels.

 Talk with your doctor about modifying your lifestyle or your potential risk factors. If you do have high cholesterol, follow all your doctor's instructions, and have your cholesterol retested as your doctor recommends. See Chapter 2 for more info on high cholesterol.

High Blood Pressure Is Caused by High Stress

Everyone feels stress at one time or another, but stress isn't the cause of ongoing high blood pressure. In fact, doctors aren't completely sure what causes high blood pressure. Many risk factors have been cited and stress is often included in the list, but there hasn't been a direct link between the two.

With that said, stressors can elevate the heart rate and blood pressure, but they then return to baseline. There are many people that are placed under stress and don't have elevations in their blood pressure. Often, the stressed individuals that do see ongoing elevations have also added several other blood pressure elevating factors into their lifestyle, such as smoking, being sedentary, weight gain, and poor diet.

Women Shouldn't Worry About Heart Disease

If you tell a woman that she's more likely to die of a heart attack or stroke than breast cancer, she may not believe you. Why? According to a recent study, women think heart disease is a man's disease and cancer is the disease that most women die from. Not true. Heart disease is the *leading* cause of death in women and is responsible for nearly twice as many deaths in women than all cancers combined, including breast cancer. Some of the reasons why this myth isn't true are that women are smoking more, working more, and often aren't as aggressively screened for heart disease.

Since the initiation of some national programs targeting heart disease in women, there has been a large jump in the number of women that now know that heart disease is a deadly disease for women and that they need to be pro-active in their care. Refer to Chapters 2 and 12 for more information on cardiovascular disease and how to avoid it.

Osteoporosis Is a Normal Part of Aging

Brittle bones, fractured hips, and humpbacks aren't part of normal aging. Not everyone develops osteoporosis, and even if you're at risk (see Chapter 6), there are measures you can take to prevent it. The earlier in life you start preventing, the better, because you hit your maximum bone mass in your 30s.

Stacking up on bone-building activities like strength and resistance training as well as weight-bearing exercise enables you to use the force of gravity against your muscles to push the calcium into your bones. This can reduce the rate of bone loss. See Chapter 10 for specific ways to increase bone density through weight training.

Only Smokers Get Lung Cancer

The rate of people being diagnosed with lung cancer who've never smoked is increasing, particularly among women. According to the American Cancer Society (ACS), about 10 percent of men and 20 percent of women with lung cancer never smoked. Two possible reasons are secondhand smoke and genetics.

Stanford University medical oncologist Heather Wakelee's research indicated that a nonsmoker who's married to a smoker has a 30 percent greater risk of developing lung cancer than the spouse of a nonsmoker. While it's possible that the reason women have a greater risk than men is because it's more common for men to smoke than women, women would still be exposed to the secondhand smoke of their spouses.

Genetics may be another factor for developing lung cancer in people who never smoked, as in the case of actress Dana Reeves (widow of actor Christopher Reeves) who was diagnosed with lung cancer at the age of 44. According to the ACS, only 3 percent of lung cancers occur in people under 45, regardless of smoking status.

People with Darker Skin Don't Need to Wear Sunscreen

You may have heard that people with dark skin are naturally protected from the sun's ultraviolet A and B (UVA and UVB) rays, so they don't need to wear sunscreen. Although dark skin does contain more *melanin* — the pigment responsible for determining skin color — it's not true that dark skin can't be burned or damaged. Melanocytes are pigment-producing cells that make more melanin (and thus create a tan) when you expose your skin to the sun. Melanin is your skin's natural defense system against burning, so there is some truth that dark skin provides some protection against sun damage.

So regardless of your skin type, remember to protect your skin in the sun by liberally applying a broad-spectrum sunscreen of sun protection factor (SPF) 15 or more and by wearing sun-protective clothing. Check out Chapter 5 for more information about protecting your skin.

If you think that SPF 1000 is better than SPF 30, here's the truth about the numbers: An SPF over 30 doesn't increase the amount of blockage; it increases the length of time you can stay in the sun without burning. Once you get past SPF 30, the higher SPF creams are more expensive, so save your money and stop at SPF 30.

Herbs Are Natural, So They Can't Hurt You

Just because something's natural, doesn't mean that it's guaranteed to be safe. Many herbs can be harmful or even deadly if ingested. And herbal products and supplements that are advertised as *natural* aren't necessarily natural to the human body. Many herbs interact with over-the-counter (OTC) and prescription medications, making it difficult for your doctor to manage medications.

Find a good pocket consumer guide that explains terminology. Also, read labels and talk with your doctor before taking these natural products, especially if you're taking other medications.

The Older You Get, The Less Sleep You Need

Did you ever wonder why Grandma was up at 4 a.m. when you had no trouble sleeping in until 10 a.m.? Well, Grandma may have gotten used to waking before the dawn, but she still needs sleep — she just can't get all she needs.

As you age, you tend to lose the *ability* to sleep as deeply at nighttime. Your sleep cycles naturally change, causing a gradual degradation of the sleep/wake process (see Chapter 14 for details). So, you may sleep more lightly and for shorter time spans as you get older, but you generally need about the same amount of sleep as you need in early adulthood.

This fact explains why older people take naps — in an attempt to catch up on their sleep, which unfortunately isn't possible. About half of all people over 65 have frequent sleeping problems like insomnia. This change is mainly due to aging, but other factors that may contribute are medical problems and the medications to treat those problems. See Chapter 14 for more details about the different stages of sleep.

As You Age, You Can't Build Muscle

While body building may not be high on most seniors' "to do" list, building muscle is more important than ever as a person ages and it is possible. Muscle mass declines with age — with each decade after age 25, 3 to 5 percent of muscle mass is lost. However, studies also have shown that there can be significant improvements in muscle strength in previously sedentary older adults that follow a regular exercise program.

The American College of Sports Medicine now recommends weight training for people over 50 — even people well into their 90s can benefit. A group of nursing home residents ranging in age from 87 to 96 recently improved their muscle strength by almost 180 percent after just eight weeks of strength training. Adding that much strength gave these folks significant functionality that they thought they had permanently lost. See Chapter 10 for more on building lean muscle mass.

Eating Late at Night Is Less Healthy Than Eating Early

If you eat a bowl of chocolate ice cream at midnight, it has the same number of calories no matter when they're consumed. But it's not the full stomach at bedtime that puts on the extra pounds; it's the extra calories — no matter when you eat them.

You're likely to experience discomfort at night and the next morning if you eat late at night. Here's why:

- ✔ **Your food may only partially digest:** Food left in the stomach leads to heartburn, indigestion, and, as a result, the inability to fall sleep. Lying in a prone position doesn't allow gravity to pull food down the digestive track. Late-night eating can also cause morning gas and stomach cramps.

- ✔ **Your body is using its energy on digestion when it should be in energy-save mode:** One primary function of sleep is to help you recuperate from the day. You want your body to be as relaxed as possible so you can wake up energized.

Generally, don't eat two to three hours before bed to allow your body sufficient time for digestion. If you're not starving, the best option is to have some water and call it a night, but don't go to bed hungry, because you can have a restless night of sleep, too. If you're hungry and you do eat, try something small and healthy like a snack with protein to help you feel more full such as an ounce of mixed nuts, a salad, or a cup of yogurt. This way you don't overeat or significantly raise your caloric count while risking a long night of heartburn. The best way to avoid being hungry at night is to drink enough water and eat at least five small meals during the day rather than the normal 2 to 3 meals. This helps maximize your metabolism and also your blood sugars.

Chapter 17

Ten Foods to Help You Age Healthfully

● ●

In This Chapter

▶ Packing a wallop with fruits, veggies, nuts, and yogurt
▶ Counting on the benefits of fish, grain, soy, and nuts
▶ Satisfying more than your sweet tooth with healthy dark chocolate

● ●

Is there a magic food that can act as a fountain of youth? Of course not. But some foods are *really* good for you and keep your body functioning at its best. In this chapter, we list ten important, healthful foods that can help you stay young, provided that you also adopt the other lifestyle changes that we guide you through in this book. Whether these foods target your heart, bones and joints, free radicals, or cancer, they are supported by research to promote healthy aging. These foods — when combined — provide the most nutritional bang for your bite. *Bon appetite!*

Blueberries

Blueberries are one of the highest food sources of vitamins

A, C, dietary fiber, iron, folic acid, and *ellagic* acid (a disease-fighting phytochemical that slows down tumor formation). They contain specific phytonutrients that maximize the use of vitamin C in your body and contain more disease-fighting antioxidants than most other foods. In fact, their Oxygen Radical Absorbance Capacity (ORAC — a lab test analysis that measures the total antioxidant properties of foods and other chemical substances) score is a very high 2,400 units! To compare, the recommended "5-a-day" fruits and veggies gives you an ORAC score of 1750 units. By eating plenty of high-ORAC fruits and vegetables, you may help slow the aging processes in your body and your brain. One cup of blueberries is only 84 calories and contains no cholesterol or fat.

The blueberry has these additional benefits:

- The deep blue skin contains *anthocyanin*, a plant flavonoid (plant metabolite that has high antioxidant activity) that contributes to heart and brain health by protecting blood vessels from oxidation and helping maintain a healthy cholesterol balance.

- It may improve your coordination, strength, and memory.

Broccoli

Broccoli is a member of the cabbage family of vegetables and contains two significant cancer-fighting phytonutrients: *sulforaphane* and *indole*. This green veggie is packed with powerful antioxidants such as vitamin A, C, beta carotene, querectin, glutathione, and lutein. Broccoli actually has more vitamin C than an orange!

In addition, broccoli

✔ Is one of the richest food sources of trace metal chromium, a hard-to-find nutrient that has the ability to normalize blood-sugar concentrations, which could be effective in preventing adult-onset diabetes in some people

✔ Helps a woman's body inactivate the harmful type of estrogen that promotes cancer

✔ Is a great source of calcium for bone health — it contains as much calcium as milk, ounce for ounce

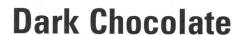

One cup of cooked broccoli contains 74 mg of calcium plus 123 mg of vitamin C, which significantly improves calcium's absorption — all for only 44 calories.

Dark Chocolate

Dark chocolate (as in, 70 percent cocoa or more, so milk chocolate doesn't count!) has many benefits:

✔ Contains *epicatechin,* a flavonoid, that increases blood flow through your arteries. Better blood flow is good for your heart.

✔ Contains essential trace elements and nutrients such as iron, calcium, phosphorus, and potassium, as well as the vitamins A, B1, C, D, and E

✔ Has the highest natural source of magnesium, which protects against hypertension, diabetes, and heart disease

✔ Contains oleic acid, which raises HDL (good cholesterol)

✔ Contains phenylethylamine (PEA), a mild mood elevator (your brain naturally produces PEA when you feel joy or love)

- Boosts serotonin (your brain's antidepressant) and endorphin levels

- Produces smoother-looking, thicker, and better-hydrated skin

- Helps protect your skin from sun damage (when it's fortified with cocoa flavonols) by making your skin more tolerant of UV sunlight

How much chocolate can you eat? Some studies that looked at cocoa phenols recommend eating as much as 100 grams of dark chocolate a day to get the blood-pressure-lowering potential (there's not enough research to support throwing away the blood pressure medications just yet), but watch out for the calories. That amount can have as many as 500 calories!

Green Tea

Green tea comes from the leaves of the tea plant, *Camellia sinensis,* a bush native to Asia. The leaves of green tea plants are less processed than regular black tea and carry a bigger supply of antioxidants and phytochemicals, which can decrease plaque forming in arteries. The main body booster in green tea is catechin (epigallocatechin-3-gallate), a powerful antioxidant that does the following:

- Protects against digestive and respiratory infections

- Blocks the actions of carcinogens (substances that promote cancer)

- Acts as an antibacterial (some people use as a mouth rinse)

- Helps lower triglycerides and raises your HDL

✔ Blocks the production of *prostaglandin E2,* a hormone-like substance that is responsible for joint inflammation

 To receive maximum health benefits, drink four to five cups of green tea a day (80 to 107 mg of polyphenols per cup). Green tea extract is available in capsule form for doses of 100 to 150 mg three times a day. Remember that green tea contains caffeine and might not be appropriate for everyone, so talk to your doctor to see if drinking this much tea is okay for you. Decaffeinated green tea is also available.

Nuts

Nuts are packed full of healthy monounsaturated fats (which can reduce coronary heart disease), antioxidants, vitamin E, protein, fiber, calcium, iron, selenium, and magnesium. A little goes a long way — eat one ounce a day to fill you up and reap the benefits. Nuts contain about 150 to 170 calories per quarter cup, so make sure to measure.

Vitamin E in nuts may help protect your cell membranes from free radical damage. Cardiac benefits include decreased oxidation of LDL cholesterol (bad) and improved functioning of the blood vessels.

Walnuts, the nut studied the most, give you a healthy dose of omega-3 essential fatty acids (see that section later in the chapter). Almonds are the richest source of calcium and are great for vegans and people with dairy allergies.

Oatmeal

Oats are full of antioxidants, vitamin E, selenium, magnesium, fiber, and many other bioactive compounds. High fiber oats lower cholesterol, aid in good digestion, and may help your memory performance. The high fiber and protein content in oatmeal helps to slow down digestion and promote a slower and more sustained release of glucose into your bloodstream. This controlled release of glucose keeps you feeling satisfied from hunger longer.

In addition, high fiber oats seem to improve insulin sensitivity (which often worsens prior to the onset of diabetes) by keeping blood sugars stable and reduce your risk factors for cardiovascular disease by lowering your LDL cholesterol.

A cup of cooked oatmeal provides 4 grams of total fiber, which includes 2 grams of *soluble fiber.* Soluble fiber binds with fatty acids (such as *trans fatty acids* — trans fat, which raises your LDL and lowers your HDL), and removes them from your body.

Mix 1 to 2 tablespoons of flax seed in your oatmeal for a great cholesterol-lowering breakfast that's packed with fiber and omega-3 fatty acids.

Omega-3 Fatty Acids

As you age, your brain function gradually slows due to slower transmission of nerve impulses and worn-out brain cell membranes. Because omega-3 fatty acids are the primary components of your brain cell membrane, the omega-3 oils in fish can slow down brain aging by helping to make the myelin (the insulation around the nerves) stronger so nerve impulses travel faster.

Research supports that these fatty acids reduce the risk of cardiovascular disease. They've been found to directly reduce risks by their beneficial effects on cholesterol, heart rhythm, and clotting. Eating fish and getting more omega-3s also indirectly helps reduce heart disease, because fish is a healthy alternative to other protein choices with higher saturated fat content, such as beef.

But for the most part, omega-3 fats provide these benefits:

- ✔ Help neurotransmitters (the brain's chemical messengers) function optimally

- ✔ Help improve memory and clear thinking

- ✔ Can reduce your risk of Alzheimer's disease

- ✔ Lower triglycerides, increase HDL, lower blood pressure, and reduce risk of blood clots that can lead to stroke

- ✔ May ease arthritis, asthma, and even depression

- ✔ Help reduce wrinkles from sun exposure

You can get omega-3s by eating fish (like mackerel, tuna, and salmon) or taking fish oil supplements. High-quality supplements are harvested from oils in the fishes' bodies and then purified and deodorized.

Soy

Soy is a unique combination of complex carbohydrates and protein that can be eaten in a variety of ways (think soy burger, soy beans, soy milk, and so on). Regular soy intake can lower and balance cholesterol, reducing your risk of coronary heart disease.

Note: Soy foods that claim to help reduce the risk of heart disease must contain at least 6.25 grams of soy protein per serving. The label has to specify that you need at least 25 grams of soy protein every day (four servings) to see any benefit.

Other benefits of soy include the following:

- A high soy diet increases bone density after six months.

- Twenty grams a day decreases hot flashes.

- Soy foods lower blood pressure.

- *Isoflavonoids* (antioxidants), such as genistein and daidzein, are weak estrogens that may lessen the risk of osteoporosis and heart disease.

Tomatoes

Tomatoes are rich in several nutrients: potassium, which decreases calcium loss; vitamin A, which maintains skin tissue; vitamin C; calcium; and iron. Tomatoes (particularly cooked tomatoes, such as tomato sauce and even ketchup) are also the best food source for *lycopene,* a phytochemical with potent antioxidant effects that has been linked to reducing cancer of the cervix, colon, bladder, stomach, and prostate and promoting heart health. This food actually is better when processed. The cooking of the tomatoes releases more lycopene from the skin.

Yogurt

As you age, your digestion and intestinal immunity slow down and bones weaken. Yogurt contains vital nutrients (protein and calcium) to combat these natural declines. Many yogurts also add vitamin D to further support your bones. The *probiotics* (see Chapter 8) in yogurt are beneficial bacteria, and they enhance the growth of healthy bacteria throughout your digestive system and keep harmful bacteria in balance.

When choosing a yogurt, look for one with the most live and active cultures (some have as many as six). Check out Chapter 8 for more information on probiotics.

Chapter 18

Ten Mind Games to Boost Your Brainpower

....

In This Chapter

▶ Challenging your verbal and numeric skills

▶ Getting the picture right: Visual workouts

▶ Exercising your powers of strategizing and reasoning

....

Want to improve your brain? Give it something to think about! Your brain, like every other part of your body, could use a little exercise to stay in shape — mental exercise, in this case. Exercising your brain is easy and fun. Puzzles, board games, and word play can sharpen your memory, heighten your verbal and numeric skills, and increase your spatial ability. Better yet, keeping your brain in shape can help stave off memory loss and dementia in your later years.

In this chapter, we discuss ten types of puzzles and games that give your brain a great, balanced workout. We don't provide actual puzzles here because concocting those isn't our strong suit — but the *For Dummies* series has a whole slew of great puzzle and game books that tell you how to play the games and provide the strategies to boot. We also provide the Web addresses of several mind-building games online in case you're the technical sort.

Crossword Puzzles

Crosswords challenge your memory skills as well as your verbal language acuity. Doing crossword puzzles stimulates the temporal lobes of your brain, which helps you identify sounds and understand speech. The temporal lobes also contain the hippocampus, which is important for short-term memory.

 You can find these classic brain trainers in newspapers, but they're also available on the Internet, in books, magazines, and on CDs. You can even create your own. There are even crosswords devoted to specific subjects as well as in varying degrees of difficulty. A few of our favorite sources include the following:

- ✔ *USA TODAY:* You can work the hard copy or the one online at http://puzzles.usatoday.com.

- ✔ *The Washington Post:* The Sunday and daily puzzles are good choices.

- ✔ *The New York Times:* To access this crossword puzzle, you must subscribe to receive the paper, and you'll get one free per week.

- ✔ **Newsday Crossword:** Visit online at www.newsday.com/crossword.

- ✔ **Thinks.com:** Try this daily crossword at www.thinks.com/crosswords/crosswords.htm.

Here are two more Web links to check out:

✔ www.bestcrosswords.com

✔ www.webcrosswords.com

Sudoku Puzzles

Sudoku is a highly addictive strategic number placement game that relies on logic and reasoning. The puzzles consist of a 9-x-9 square grid subdivided into nine 3-x-3 square grids. The object of the game is to place a number in each square; each row, column, and 3-x-3 square must contain all the numbers 1 through 9, with no duplicates. The puzzles come with a handful of squares already filled in, so you have to look ahead and follow trails of consequences.

This activity is a "left brain" kind of game because it deals with logic and reasoning skills. Sudoku uses *working memory* (memory for temporarily storing and manipulating information). Check out *The Big Book of Sudoku For Dummies* by Andrew Heron (Wiley) for a fun memory challenge.

Strategy Games

Strategy board games like chess, checkers, backgammon, and battle games, and card games like pinochle, Hearts, and Bridge, have long been popular ways of developing and challenging a person's decision-making abilities, reasoning skills, and critical thinking skills. These games focus on the outcome, so the thought process requires forward thinking. They help stretch the mind by requiring you to concentrate on the next several moves ahead.

Because strategy games require at least two players (one of which can be a computer), you have to consider not only your next move but also your opponent's. Part of knowing what your opponent is going to do may involve reading their body language, which utilizes your temporal lobes to "read" facial expression, and the parietal lobes, which react to changes in speech tone. The more players, the more different personalities and competitive expressions that can be observed, studied, and then used in your strategy for winning.

There are local and national tournaments for many of these strategy games; you'll see that there are often repeat winners. These people have honed their strategic and observational skills, and you can do the same! Take a look at *Card Games For Dummies,* 2nd Edition (Wiley) by Barry Rigal and Omar Sharif to find out more about a variety of card games.

Jigsaw Puzzles

Jigsaw puzzles work with spatial relations and memory skills as well as fine motor skills for picking up and putting together the pieces. There is also a creative element to solving jigsaw puzzles because you're constructing pictures.

Create your own puzzles. Buy the blank puzzles at craft stores or teachers' supply stores, and make your own design (you can even print a photo right from your own printer). When you have finished that, you break apart the pieces and put them back together. This way of getting your creative juices flowing uses your right brain and costs less than a couple of bucks.

Word Games

Do you have a way with words? If you do, there are dozens of games to test your word recognition, vocabulary, and ability to decipher words, all which stimulate your hippocampus, frontal lobes, parietal lobes, and temporal lobes (see Chapter 12 for info on the brain). Cryptograms, anagrams, and Jumbles are all puzzles that involve substituting or unscrambling letters and are often found in daily newspapers, as well as online.

There are also some great word board games you can play, such as Boggle, Scrabble, and Balderdash. Go to www.wordplays.com for a variety of word puzzles that can keep your brain sizzling for hours.

Short-Term Memory Quizzes

The average person's short-term memory can hold about seven pieces of information. Short-term memory games help you determine and even stretch that limit. These games have many practical applications including remembering to take medicine and making a list of items to buy at the grocery store.

You may remember playing games like this as a child; often they utilize letters of the alphabet to help you remember a list of items. One example would be, "I'm going on a trip and taking . . ." and then saying something beginning with the letter A. The next person then adds something beginning with B but including the A item too, and so on. The person who remembers the longest without mistakes wins.

Online games allow you to make up your own variation and play with a friend. Try www.allstarpuzzles.com, which has a number of memory puzzles with different themes.

Some games have someone say three numbers like *13, 4,* and *26.* After a certain amount of time, you have to repeat them back to the person. Increase the degree of difficulty by adding more numbers in the series (up to seven), by mixing categories like *apple, telescope, car keys, waiter,* or by increasing the amount of time before recalling the items (from five minutes to one hour). You can also play this game with pictures or flash cards to incorporate the visual element — better yet, use old family photos to match up or quiz over (ever wonder what you were going to do with that second set of pictures that you got for free?).

Sports

Many athletes say that a game is more mental than physical. For example:

- **Basketball:** Playing basketball takes strategic thinking to analyze what opposing players will do to try and prevent you from getting to the basket.

- **Baseball or softball:** A baseball or softball player must focus on the pitch, see what type of throw is coming, at what rate of speed, any curve, and calculate all these aspects together to determine how and when to swing.

- **Golf:** Golf is thought to be one of the best combinations of physical and mental skill. When you golf, you're trying to get the best score you can, which is independent of the others you're playing with. Every shot takes thought, planning, focus, and relaxation. If any one of these lapses, you risk a bad shot and the negativity that comes with it. After a bad shot you must refocus and overcome the negativity and anger that usually leads to lack of concentration and a quick downhill slide. The physical skill is hard enough to master, but to manage the mental components on every shot for 18 holes can be a real mental challenge!

Based on your current fitness level, lifestyle, and interests, look for a sport that benefits your mind and body, whether it's a game of golf, tennis, ping-pong, or playing catch with the grandkids. *Note:* Cheering on your favorite team from the couch doesn't count!

There are mental benefits that come with physical activity. The <u>aerobic activity</u> in sports <u>increases</u> oxygen to the brain and also causes the <u>release</u> of endorphins (chemicals released by the brain), which give you energy and a sense of well-being. We discuss them in more detail in Chapter 12 where we discuss endorphin release.

Optical Illusions

As you get older, it's easy to fall into a rut — looking at things from the same perspective. Optical illusions are a fun way to train your brain to look at things from different angles and to see more than what's immediately obvious. The more optical illusions you look at, the better you get at spotting the "hidden pictures." You can buy books of optical illusions, or try your eye at the illusions found at the following sites:

- ✔ www.brainden.com/optical-illusions.htm
- ✔ www.eyetricks.com

Visualization and Meditation

Visualizing is a great workout for your brain. Pick a specific memory and recall everything you can. Think about smells, what you were wearing, what you were thinking about, and so on. For example, visualize a sunset you remember. Then picture the beach, the sand, the fading sun rays on your face, the water on your toes, and smell the salt air.

Spend at least 15 minutes just visualizing every detail with each of your senses. This simple workout exercises almost all functions of the brain: the five senses, your memory, the ability to consciously relax, and so on. Repeat daily (with different memories) for a great brain-fitness routine.

Philosophical Reasoning

Reasoning is an important — and practical — function of the brain. Practice reasoning by asking the question "Why?" Children are great at this process and begin at about age three. Every question is "Why?" Why does the dog have spots? Why are leaves green? Why are pillows soft? Children learn and discover the world this way, and you can stimulate your reasoning skills by doing the same.

Just thinking about the possible answers to these questions forces your brain to use logic and intuition. Be just as curious about the world around you as a child, no matter how silly or reasonable your questions are.

Try this simple exercise:

1. **Pick an object, action, or topic to think about, and lie back and contemplate it for 30 minutes to an hour, working through all possible answers.**

2. **When you're tired of thinking, let it go and move on.**

   Some questions don't have answers, but they're still good to think about because of the strengthening effect they have on your mind and your ability to communicate reason.

 Be careful not to let your thoughts drift toward a resentment or bad feelings you may be carrying when you're doing this exercise. Problem-solving is great mental work, but the goal is to grow your mind, not wear it down.

Chapter 19

Ten Ways to Make Your Home Safer as You Age

Home may be the place you feel safest, but statistically, it's the place you're most likely to be injured. People age 65 and older consistently experience the highest numbers of home-injury-related deaths. Preventing injuries at home is common sense, but most people don't think about dangerous situations until they get injured. In this chapter, we offer some hints to stay safe at home at *any* age.

Preventing Falls

Falls are the leading cause of injury deaths and the most common cause of nonfatal injuries and hospital admissions for trauma. Each year in the U.S. nearly one-third of older adults experience a fall. Check out these suggestions to keep yourself from becoming a statistic:

- ✔ Install a hand rail — that extends the full length of the stairs — on each side of all stairs in your house.

- ✔ Keep all stairways, pathways, and walkways well lit and free of clutter.

- ✔ Get rid of all throw rugs and carpets with corners that can flip up or have them taped down tight to the floor.

- ✔ Install grab bars along the toilets and showers, and use a non-slip mat or adhesive safety strips inside the bath or shower.

- ✔ Wear sturdy shoes with thin, non-slip soles.

- ✔ Stay off ladders and don't climb on chairs, because poor vision and balance contribute to falls.

 You also want to do your part to keep your sense of balance and flexibility. Maintain an active lifestyle that includes exercise as part of your daily routine with a focus on balance, strength, and flexibility. And if you experience dizziness, consult your doctor to see what's at fault.

In Case of Fire . . . Plan Ahead

A home fire is dangerous at any age, but the odds of injury increase when you get older. To prevent injury from fire, do the following:

- ✔ Install smoke alarms on every level of your home and test them monthly. Change smoke alarm batteries at least once a year. New systems available can be wired so if one alarm goes off it sets off all the alarms.

- Develop and practice a fire escape plan with your family that identifies two exits out of every room with a place to meet outside.

- Buy a hanging escape ladder for rooms on the second story.

- Install alarms on the stove or an automatic shut-off for the times when the stove is accidentally left on. Never leave food cooking on the stove while you leave the room.

- Don't smoke in bed. If possible, don't smoke in the house at all — a cigarette left burning outside is much less likely to cause a house fire.

Be Sure Your Meds Are Safe

With every year, the number of prescription and nonprescription medications you take is likely to grow. Keeping the pills you take straight can be a real challenge, even if you aren't suffering from memory loss. Taking the wrong medication is more common than you may think and depending on the med and how much you took, can be very dangerous.

If you suspect you have taken the wrong medication or took a dose twice by mistake, call your doctor first. If your doctor isn't available, call the Poison Control Hotline at (800) 222-1222 or 911.

Other safety precautions include the following:

- **Use a medications tracker.** This tool indicates which medication to take when and what dose with instructions, such as taking pills with food. This tracker helps minimize error. You can register for some services to call and remind you to take your meds.

✔ **Get a pill box.** This method is one of the cheapest and easiest ways to keep your meds straight. There's a covered compartment for each day of the week, so you have your medication for a week organized, and you can see if you remembered to take your pills because, if you didn't, they're still in the compartment.

✔ **Ask your doctor if there's a way to simplify your schedule.** Can you take any of your meds just once a day, in a higher dose, rather than twice a day? Never change your medication schedule on your own.

✔ **Get rid of old medication.** Call your local hospital or doctor to find out how to dispose of unwanted or expired medications to eliminate the possibility of taking the wrong medications or expired medications that may be harmful rather than helpful.

✔ **Post emergency numbers.** Next to every phone in the home, list the numbers of Poison Control and other numbers you or someone else assisting you may need in an emergency.

Stock Your Emergency Supply Kit

No matter what your age, a first aid kit in a convenient and memorable location (next to your kitchen fire extinguisher, for example) is a must. Refresh and restock your first aid kit twice a year, replacing any expired or missing supplies. Have enough supplies to survive for three days. Include the following:

✔ Sterile adhesive bandages and Band-Aids in assorted sizes

- Hypoallergenic adhesive tape and sterile roller bandages (2- and 3-inch)
- Acetaminophen, Ibuprofen
- Benadryl
- Calamine lotion
- Antibiotic ointment
- Hydrocortisone cream
- Antiseptic wipes
- Hot/cold packs
- Thermometer
- Tweezers
- Small scissors or other cutting tool
- Light source (flashlight) with extra batteries
- CPR mouthpiece
- Disposable rubber gloves
- Phone numbers for poison control and emergency contacts

Update Your Life-Saving Skills

Do you know what to do if someone is having a heart attack? Acting quickly can save a life. One way is through cardio-pulmonary resuscitation (CPR). When you're able to perform CPR on someone during a heart attack, you can help save her life until emergency help arrives. Look for a CPR class near you through the American Heart Association, your local fire department, or a hospital.

Consider purchasing your own automated external defibrillator (AED), an instrument specifically designed for home use to help save a life. The FDA may require someone who purchases an AED to present a physician's prescription for the device. They cost between $1,500 to $2,000.

While you're at it, learn the Heimlich maneuver. According to the U.S. Department for Housing and Urban Development (HUD), the death rate due to choking is highest among people over age 75.

Let Lighting Lead Your Way

Too often people overlook the importance of good lighting; it's one of the best and least-expensive insurances against home injuries. As age progresses, vision changes. In general, after age 40, your eyes function best for distant viewing, so exceptionally good light is important in all areas of the home, especially the kitchen, laundry, other work areas, and over steps.

 The following suggestions can get you started toward a safer environment:

- Install a night light in your bathroom.

- Install overhead lights to illuminate all areas of a room.

- Install task lighting under counters in the kitchen.

- Install overhead lights over the entryway so visitors can be seen.

- Consider outside motion sensors that automatically turn on when visitors (expected or unexpected) make an appearance.

Reach Easily

As you age, your body has a harder time maintaining balance and finding its equilibrium, so reaching for objects becomes more of a challenge, increasing the likelihood of an injury in the process. These suggestions may help:

- Incorporate adjustable upper shelves, pull-out lower shelves, and Lazy Susans into your cabinets and closets.

- Replace cabinet knobs or pulls and sink faucets with levers for easier handling.

- Keep the items you use often low and within reach to avoid climbing on ladders and stools.

- Enlist the help of family or neighbors to move items so they're within your reach.

Bathe Safely

The bathroom seems one of the most popular places for home accidents. To minimize the possibilities there, follow these guidelines:

- Install grab bars and rails to reduce falls around the tub and toilet.

- Consider a stall shower with a low threshold and shower seat instead of a tub if you're planning to remodel.

- Remove bath mats or double-tape them down and place non-slip surfaces in the tub or shower.

- Clean up water spills immediately.

> ✔ Wear an in-home personal emergency response system that automatically calls for help in case you injure yourself and can't get to the phone.

 The elderly are in the top 90 percent risk group for being burned by hot water (the others are children under 4 and the mentally disabled). The thermostat on the hot water heater should be set below 120 degrees Fahrenheit.

Prevent Poisoning

Poisoning is the third-leading cause of unintentional injury-related death in the home among older adults, and certainly one of the most preventable. Take a look at these three poison sources:

- ✔ **Carbon monoxide (CO):** Carbon monoxide poisoning is the leading cause of accidental poisoning deaths in America. Install at least one carbon monoxide detector near your sleeping areas. A CO detector sounds an alarm if too much CO is present. Major sources of CO come from tobacco smoke, an idling car in the garage, combustion appliances (gas or kerosene heaters), and fireplaces.

- ✔ **Food poisoning:** Many elderly people have the inability to do everyday tasks, such as preparing meals and grocery shopping. As a result, many may eat food that's past its expiration date, resulting in food poisoning. In some cases, this can lead to dehydration from gastrointestinal distress.

- ✔ **Chemical poisoning:** Keep all chemicals (including common household cleaners) away from food and stored in different containers than non-food items. Choose non-toxic products when you can. Avoid mixing chemicals because some chemical reactions can cause watery eyes, nausea, and vomiting. Only use chemicals in well-ventilated areas. Older people are more prone to accidental spillage due to loss of muscle strength and can't tolerate or escape the fumes as quickly.

Make Sure that You Can See Clearly Now

Vision loss is very common as you age. An entire industry is devoted to making things easier to see to prevent problems as you get older. Some of the visual aides that can help include

- ✔ Talking blood pressure cuffs, blood glucose monitors, and thermometers

- ✔ Marked stove dials so you can tell the temperature setting by feel

- ✔ Large magnifying glasses to enlarge instructions on pill bottles

- ✔ Boil alert gadgets that fit on a pan and rattle when the water is boiling

- ✔ Liquid level indicators that fit on your cup and buzz when the liquid is an inch from the top

 One good source of low-vision aids is www.lhb.org, the Web site for Lighthouse for the Blind. The toll free number is (888) 792-0163.

Appendix

Health, Lifestyle, and History Self-Assessment

Have you ever wondered how healthy you really are? To answer this question you have to compile information not only on your current state of health, but also on your past medical history, the medical history of your first degree relatives (parents, siblings, and children), and your lifestyle choices. All these factors piece together to form your total health picture.

Answer all questions in this Appendix honestly. The information you provide helps your healthcare provider compile a picture of your health. Your doctor may then ask more questions or schedule tests to reveal further info about your health. See Chapter 3 for more on health assessments.

Personal Information

A doctor uses several pieces of personal information before she actually sees you. She can discover important aspects of your healthcare based on the following questions:

✔ What's your age? _____

✔ What's your gender (check one)?

❑ Male
❑ Female

✔ What state do you live in? _____

✔ What's your ethnicity? _____

✔ What's your height (without shoes, no fractions)?
_____ feet _____ inches

✔ What's your weight (without shoes, no fractions)?
_____ pounds

✔ What's your body frame size (check one)?

❑ Small
❑ Medium
❑ Large

✔ What's your BMI? _____

See Chapter 11 for more on your BMI.

General Health Survey

Some people have a good sense of the condition their bodies are in and often will be the first to admit when they're not in good health. On the other side of the coin, many people like to deny health issues such as weight. Many people don't seek medical attention even when they think something may be wrong. This section gives you the opportunity to grade yourself on the current state of your health. Answer the following questions:

1. In general, how would you rate your health?

❑ Excellent

- ❑ Very good
- ❑ Good
- ❑ Fair
- ❑ Poor
- ❑ Very poor

2. Compared to one year ago, how would you rate your current health?

- ❑ Much better now than one year ago
- ❑ Somewhat better now than one year ago
- ❑ About the same
- ☒ Somewhat worse now than one year ago
- ❑ Much worse than one year ago

3. Please answer each question by checking all boxes that apply:

- ❑ I am sexually satisfied.
- ❑ I get sick more easily than other people.
- ☒ I am as healthy as anybody I know.
- ☒ I expect my health to get worse.

4. During the past three months, have you had any of the following problems with your work or other regular daily activities as a result of your physical health? (Check boxes that apply)

- ❑ Cut down the amount of time you spend on work or other activities
- ❑ Accomplished less than you would like
- ❑ Were limited in the kind of work or other activities
- ❑ Had difficulty performing work or other activities (for example, it took extra effort)
- ❑ Took any prescribed medicines

❑ Took three or more different prescribed or over-the-counter drugs a day

5. Do you have any of the following conditions?
(Check boxes that apply)

❑ Angina
❑ Arthritis or rheumatism
❑ Asthma
❑ Blindness or trouble seeing, even when wearing glasses
❑ Cancer (not including skin cancer)
❑ Chronic lung disease (including bronchitis or emphysema)
❑ Congestive heart failure
☒ Deafness or trouble hearing
❑ Heart attack or myocardial infarction
❑ Heart murmur or artificial valve
❑ Hypertension or high blood pressure
❑ Kidney disease
❑ Sciatica or chronic back problem
❑ Stroke
❑ Sugar diabetes (diabetes mellitus)
❑ Ulcer or gastrointestinal bleeding (not counting hemorrhoids)

6. If you've had your blood pressure checked in the last week, please provide it. _____/_____

7. If you've had any blood tests, whether routine or for specific reasons, within the last six months, please provide what the test was for and the test results. _____/_____

8. What's your fasting blood sugar? _____

9. What's your total cholesterol level?

    a. _____ mg/dl   b. _____ Don't know

10. What's your HDL (good) cholesterol level?

    a. _____ mg/dl   b. _____ Don't know

11. What's your LDL (bad) cholesterol level?

    a. _____ mg/dl   b. _____ Don't know

12. Do you smoke tobacco (check one)?

❑ Yes
☒ No

***If yes:* How many cigarettes per day do you smoke?**

❑ Less than a pack a day
❑ 1 pack a day
❑ 2 or more packs a day

13. If you used to smoke, how many years has it been since you smoked regularly? _____

What was the average number of cigarettes per day that you smoked in the two years before you quit?

❑ Less than a pack a day
❑ 1 pack a day
❑ 2 or more packs a day

14. If you use smokeless tobacco (chewing tobacco, snuff, pouches, and so on) how often do you use it? _____ times per day

15. Have you ever had blood in your stool? In the toilet? On the toilet paper?

❑ Yes
❑ No

16. Have you ever had a colonoscopy?

☒ Yes
❑ No

17. Have you ever used any illicit drugs?

❑ Yes
☒ No

If yes, which drugs and when did you last use them?

_____

18. Did you use IV drugs?

❑ Yes
☒ No

If yes, which drugs and when did you last use them?

_____

19. Have you ever had a sexually transmitted disease (STD)?

❑ Yes
☒ No

If yes, which ones and when? _____

20. Are you sexually active now?

❑ Yes
❑ No

If yes, do you have more than one partner?

❑ Yes
❑ No

How many? _____

Just for Women

Women have specific preventative healthcare needs to be addressed during different stages of their lives. Whether you're in your reproductive years, menopausal, or post menopausal, yearly gynecologic exams are important. The following questions should be part of every woman's health assessment:

1. How long has it been since your last mammogram?

❑ Less than 1 year ago
❑ 1 year ago
❑ 2 years ago
☒ 3 or more years ago
❑ Never

2. How many women in your immediate family (mother or sisters only) have had breast cancer?

___0___ women

3. Have you had a hysterectomy?

❑ Yes
☒ No

4. How long has it been since you had a pap smear?

❑ Less than 1 year ago
❑ 1 year ago

☐ 2 years ago

☒ 3 or more years ago

☐ Never

5. At what age did you experience your first period (menarche)? _12_

6. Have you ever been pregnant?

☒ Yes

☐ No

If yes, how many resulted in children? _5_

7. Have you started menopause?

☒ Yes

☐ No

If no, at what age did your mother start menopause?

_____

Just for Men

Men aren't off the hook when it comes to specific tests, either. Men are notorious for waiting until symptoms are present or even unbearable before seeing a doctor. Don't feel embarrassed because men's conditions are common and getting them resolved may prevent further embarrassing situations. See Chapter 2 for info on the prostate and prostate cancer and other issues related to men.

The following questions are just for men:

1. Are you 40 years of age or older?

☐ Yes

☐ No

2. About how long has it been since you had a rectal or prostate exam?

- ❑ Less than 1 year ago
- ❑ 1 year ago
- ❑ 2 years ago
- ❑ 3 or more years ago
- ❑ Never

3. About how long has it been since your last blood prostate specific antigen (PSA)?

- ❑ Less than 1 year ago
- ❑ 1 year ago
- ❑ 2 years ago
- ❑ 3 or more years ago
- ❑ Never

Result: _____

4. Do you have any of the following problems?
(Check boxes that apply)

- ❑ Getting an erection
- ❑ Maintaining an erection
- ❑ Frequent urination
- ❑ Urination often at night time

Physical Fitness

Exercise has many benefits and it only requires 150 minutes a week. Why is something so easy often so neglected? Exercise should be mentioned in every health-related assessment, because it has either a direct or indirect influence on your health. See Chapters 9 and 10 on fitness to find out more about this topic. Here are some questions to look into for your fitness health:

1. **The following items are about activities you may do on a normal day. Does your health now limit you in these activities? If so, how much?** (Circle one number on each line.)

   1 = Limited a lot   2 = Limited a little   3 = Not limited at all

   - Vigorous activities, such as running, lifting heavy objects, or participating in strenuous sports: 1   2   3
   - Moderate activities, such as moving a table, pushing a vacuum cleaner, bowling, or playing golf: 1   2   3
   - Lifting or carrying groceries: 1   2   3
   - Climbing several flights of stairs: 1   2   3
   - Climbing one flight of stairs: 1   2   3
   - Bending, kneeling, or stooping: 1   2   3
   - Walking more than a mile: 1   2   3
   - Walking several blocks: 1   2   3
   - Walking one block: 1   2   3
   - Bathing or dressing yourself: 1   2   3

2. **In an average week, how many times do you engage in physical activity?** (Physical activity = 30 minutes of nonstop exercise or work that makes you breathe heavier and gets your heartbeat faster.)

   - ❑   Less than 1 time per week
   - ❑   1 or 2 times per week
   - ❑   3 or more times per week

3. **Please answer each question by checking all boxes that apply:**

   - ☒   My energy level is too low.
   - ☒   I am happy with my general appearance.
   - ☒   I am happy with my body.

Nutritional Health

Being overweight and sedentary is a trend that's spreading across the globe. Poor nutrition is linked to many medical conditions. Understanding where you can improve nutritionally has one of the greatest impacts on your ability to age well. See Chapters 7 and 8 on nutrition and Chapter 11 on obesity for more info. The following questions should alert you to your nutritional strengths and weaknesses:

1. How many full meals do you eat daily?

- ❑ 1 meal
- ☑ 2 meals
- ❑ 3 meals
- ❑ 4 meals
- ❑ 5 or more

2. Do you eat foods every day that are high in cholesterol or fat, such as fatty meat, cheese, fried foods, or eggs?

- ❑ Yes
- ❑ No

3. Do you have any medical condition that would change the kind and/or amount of food that you eat?

- ❑ Yes
- ❑ No

4. Do you eat few fruits or vegetables?

- ❑ Yes
- ❑ No

5. Do you have 1 to 2 drinks of beer, liquor, or wine almost every day?

- ☐ Yes
- ☒ No

6. Have you unintentionally lost or gained 10 pounds in the last 6 months?

- ☐ Yes
- ☒ No

7. Are you currently on a diet or have you dieted in the last 3 months? (This includes any cultural or religious diets)

- ☐ Yes
- ☐ No

8. Do you consume any dairy products (a glass of milk, cheese in a sandwich, or serving of yogurt) every day?

- ☒ Yes
- ☐ No

9. Do you eat meat, fish, or chicken every day?

- ☐ Yes
- ☒ No

10. How much water do you drink per day?

- ☐ Less than 20 ounces
- ☒ 20 to 40 ounces
- ☐ 40 to 80 ounces
- ☐ Greater than 80 ounces

11. Do you drink any diet or regular soda?

- ❏ Yes
- ☒ No *seldom*

12. Do you eat food after 8 p.m.?

- ❏ Yes
- ☒ No

Family History

Knowing about your family history is more complicated than just putting together your family tree, although this is a good start. Your family's medical history is very important in determining your health maintenance examinations, screenings, and other necessary testing.

Just because certain ailments or diseases may run in the family doesn't guarantee that you'll have them, too. Lifestyle habits can affect risks as well as prevent several conditions. So don't give up on good health if your family history reveals "bad" genes, just work harder to overcome them with good nutrition, healthy exercise habits, and smart lifestyle choices.

The following answers help determine your genetic risks:

1. **Please indicate family members (parent, sibling, grandparent, aunt, or uncle) with any of the following conditions:** (Check all boxes that apply and list relationship)

   - ❏ Alcoholism _____
   - ❏ Asthma/COPD _____
   - ❏ Bleeding or clotting disorder *mother sister* _____
   - ❏ Cancer: specify type _____; age of diagnosis _____

❑ Cardiovascular disease (stroke or heart attacks) before the age of 55 _____ Before the age of 70 ____mother____

❑ Depression/suicide __—_____

❑ Diabetes ____mother_____

❑ Genetic disorders, such as birth defects or learning disabilities ___—_____

❑ High blood pressure _____

❑ High cholesterol ___mother_____

❑ Migraines ____mother_____

❑ Obesity ___mother_____

❑ Thyroid disease _____

❑ Tobacco use ___father_____

2. Does anyone in your family have any severe reactions to medications?

❑ Yes   *If yes, who?* _____
☑ No

3. Has anyone in your family had multiple miscarriages?

☑ Yes   *If yes, who?* ___me (2)_____
❑ No

4. Has anyone had any reactions to anesthesia?

❑ Yes   *If yes, who?* _____
❑ No

Index

autosomal dominant disease, 418

D

lung cancer, 64–70, 372, 512

M

macronutrients, 244, 258–69

macular degeneration. *See* age-related macular degeneration (AMD)

magnetic resonance imaging (MRI) scans, 49, 78

makeup, 186, 199

male characteristics side effects, 60

mammograms, 77–78, 125–26

managed care limitations, 56

marital status, 498–99

massage, 390

meal hour myths, 515–16

meal size/frequency, 422, 472

measles, 47

measurement accuracy, 329–32

meat, 252, 261–61, 278–79

medical benefit, 300

medical clearance, 325–27

medical complaints (to doctor), 117–19

medical conditions, 119

medical myths, 509–16

medical technology improvements, 48–49

medication-related muscle loss, 369

medications. *See also specific medications*

  for Alzheimer's disease, 411, 412, 418–19

  anti-inflammatory, 390

  calcium absorption, 219

  challenges, 407

  immunosuppressive, 306

  for Parkinson's disease, 419

  periodontal disease, 152

  reviewing, 119

  safety, 536

optical illusions, 532
optimism, 137
oral cancer, 154–57
organ damage, 251
organ transplants, 48
organic products, 271–72, 285, 312
orgasm, 501, 504
osteoarthritis, 232, 320
osteonecrosis of the jaw, 227
osteoporosis
  overview, 106–9, 219–20
  diet, 51, 249
  myths, 511–12
  screening tests, 54–55
  smoking, 50
  strength training, 376
  treatment, 108, 109, 226–28
overworking (muscles), 387–88
Oxidation, 245
oxygen consumption, 355–56
Oxygen Radical Absorbance Capacity (ORAC), 518
oxytocin, 500, 502

P
Paget disease of the nipple, 73
pain, 85–86, 91, 463. *See also specific diseases*
palpitations, 104
pancreatic cancer, 93
pandemics, 44–46
pap smears, 125
parasympathetic systems, 428, 430
parathyroid hormone (PTH), 215
parietal lobe, 399
Parkinson's disease, 400, 402, 414–15, 417, 419
penicillin, 48

pulmonary vein, 352
pulse, 122

Q
QCT (quantitative computed tomography), 225
quadriceps, 373

R
RA (rheumatoid arthritis), 232–33
radiation, 70, 82, 86
radon, 66
raloxifene (Evista), 228
raw foods, 291, 294
recommended daily allowance (RDA), 281, 282–83, 286
rectal bleeding, 89–90, 91
Red 40 food dye, 277
red meat, 259, 260
red wine, 51
refractory period, 502–3
relaxation, 445, 476, 477
religious faith, 493
REM (rapid eye movement), 457–58, 460–61
remembering, techniques for, 425–26
remodeling, bone, 216–17
renal changes, 274
repeating learned items, 426
repetitive stress injuries, 233
reproductive history, 120
residue (smoking) on face, 190
resistance bands, 339, 379
resistance training, 356, 378, 379–80
respiratory system
   health examinations, 118, 122, 124
   illness/infections, 49, 153–54
   lung cancer symptoms, 69

592

X

xerostomia (dry mouth), 151, 160–61, 163
x-rays, 67

Y

yeast infections, 246, 302
Yellow 5 food dye, 277
yoga, 354–55, 380–81, 382, 448
yogurt, 305–6, 524–25